S0-ACY-544

Study Guide for

Clinical Procedures for Medical Assistants

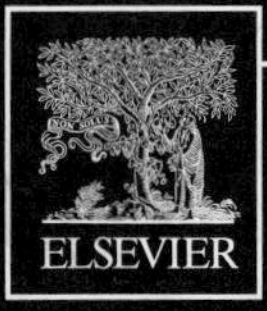

evolve

To access your Resources, visit:

http://evolve.elsevier.com/Bonewit/

Evolve® Resources for *Clinical Procedures for Medical Assistants,* 7th Edition offfer the following features:

Resources

- **WebLinks**
  Links to places of interest on the web specific to medical assisting.
- **Content Updates**
  Find out the latest information on relevant issues in the field of medical assisting.

Study Guide for

Clinical Procedures for Medical Assistants

Seventh Edition

Kathy Bonewit-West, BS, MEd
Coordinator and Instructor
Medical Assistant Technology
Hocking College
Nelsonville, Ohio

Former Member, Curriculum Review Board
of the American Association of Medical Assistants

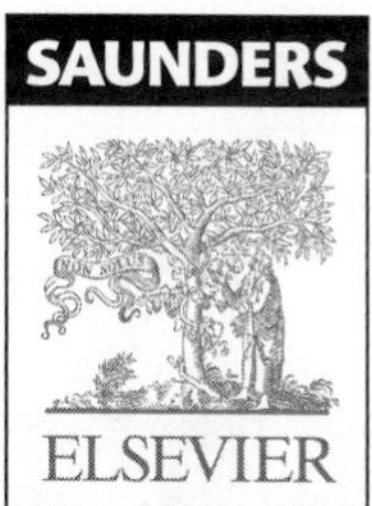

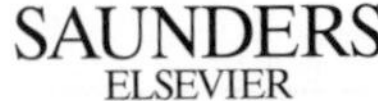

SAUNDERS
ELSEVIER

11830 Westline Industrial Drive
St. Louis, Missouri 63146

STUDY GUIDE FOR CLINICAL PROCEDURES FOR MEDICAL ASSISTANTS, SEVENTH EDITION

ISBN: 978-1-4160-4766-7

Copyright © 2008, 2004, 2000, 1995, 1990 by Saunders, an imprint of Elsevier Inc.

All rights reserved. No part of this publication may be reproduced or transmitted in any form or by any means, electronic or mechanical, including photocopying, recording, or any information storage and retrieval system, without permission in writing from the publisher. Permissions may be sought directly from Elsevier's Rights Department: phone: (+1) 215 239 3804 (US) or (+44) 1865 843830 (UK); fax: (+44) 1865 853333; e-mail: healthpermissions@elsevier.com. You may also complete your request on-line via the Elsevier website at http://www.elsevier.com/permissions.

Notice

Knowledge and best practice in this field are constantly changing. As new research and experience broaden our knowledge, changes in practice, treatment and drug therapy may become necessary or appropriate. Readers are advised to check the most current information provided (i) on procedures featured or (ii) by the manufacturer of each product to be administered, to verify the recommended dose or formula, the method and duration of administration, and contraindications. It is the responsibility of the practitioner, relying on their own experience and knowledge of the patient, to make diagnoses, to determine dosages and the best treatment for each individual patient, and to take all appropriate safety precautions. To the fullest extent of the law, neither the Publisher nor the Editors assume any liability for any injury and/or damage to persons or property arising out or related to any use of the material contained in this book.

Previous editions copyrighted 2004, 2000, 1995, 1990

ISBN: 978-1-4160-4766-7

Publisher: Michael S. Ledbetter
Senior Developmental Editor: Melissa K. Boyle
Publishing Services Manager: Pat Joiner-Myers
Project Manager: Jennifer Bertucci
Design Direction: Julia Dummitt

Printed in the United States of America

Last digit is the print number: 9 8 7 6 5 4 3 2 1

Working together to grow
libraries in developing countries
www.elsevier.com | www.bookaid.org | www.sabre.org
ELSEVIER BOOK AID International Sabre Foundation

Preface

Outcome-based education is education directed toward preparing individuals to perform the pre-specified tasks of an occupation under "real world" conditions at a level of accuracy and speed required of the entry-level practitioner of that profession. Outcome-based education plays an important role in medical assisting programs to assist in preparing qualified individuals for careers in medical offices, clinics, and related health care facilities. The *Study Guide for Clinical Procedures for Medical Assistants* has been developed using a complete and thorough outcome-based approach. It meets the criteria stipulated by the AAMA/CAAHEP Standards and Guidelines for the Medical Assisting Educational Programs. Instructors should find this Study Guide a valuable teaching aid for preparing well-trained students who are able to think critically and to perform competently in the clinical setting.

Each study guide chapter is organized into the following eight sections:

1. **ASSIGNMENT SHEETS**: The textbook and Study Guide Assignment Sheets indicate the assignments required for each chapter along with a space for the student to document the following: (a) the date each assignment is due, (b) completion of the assignment, and (c) points earned for each assignment. The Laboratory Assignment Sheet presents the procedures required for each chapter along with the textbook and Study Guide reference pages, the number of practices required to attain competency, and a space for documenting the score earned on the Performance Evaluation Checklist.
2. **PRETEST AND POSTTEST:** A Pretest and Posttest have been included for each chapter using true/false questions that allow the student to test his/her acquisition of knowledge for each chapter before and after completing the chapter. These tests can be used as a study guide to prepare for chapter tests.
3. **KEY TERM ASSESSMENT:** The Key Term Assessment section provides the student with an assessment of his/her knowledge of the medical terms relating to each chapter.
4. **EVALUATION OF LEARNING:** The Evaluation of Learning questions help the student evaluate his/her progress throughout each chapter. Once the student has completed these questions and checked them for accuracy, they will serve as an ongoing review of the cognitive knowledge presented in the textbook. Individuals preparing for a national certification examination will find the completed Evaluation of Learning sections a useful study aid for the clinical aspect of the examination.
5. **CRITICAL THINKING ACTIVITIES:** In the Critical Thinking Activities section, the student performs activities that enhance his/her ability to think critically. Some situations require that the student become involved in a game or role-playing situation; others require that the student use independent study in order to answer questions posed by a patient. Independent study helps the student become familiar with resources available to acquire additional knowledge and skills outside the classroom. By learning techniques of self-development, the medical assisting student may become aware of the necessity for continuing education after graduation and entrance into the medical assisting profession.
6. **PRACTICE FOR COMPETENCY:** The Practice for Competency section consists of worksheets that provide the student with a guide for the practice of each clinical skill presented in the textbook.
7. **EVALUATION OF COMPETENCY:** The Evaluation of Competency section is divided into two parts. The first part is the Performance Objective. Its purpose is to provide an exact description of what the learner must be able to demonstrate to attain competency. A performance objective consists of the following three components: (1) the outcome, (2) conditions, and (3) standards. Each Performance Objective in this Study Guide has been developed to correspond with the procedures presented in the textbook.

   The second part of the Evaluation of Competency section is the Performance Evaluation Checklist. The Performance Evaluation Checklist provides quality control by comparing the student's performance against an established set of performance standards.

Copyright © 2008, 2004, 2000, 1995, 1990 by Saunders, an imprint of Elsevier Inc. All rights reserved.

8. **SUPPLEMENTAL EDUCATION:** Due to the nature of the material, several medical assisting content areas are more difficult than others for the student to comprehend and perform. In particular, students have difficulty in taking patient symptoms and in calculating drug dosage. Because of this, two supplemental education sections have been incorporated into this manual. The section "Taking Patient Symptoms" provides supplemental education for Chapter 1 (The Medical Record) in the textbook; the section "Drug Dosage Calculation" provides supplemental education for Chapter 11 (Administration of Medication). In these two sections, a step-by-step, self-directed approach has been used, beginning with basic concepts and advancing to more difficult ones. The student should find that this type of approach facilitates the process of becoming proficient in these areas.

I would like to thank the staff at Elsevier for their assistance and support in preparing this Study Guide. I would also like to express my appreciation to the following individuals who provided encouragement and friendship throughout this endeavor: Dave Brennan, Marlene Donovan, Dawn Bennett, Deborah Murray, Rob Bonewit, Hollie Bonewit, Tristen West, and Caitlin Brennan.

Kathy Bonewit-West, BS, MEd

AAMA/CAAHEP competencies used on the "Evaluation of Competency" checksheets with permission from the American Association of Medical Assistants, Chicago, Illinois, and the Commission on Accreditation of Allied Health Education Programs, Clearwater, Florida.

Copyright © 2008, 2004, 2000, 1995, 1990 by Saunders, an imprint of Elsevier Inc. All rights reserved.

Message to the Student

This Study Guide has been designed to facilitate the attainment of competency in the clinical theory and procedures in your textbook. Each chapter of the manual has been organized into the eight components outlined below. By completing each component, it is hoped that your ability to assimilate the theory and perform the clinical skills will be greatly enhanced.

1. TEXTBOOK AND STUDY GUIDE ASSIGNMENT SHEETS
   A. Each time your instructor makes an assignment from the textbook, Study Guide, or Companion CD, document the date due in the appropriate space on the Textbook or Study Guide Assignment Sheet.
   B. Complete each assignment by the due date. Place a checkmark in the appropriate space on the Textbook or Study Guide Assignment Sheet after completing each assignment.
   C. Grade your assignment according to the directions stipulated by your instructor.
   D. Record your points earned in the appropriate space on the Textbook or Study Guide Assignment sheet.

2. LABORATORY ASSIGNMENT SHEET
   A. Your instructor will assign the procedure (or procedures) to be completed for each laboratory practice session. Check which procedures are assigned in the appropriate space on the Laboratory Assignment Sheet.
   B. Refer to the page numbers on the Laboratory Assignment Sheet for the Practice for Competency and Evaluation of Competency worksheets required for each procedure your instructor assigned.
   C. Locate and tear out the worksheets required for each procedure to be performed and bring them to your laboratory practice session.
   D. Record the score you earned on the Evaluation of Competency Performance Evaluation Checklist in the appropriate space on the Laboratory Assignment Sheet. This will provide you with an ongoing record of your progress on your clinical procedures.

3. PRETEST AND POSTTEST
   A. Complete the Pretest before beginning a study of each chapter. Complete the Posttest after completing the study of the chapter. Place a checkmark in the appropriate space on the Study Guide Assignment Sheet after completing each test.
   B. Check your work for accuracy with the textbook and correct any errors.
   C. Grade your Pretest and Posttest according to the directions stipulated by your instructor.
   D. Record the points you earned in the appropriate space on the Study Guide Assignment Sheet.
   E. Review the Pretest and Posttest before taking your chapter test.

4. KEY TERM ASSESSMENT
   A. Study the Terminology Review section located at the end of each chapter in the textbook.
   B. Match the medical terms with the definitions. Place a checkmark in the appropriate space on the Study Guide Assignment Sheet after completing.
   C. Check your work for accuracy, using your textbook, and correct any errors.
   D. Grade your Key Term Assessment according to the directions stipulated by your instructor.
   E. Record the points you earned in the appropriate space on the Study Guide Assignment Sheet.
   F. Review the Key Term Assessment before taking your chapter test.

Copyright © 2008, 2004, 2000, 1995, 1990 by Saunders, an imprint of Elsevier Inc. All rights reserved.

5. EVALUATION OF LEARNING QUESTIONS
   A. Read the textbook chapter.
   B. Complete the Evaluation of Learning questions. Place a checkmark in the appropriate space on the Study Guide Assignment Sheet after completing the questions.
   C. Check your work for accuracy, using the textbook, and correct any errors.
   D. Grade your Evaluation of Learning questions according to the directions stipulated by your instructor.
   E. Record the points you earned in the appropriate space on the Textbook Assignment Sheet.
   F. Review the Evaluation of Learning questions before taking your chapter test.

6. CRITICAL THINKING ACTIVITIES
   A. Review the information required to complete the Critical Thinking Activities.
   B. Obtain any additional materials or resources required.
   C. Complete each Critical Thinking Activity. Place a checkmark in the appropriate space on the Study Guide Assignment Sheet after completing each assigned activity.
   D. Grade each Critical Thinking Activity according to the directions stipulated by your instructor.
   E. Record the points you earned in the appropriate space on the Textbook Assignment Sheet.

7. PRACTICE FOR COMPETENCY
   A. Your instructor will assign the procedure (or procedures) to be completed for each laboratory practice session. For each procedure assigned, place a checkmark in the appropriate space on the Laboratory Assignment Sheet.
   B. Refer to the page numbers on the Laboratory Assignment Sheet for the Practice for Competency and Evaluation of Competency sheets required for each procedure your instructor assigned. Locate and tear out the sheets required for each procedure to be performed and bring them to your laboratory practice session.
   C. Practice each assigned procedure the required number of times indicated on the Laboratory Assignment Sheet or as designated by your instructor. Use the following as a guide when practicing the procedure to attain competency over each procedure:
      (1) Information indicated on the Practice for Competency sheet
         - Record your practices in the chart provided on the Practice for Competency sheet.
      (2) Procedure as presented in your textbook
      (3) Video of the procedure (located on the Companion DVDs accompanying your textbook)
         - It is often helpful to view the procedure on the Companion DVD several times to make sure you understand the correct technique and theory for each procedure.
      (4) Evaluation of Competency Performance Checklist
         - Make sure that you are able to perform each procedure according to the criteria stipulated under conditions and standards.
      (5) Peer Evaluation
         - If directed by your instructor, obtain a peer evaluation using the Evaluation of Competency Performance Evaluation Checklist.
   D. Bring the completed Practice for Competency sheet to your laboratory testing session and present it to your instructor for his/her review before testing over the procedure.

8. EVALUATION OF COMPETENCY PERFORMANCE CHECKLIST
   A. Write your name and date in the space indicated on the Evaluation of Competency Performance Evaluation Checklist.

   *Important Note: Do not chart the procedure (in advance) on the Evaluation of Competency sheet. You will do this after you have tested over the procedure.
   B. For each procedure you are being evaluated over, bring the following to your laboratory testing session and present them to your instructor:
      (1) Completed Practice for Competency sheet
      (2) Evaluation of Competency Performance Checklist
      (3) Outcome Assessment Record
   C. Demonstrate the proper procedure for performing the clinical skill for your instructor.
   D. Record results (if required) in the chart provided on the Evaluation of Competency Checklist.
   E. Obtain your instructor's initials on your Outcome Assessment Record indicating you have performed the procedure with competency.
   F. Record the score you earned in the appropriate space on your Laboratory Assignment Sheet.

Copyright © 2008, 2004, 2000, 1995, 1990 by Saunders, an imprint of Elsevier Inc. All rights reserved.

Once you have completed each chapter in this Study Guide, it is suggested that you place the perforated sheet into a three-ring notebook. This will provide you with an ongoing record of your academic progress. In addition, the notebook will be useful both as a classroom reference and as a certification examination review resource. The author hopes that this Study Guide will assist your attainment of competency in clinical medical assisting procedures, and in turn, facilitate your transition from the classroom to the workplace.

Kathy Bonewit West, BS, MEd

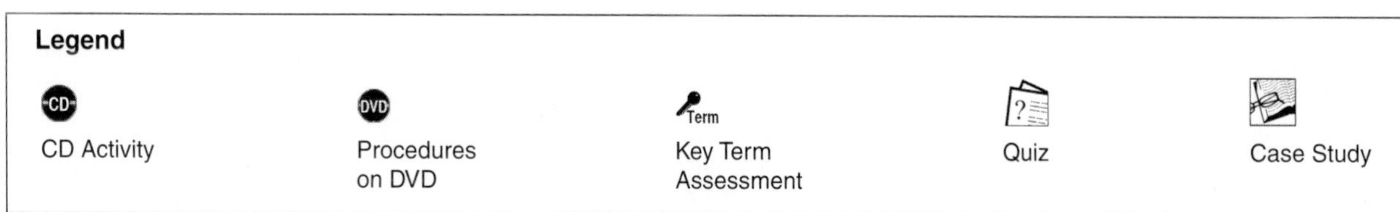

Copyright © 2008, 2004, 2000, 1995, 1990 by Saunders, an imprint of Elsevier Inc. All rights reserved..

Outcome Assessment Record

Guidelines: This list of outcomes is used to maintain an ongoing record of classroom and externship outcome assessment. Your instructor should initial each outcome when you have performed it with competency in the classroom. When you have performed the outcome with competency at your externship facility, it should be initialed by your externship supervisor. (Note: Space is provided for three externship experiences in the event that you extern at more than one externship site.)

Name ______________________________	Classroom Performance	Externship	Externship	Externship
THE MEDICAL RECORD				
Prepare a medical record for a new patient.				
Obtain patient consent for treatment.				
Assist a patient in the completion of a consent to release medical information form.				
Release information according to a completed release of medical information form.				
Complete or assist the patient in completing a health history form.				
Obtain and record patient symptoms.				
MEDICAL ASEPSIS AND THE OSHA STANDARD				
Wash hands.				
Apply an alcohol-based hand-rub.				
Apply and remove clean disposable gloves.				
Adhere to the OSHA Standard.				
STERILIZATION AND DISINFECTION				
Sanitize instruments.				
Wrap and label an article for autoclaving.				
Sterilize articles in the autoclave.				
Chemically disinfect contaminated articles.				

Copyright © 2008, 2004, 2000, 1995, 1990 by Saunders, an imprint of Elsevier Inc. All rights reserved.

Name ______________________________	Classroom Performance	Externship	Externship	Externship
VITAL SIGNS				
Measure oral body temperature.				
Measure axillary body temperature.				
Measure rectal body temperature				
Measure aural body temperature.				
Measure temporal artery body temperature.				
Measure radial pulse.				
Measure apical pulse.				
Perform pulse oximetry.				
Measure blood pressure.				
THE PHYSICAL EXAMINATION				
Prepare the examining room.				
Prepare the patient for a physical examination.				
Measure weight and height.				
Position and drape an individual.				
Assist the physician with a physical examination.				
EYE AND EAR PROCEDURES				
Assess distance visual acuity.				
Assess color vision.				
Perform an eye irrigation.				
Perform an eye instillation.				
Perform an ear irrigation.				
Perform an ear instillation.				
PHYSICAL AGENTS TO PROMOTE TISSUE HEALING				
Apply a heating pad.				
Apply a hot soak.				
Apply a hot compress.				
Apply an ice bag.				
Apply a cold compress.				
Apply a chemical cold and hot pack.				
Administer an ultrasound treatment.				
Measure an individual for axillary crutches.				
Instruct an individual in mastering crutch gaits.				
Instruct an individual in the use of a cane.				
Instruct an individual in the use of a walker.				

Copyright © 2008, 2004, 2000, 1995, 1990 by Saunders, an imprint of Elsevier Inc. All rights reserved.

Name ________________	Classroom Performance	Externship	Externship	Externship
THE GYNECOLOGICAL EXAMINATION AND PRENATAL CARE				
Provide instructions for a breast self-examination.				
Prepare the patient for a gynecologic examination.				
Assist with a gynecologic examination.				
Prepare the patient for a prenatal examination.				
Assist the physician with a prenatal examination.				
THE PEDIATRIC EXAMINATION				
Carry an infant in the following positions: cradle and upright.				
Measure the weight and length of an infant.				
Measure the head circumference of an infant.				
Measure the chest circumference of an infant.				
Plot pediatric measurements on a growth chart.				
Apply a pediatric urine collector.				
Collect a specimen for a newborn screening test.				
MINOR OFFICE SURGERY				
Apply and remove sterile gloves.				
Open a sterile package.				
Add a sterile article to a sterile field using a peel-apart package.				
Pour a sterile solution into a container on a sterile field.				
Change a sterile dressing.				
Remove sutures.				
Remove staples.				
Apply and remove adhesive skin closures.				
Set up a surgical tray for minor office surgery.				
Assist the physician with minor office surgery.				
Apply the following bandage turns: circular, spiral, spiral-reverse, figure-eight, and recurrent.				
Apply a tubular gauze bandage.				

Copyright © 2008, 2004, 2000, 1995, 1990 by Saunders, an imprint of Elsevier Inc. All rights reserved.

Name ______________________	Classroom Performance	Externship	Externship	Externship
ADMINISTRATION OF MEDICATION				
Administer oral medication.				
Prepare an injection from a vial.				
Prepare an injection from an ampule.				
Reconstitute a powdered drug.				
Administer a subcutaneous injection.				
Locate the following intramuscular injection sites: dorsogluteal, deltoid, vastus lateralis, and ventrogluteal.				
Administer an intramuscular injection.				
Administer an injection using the Z-track method.				
Administer an intradermal injection.				
Administer a Mantoux test.				
Read and interpret Mantoux test results.				
CARDIOPULMONARY PROCEDURES				
Record a 12-lead ECG.				
Instruct a patient in the guidelines for wearing a Holter monitor.				
Apply a Holter monitor.				
Perform spirometry testing.				
COLON PROCEDURES				
Provide instructions for a fecal occult blood test.				
Develop a fecal occult blood test.				
Prepare the patient for a sigmoidoscopy.				
Assist the physician with a sigmoidoscopy.				
Provide instructions for a testicular self-examination.				
RADIOLOGY AND DIAGNOSTIC IMAGING				
Instruct a patient in the proper preparation required for each of the following x-ray examinations: mammogram, upper GI, lower GI, and intravenous pyelogram.				
Instruct a patient in the proper preparation required for each of the following: ultrasonography, computed tomography, magnetic resonance imaging, and nuclear medicine.				

Copyright © 2008, 2004, 2000, 1995, 1990 by Saunders, an imprint of Elsevier Inc. All rights reserved.

Name ______________________________	Classroom Performance	Externship	Externship	Externship
INTRODUCTION TO THE CLINICAL LABORATORY				
Use a laboratory directory.				
Complete a laboratory request form.				
Prepare a laboratory report for review by the physician.				
Instruct the patient in advance preparation requirements for a specimen collection.				
Collect a specimen.				
Properly handle and store a specimen.				
Review a laboratory report.				
URINALYSIS				
Instruct a patient in clean-catch midstream urine specimen collection.				
Instruct a patient in 24-hour urine specimen collection.				
Assess the color and appearance of a urine specimen.				
Measure the specific gravity of a urine specimen.				
Perform a chemical assessment of a urine specimen.				
Prepare a urine specimen for microscopic analysis.				
Perform a rapid urine culture test.				
Perform a urine pregnancy test.				
PHLEBOTOMY				
Perform a venipuncture using the vacuum tube method.				
Perform a venipuncture using the butterfly method.				
Perform a venipuncture using the syringe method.				
Separate serum from whole blood.				
Obtain a capillary blood specimen.				
HEMATOLOGY				
Perform a hemoglobin determination.				
Perform a hematocrit determination.				
Prepare a blood smear.				

Copyright © 2008, 2004, 2000, 1995, 1990 by Saunders, an imprint of Elsevier Inc. All rights reserved.

Name ______________________	Classroom Performance	Externship	Externship	Externship
BLOOD CHEMISTRY AND SEROLOGY				
Perform blood chemistry testing.				
Perform a fasting blood sugar using a glucose monitor.				
Perform a rapid mononucleosis test.				
MICROBIOLOGY				
Use a microscope.				
Collect a specimen for a throat culture.				
Obtain a specimen using a collection and transport system.				
Perform a rapid strep test.				
Prepare a wet mount slide.				
Prepare a microbiologic smear.				
ADDITIONAL OUTCOMES (List)				

Copyright © 2008, 2004, 2000, 1995, 1990 by Saunders, an imprint of Elsevier Inc. All rights reserved.

Contents

Copyright © 2008, 2004, 2000, 1995, 1990 by Saunders, an imprint of Elsevier Inc. All rights reserved.

1

The Medical Record

CHAPTER ASSIGNMENTS

√ After Completing	Date Due	Textbook Page(s)	TEXTBOOK ASSIGNMENTS	Possible Points	Points You Earned
		1-48	Read Chapter 1: The Medical Record		
		5 44	Read Case Study 1 Case Study 1 questions	5	
		23 44	Read Case Study 2 Case Study 2 questions	5	
		29 44-45	Read Case Study 3 Case Study 3 questions	5	
		45-46	Apply Your Knowledge questions	11	
			TOTAL POINTS		
√ After Completing	**Date Due**	**Study Guide Page(s)**	**STUDY GUIDE ASSIGNMENTS (CTA: Critical Thinking Activity)**	**Possible Points**	**Points You Earned**
		5	Pretest	10	
		6	Key Term Assessment	20	
		7-11	Evaluation of Learning questions	48	
		12	CTA A: Medication Administration Record	4	
		12	CTA B: Consultation Report	4	
		12	CTA C: Radiology Report	3	
		12	CTA D: Diagnostic Imaging Report	4	
		12	CTA E: Discharge Summary Report	5	
		13	CTA F: Release of Medical Information	4	
		13	CTA G: Chief Complaint	6	
		14	CTA H: Crossword Puzzle	23	

Copyright © 2008, 2004, 2000, 1995, 1990 by Saunders, an imprint of Elsevier Inc. All rights reserved.

√ After Completing	Date Due	Study Guide Page(s)	STUDY GUIDE ASSIGNMENTS (CTA: Critical Thinking Activity)	Possible Points	Points You Earned
		16	CTA I: Road to Recovery: Medical Abbreviations (Team Players) (Record points earned)		
			CD Activity: Road to Recovery: Medical Abbreviations (Individual Player) (Record points earned)		
		44-51	Taking Patient Symptoms: Supplemental Education for Chapter 1 (10 points for each problem)	60	
		5	Posttest	10	
			ADDITIONAL ASSIGNMENTS		
			TOTAL POINTS		

Copyright © 2008, 2004, 2000, 1995, 1990 by Saunders, an imprint of Elsevier Inc. All rights reserved.

√ When Assigned By Your Instructor	Study Guide Page(s)	Practices Required	LABORATORY ASSIGNMENTS (Procedure Number and Name)	*Score
	29-31	1	**Practice for Competency** Health History Form Textbook reference: pp. 30-32	
	32	1	**Practice for Competency** 1-1: Completion of a Consent to Treatment Form Textbook reference: p. 21	
	35-36		**Evaluation of Competency** 1-1: Completion of a Consent to Treatment Form	*
	33	1	**Practice for Competency** 1-2: Release of Medical Information Textbook reference: p. 22	
	37-38		**Evaluation of Competency** 1-2: Release of Medical Information	*
	33		**Practice for Competency** 1-3: Preparing a Medical Record Textbook reference: pp. 27-28	
	39-40		**Evaluation of Competency** 1-3: Preparing a Medical Record	*
	33		**Practice for Competency** 1-4: Obtaining and Recording Patient Symptoms Textbook reference: p. 41	
	41-42		**Evaluation of Competency** 1-4: Obtaining and Recording Patient Symptoms	*
			ADDITIONAL ASSIGNMENTS	

Copyright © 2008, 2004, 2000, 1995, 1990 by Saunders, an imprint of Elsevier Inc. All rights reserved.

Notes

Copyright © 2008, 2004, 2000, 1995, 1990 by Saunders, an imprint of Elsevier Inc. All rights reserved.

Name GRACE V. MAURICIO Date ____________

PRETEST

True or False

T 1. The medical record serves as a legal document.

T 2. The purpose of progress notes is to update the medical record with new information.

F 3. The patient registration record consists of a list of the problems associated with the patient's illness.

T 4. All OTC medications taken by the patient should be charted on the medication record form.

T 5. A consultation report is a narrative report of a clinical opinion about a patient's condition by a practitioner other than the primary physician.

F 6. A report of the analysis of body specimens is known as a diagnostic report.

T 7. Medical impressions are conclusions drawn from an interpretation of data.

_____ 8. A consent to treatment form is required for tuberculin skin testing.

T 9. Diabetes mellitus is an example of a familial disease.

F 10. Pain is an example of an objective symptom.

POSTTEST

True or False

T 1. The purpose of HIPAA is to provide patients with more control over the use and disclosure of their health information.

T 2. The health history provides subjective data about a patient to assist the physician in arriving at a diagnosis.

F 3. Physical therapy helps a patient with a disability learn new skills to perform the activities of daily living.

T 4. A copy of the patient's emergency room report is sent to the patient's family physician.

T 5. When a medical assistant witnesses a patient's signature on a form, it means that the medical assistant is verifying that the patient understands the information on the form.

T 6. SOAP is the acronym for the format used to organize POR progress notes.

T 7. The chief complaint is the symptom causing the patient the most trouble.

T 8. The purpose of progress notes is to update the medical record with new information.

F 9. The patient's name must be included at the beginning of each entry charted in the patient's medical record.

F 10. A decrease in the amount of water in the body is known as edema.

Copyright © 2008, 2004, 2000, 1995, 1990 by Saunders, an imprint of Elsevier Inc. All rights reserved.

KEY TERM ASSESSMENT

Directions: Match each medical term with its definition.

____ 1. Attending physician

____ 2. Charting

____ 3. Consultation report

____ 4. Diagnosis

____ 5. Diagnostic procedure

____ 6. Discharge summary report

____ 7. Electronic medical record

____ 8. Familial

____ 9. Health history report

____ 10. Informed consent

____ 11. Inpatient

____ 12. Medical impressions

____ 13. Medical record

____ 14. Objective symptom

____ 15. Patient

____ 16. Physical examination report

____ 17. Problem

____ 18. Prognosis

____ 19. Subjective symptom

____ 20. Symptom

A. A collection of subjective data about a patient

B. A narrative report of an opinion about a patient's condition by a practitioner other than the attending physician

C. Any condition that requires further observation, diagnosis, management, or patient education

D. A symptom felt by the patient but not observed by an examiner

E. The process of making written entries about a patient in the medical record

F. The consent given by a patient for a medical procedure after being informed of the procedure

G. Any change in the body or its functioning indicative that a disease is present

H. The conclusions reached by the physician from an interpretation of data

I. A medical record that is stored on a computer

J. A brief summary of the significant events of a patient's hospitalization

K. A written record of the important information regarding a patient

L. A symptom that can be observed by an examiner

M. The probable course and outcome of a disease and the prospect for recovery

N. The scientific method of determining and identifying a patient's condition

O. A report of the objective findings from the physician's assessment of each body system

P. Occurring or affecting members of a family more frequently than would be expected by chance

Q. The physician responsible for the care of a hospitalized patient

R. A procedure performed to assist in the diagnosis, management, or treatment of a patient's condition

S. A patient who has been admitted to the hospital for at least one overnight stay

T. An individual receiving medical care

Copyright © 2008, 2004, 2000, 1995, 1990 by Saunders, an imprint of Elsevier Inc. All rights reserved.

EVALUATION OF LEARNING

Directions: Fill in each blank with the correct answer.

1. List three functions of the medical record.

____

____

____

2. What is the meaning of the acronym HIPAA?

HIPAA - HEALTH INSURANCE PORTABILITY AND ACCOUNTABILITY ACT

3. What is the purpose of the HIPAA Privacy Rule?

To provide patients with more control over the use and disclosure of their health information.

4. Who must comply with HIPAA?

HEALTH CARE PROVIDERS, HEATH PLANS and HEALTH CARE CLEARING-HOUSES.

5. What is a Notice of Privacy Practices?

It is a written document develop by medical office. It must explain to patients how their PHI will be used and protected by the medical office.

6. List examples of when HIPAA does not require written consent for the use or disclosure of a patient's health information in the following categories:

   a. Treatment: _______________

   b. Payment: _______________

   c. Health care operations: _______________

7. What two general categories of information are included on a patient registration record?

1) DEMOGRAPHIC INFORMATION 2) BILLING INFORMATION

8. List three uses of the health history.

1) to determine the patient's general state of health.
2) to arrive at a diagnosis and to prescribe treatment.
3) to document any change in a patient's illness after treatment has been instituted.

9. What is the purpose of the physical examination?

To provide objective data about the patient, w/c assists the physician in determining the patient's state of health.

10. What is the purpose of progress notes?

To document the patient's health status from one visit to the next.

11. List three categories of medication that may be included in a medication record.

1) PRESCRIPTION MEDICATIONS
2) OVER-THE-COUNTER (OTC) MEDICATIONS
3) MEDICATIONS ADMINISTERED AT THE MEDICAL OFFICE

Copyright © 2008, 2004, 2000, 1995, 1990 by Saunders, an imprint of Elsevier Inc. All rights reserved.

12. What is the purpose of home health care?

To minimize the effect of disease or disability by promoting, maintaining, and restoring the patient's health.

13. List five examples of home health services.

- CARDIAC HOME CARE
- INTRAVENOUS (IV) THERAPY
- RESPIRATORY THERAPY
- PAIN MANAGEMENT
- DIABETES MANAGEMENT

14. What is the purpose of a laboratory report?

Is to relay the results of the laboratory tests to the physician to assist in diagnosing and treating disease.

15. List five examples of diagnostic procedure reports.

16. What is the purpose of a therapeutic service report?

17. What is the difference between physical therapy and occupational therapy?

18. List examples of physical agents used in physical therapy?

19. What is speech therapy?

- refers to treatment for the correction

20. What is the purpose of an operative report?

21. What is the purpose of the discharge summary report?

- To document information needed by the patient's physician to provide for the continuity of future care.
- Used to respond to authorized requests for information regarding the patient's hospitalization.

Copyright © 2008, 2004, 2000, 1995, 1990 by Saunders, an imprint of Elsevier Inc. All rights reserved.

22. What is included in a pathology report?

1) includes a microscopic (gross) and microscopic description of tissue removed from a patient

23. Why is a copy of the emergency room report sent to the patient's physician?

24. When is a consent to treatment form required?

25. What is the purpose of a consent to treatment form?

26. What information must the patient receive before signing a consent to treatment form?

27. What does "witnessing a signature" mean? What does it not mean?

It means only that the MA verified the patient's identity and watched the patient signs the form. It does not mean that the MA is attesting to the accuracy of the information provided.

28. When must a patient complete a release of medical information form?

29. When does a release of medical information form not have to be completed?

30. What is the difference between a PPR and an EMR?

31. How are documents organized in a source-oriented medical record?

32. What is reverse chronological order?

That the most recent document is placed on top or in front of the others.

33. How are documents organized in a problem-oriented medical record (POR)?

It is organized accdg. to the patient's health problems.

Copyright © 2008, 2004, 2000, 1995, 1990 by Saunders, an imprint of Elsevier Inc. All rights reserved.

34. List and describe the four parts of a POR.

35. List and describe the format used to organize progress notes in a POR.

36. What are the seven parts of the health history?

37. What is a chief complaint?

Identifies the patient's reason for seeking care.

38. What guidelines should be followed in recording the chief complaint?

39. What is the present illness, and how is it obtained?

40. List five examples of information included in the past history.

41. List three examples of familial diseases.

42. Explain the importance of the social history.

43. What is the purpose of the review of systems (ROS)?

44. List the guidelines that should be followed to ensure accurate and concise charting.

Copyright © 2008, 2004, 2000, 1995, 1990 by Saunders, an imprint of Elsevier Inc. All rights reserved.

45. List three examples of subjective symptoms.

46. List three examples of objective symptoms.

47. What is the difference between a productive and a nonproductive cough?

48. Why should the following be charted in the patient's medical record?

a. Procedures performed on the patient

b. Specimens collected from the patient

c. Laboratory tests ordered on the patient

d. Instructions given to the patient regarding medical care

Copyright © 2008, 2004, 2000, 1995, 1990 by Saunders, an imprint of Elsevier Inc. All rights reserved.

CRITICAL THINKING ACTIVITIES

A. MEDICATION ADMINISTRATION RECORD

Refer to the medication administration record (Figure 1-2) in your textbook and answer the following questions.

1. Does Kristen Antle have any allergies? ______
2. How much Rocephin was administered to Kristen? ______
3. What was the route of administration of the Rocephin injection and where was it administered? ______
4. What is the name of the company that manufactures Rocephin? ______

B. CONSULTATION REPORT

Refer to the consultation report (Figure 1-3) in your textbook and identify the following information using the corresponding letter (A, B, C, or D).

1. Documentation that the consultant reviewed the patient's health history
2. Documentation that the consultant examined the patient
3. A report of the consultants' impressions
4. A report of the consultants' recommendations

C. RADIOLOGY REPORT

Refer to the radiology report (Figure 1-5) in your textbook and answer the following questions.

1. What type of radiological examination was performed on Rose Baker? ______
2. Were the lungs clear? ______
3. Were any abnormal masses noted in the abdomen? ______

D. DIAGNOSTIC IMAGING REPORT

Refer to the diagnostic imaging report (Figure 1-6) in your textbook and answer the following questions.

1. What type of diagnostic imaging procedure was performed on Vera Ruth? ______
2. Which vertebrae of the spine were scanned? ______
3. What problem may be present with L4-5? ______
4. What additional tests might be scheduled for Vera Ruth? ______

E. DISCHARGE SUMMARY REPORT

Refer to the discharge summary report (Figure 1-10) in your textbook and answer the following questions.

1. How long was Susan Brennan hospitalized? ______
2. What was her hemoglobin level at admission? ______
3. What was the reason for the hospitalization? ______
4. Was Susan pregnant? ______
5. What was her discharge diagnosis? ______

Copyright © 2008, 2004, 2000, 1995, 1990 by Saunders, an imprint of Elsevier Inc. All rights reserved.

F. RELEASE OF MEDICAL INFORMATION

Refer to the release of medical information form (Figure 1-14) in your textbook and answer the following questions.

1. What medical information is protected by law and cannot be released unless specifically authorized by the patient? ______________________________

   ____

2. List three reasons why a patient may authorize the release of his or her medical information. __________

   ____

   ____

3. Once this form is completed and signed, how long is it valid before it expires? ________________

4. What must the patient do if he or she wants to revoke the authorization?

   ____

   ____

G. CHIEF COMPLAINT

Indicate whether each of the following statements is an incorrect (I) or correct (C) example of recording a chief complaint. If the example is incorrect, explain which recording guideline is not being followed.

__I__ 1. CC: Low back pain. ______________________________

__C__ 2. CC: Sore throat and fever for the past 2 days. ______________________________

__C__ 3. CC: Dyspnea, paleness, and fatigue, similar to that associated with anemia, which have lasted for 2 weeks.

____

_____ 4. CC: Poor health for the past several months. ______________________________

_____ 5. CC: Weakness and fatigue related to poor eating habits and lack of exercise.

____

____

_____ 6. CC: Heart palpitations occurring after drinking coffee in the morning before work.

____

____

Copyright © 2008, 2004, 2000, 1995, 1990 by Saunders, an imprint of Elsevier Inc. All rights reserved.

H. CROSSWORD PUZZLE
Symptoms

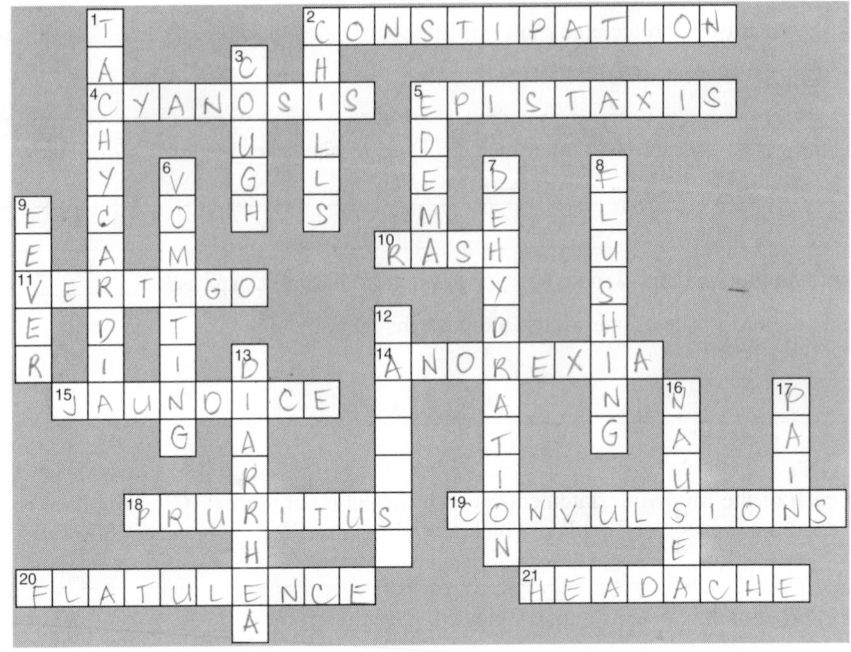

Directions: Complete the crossword puzzle using the terms presented below.

ACROSS

2 Stool is hard and dry
4 Blue skin due to lack of O_2
5 Nosebleed
10 Skin eruption rash
11 Dizziness vertigo
14 No appetite
15 Yellow skin
18 Severe itching pruritus
19 Involuntary contractions of muscles
20 Gas
21 Head pain

DOWN

1 Fast pulse rate
2 Shivering
3 May be productive or nonproductive
5 Fluid retention EDEMA
6 Ejection of stomach contents
7 Decreased H_2O levels in the body
8 Red face
9 Elevated temp
12 Bad all over
13 Loose, watery stools
16 Sensation of stomach discomfort nausea
17 Feeling of distress or suffering pain

hypothermia - low body temp.

Copyright © 2008, 2004, 2000, 1995, 1990 by Saunders, an imprint of Elsevier Inc. All rights reserved.

Notes

Copyright © 2008, 2004, 2000, 1995, 1990 by Saunders, an imprint of Elsevier Inc. All rights reserved.

I. ROAD TO RECOVERY

Object: The object of the game is to lead your "patient" to recovery by correctly providing the definition to abbreviations commonly used in the medical office.

Needed: **Road to Recovery** game board (located at the end of this manual)
Game cards
A token for each player (such as a button or coin)
Dice (1)
Score card

Directions:

1. Cut out the abbreviation cards found on the following pages.
2. Study the abbreviations and definitions in preparation for the game.
3. Place one complete set of abbreviations on the game board with the abbreviations facing up (and the definitions facing down).
4. Play **Road to Recovery** following the directions on the reverse side of the game board.
5. Keep track of your points using the Score Card provided.
6. If time permits, place the set of cards on the game board again with the definitions face-up and the abbreviations face-down; continue playing the game until all the cards have been used.

ROAD TO RECOVERY
SCORE CARD

Name: ______________________________

Recording Points:
Using the Game Card Points box, cross off a number each time you answer a game card correctly (starting with 5 and continuing in sequence). Your Total Game Card Points will be equal to the last number you crossed off. Record this number in the space provided (1). Record any extra points you were awarded during the game (2), and any points that were deducted (3). To determine your total points, add (1) and (2) together and deduct (3). Record this number in the Total Points Earned space provided. Compare your score with the other players and determine where you placed. Place a check mark next to the level of recovery your patient attained in the appropriate space.

Game Card Points:

5	75	145	215
10	80	150	220
15	85	155	225
20	90	160	230
25	95	165	235
30	100	170	240
35	105	175	245
40	110	180	250
45	115	185	255
50	120	190	260
55	125	195	265
60	130	200	270
65	135	205	275
70	140	210	280

Calculation of Points:

(1) Total Game Card Points: ________

(2) Additional Points Awarded: ________

(3) Deducted Points: ________

TOTAL POINTS EARNED: ________

LEVEL OF RECOVERY:

Patient's Name: ______________________

☐ First Place: **Fully Recovered**
☐ Second Place: **Almost Recovered**
☐ Third Place: **Still Recovering**
☐ Fourth Place: **Gasping for Air**

Copyright © 2008, 2004, 2000, 1995, 1990 by Saunders, an imprint of Elsevier Inc. All rights reserved.

Ab	abd	ac	amt
approx	appt	ASA	b/c
BC	bid	BM	BP
BS	BSE	c̄	caps
CC	chemo	c/o	d/c
disch	DOB	DSD	D & V

amount	before meals	abdomen	abortion
because	acetylsalicylic acid (aspirin)	appointment	approximately
blood pressure	bowel movement	twice a day	birth control
capsules	with	breast self-examination	blood sugar
discontinue	complains of	chemotherapy	chief complaint
diarrhea and vomiting	dry, sterile dressing	date of birth	discharge

ED	flex sig	freq	F/U
Fx	H/A	H_2O	hs
ht	IM	IV	LBP
LMP	meds	min	mod
N/C	neg	NKDA	NMP
N & V	OB	occ	OT

follow-up	frequent	flexible sigmoidoscopy	emergency department
at bedtime	water	headache	fracture
lower back pain	intravenous	intramuscular	height
moderate	minute	medications	last menstrual period
normal menstrual period	no known drug allergies	negative	no complaints
occupational therapy	occasionally	obstetrics	nausea and vomiting

OTC	OV	Pap	path
pc	peds	PEN	po
pos	PT	pt	qd
q (2,3,4) h	qid	QNS	qod
reg	Rx	s̄	SC
S/E	sl	sm	SOB

pathology	Pap test	office visit	over the counter
by mouth	penicillin	pediatrics	after meals
every day	patient	physical therapy	positive
every other day	quantity not sufficient	four times a day	every (2,3,4) hours
subcutaneous	without	prescription	regular
shortness of breath	small	slight	side effects

spec	STAT	tab(s)	tid
TPR	tr	vag	VS
wk	w/o	wt	AD
AS	AU	EENT	GI
(L)	(LA)	(LL)	LLQ
LRQ	LUQ	OD	OS

three times a day	tablet, tablets	immediately	specimen
vital signs	vagina	trace	temperature, pulse, and respiration
right ear	weight	without	week
gastrointestinal	eye, ears, nose, and throat	in each ear (both ears)	left ear
lower left quadrant	left leg	left arm	left
left eye	right eye	left upper quadrant	lower right quadrant

OU	R	RA	RL
RLQ	RUQ	Dx	Hx
PE	Sx	Tx	CAD
CHF	COPD	CVA	DM
GC	HTN	MI	OA
PID	RA	STD	TB

right leg	right arm	right	in each eye (both eyes)
history	diagnosis	right upper quadrant	right lower quadrant
coronary artery disease	treatment	symptoms	physical examination
diabetes mellitus	cerebral vascular accident	chronic obstructive pulmonary disease	congestive heart failure
osteoarthritis	myocardial infarction	hypertension	gonorrhea
tuberculosis	sexually transmitted disease	rheumatoid arthritis	pelvic inflammatory disease

URI	**UTI**	**ECG**	**PFT**
US	**Bx**	**CBC**	**C & S**
FBS	**GTT**	**Hct**	**Hgb**
UA	**WBC**	>	<
↑	↓	×	@
$\bar{x}$	$\bar{p}$	+	–

pulmonary function test	electrocardiogram	urinary tract infection	upper respiratory infection
culture and sensitivity	complete blood count	biopsy	ultrasound
hemoglobin	hematocrit	glucose tolerance test	fasting blood sugar
less than	greater than	white blood count	urinalysis
at	times	decrease	increase
negative	positive	after	except

PRACTICE FOR COMPETENCY

Health History Form. Complete the health history form (pages 29 to 31) using yourself as the patient.

PATIENT HEALTH HISTORY

A **IDENTIFICATION DATA** Please print the following information.

Today's date ______

Name ______ ___ Male ___ Female

Address ______ ___ Married ___ Separated ___ Divorced ___ Widowed ___ Single

______ Date of Birth ______

Telephone ______ ______
Home number Work number

B **PAST HISTORY**

Have you ever had the following: (Circle "no" or "yes", leave blank if uncertain)

Measles ______ no yes	Heart Disease ______ no yes	Diabetes ______ no yes	Hemorrhoids ______ no yes
Mumps ______ no yes	Arthritis ______ no yes	Cancer ______ no yes	Asthma ______ no yes
Chickenpox ______ no yes	Sexually Transmitted Disease ______ no yes	Polio ______ no yes	Allergies ______ no yes
Whooping Cough ______ no yes	Anemia ______ no yes	Glaucoma ______ no yes	Eczema ______ no yes
Scarlet Fever ______ no yes	Bladder Infections ______ no yes	Hernia ______ no yes	AIDS or HIV+ ______ no yes
Diphtheria ______ no yes	Epilepsy ______ no yes	Blood or Plasma Transfusions ______ no yes	Infectious Mono ______ no yes
Pneumonia ______ no yes	Migraine Headaches ______ no yes	Back Trouble ______ no yes	Bronchitis ______ no yes
Rheumatic Fever ______ no yes	Tuberculosis ______ no yes	High Blood Pressure ______ no yes	Mitral Valve Prolapse yes
Stroke ______ no yes	Ulcer ______ no yes	Thyroid Disease ______ no yes	Any other disease ______ no yes Please list: ______
Hepatitis. ______ no yes	Kidney Disease ______ no yes	Bleeding Tendency ______ no yes	

MAJOR HOSPITALIZATIONS: If you have ever been hospitalized for any major medical illness or operation, write in your most recent hospitalizations below.

Hospitalizations	Year	Operation or illness	Name of hospital	City and state
1st Hospitalization				
2nd Hospitalization				
3rd Hospitalization				
4th Hospitalization				

TESTS AND IMMUNIZATIONS: Mark an X next to those that you have had.

Tests:

- ☐ TB Test
- ☐ Rectal/Hemoccult
- ☐ Sigmoidoscopy
- ☐ Colonoscopy
- ☐ Electrocardiogram
- ☐ Chest X-ray
- ☐ Mammogram
- ☐ Pap Test

Immunizations:

- ☐ Influenza
- ☐ Hepatitis B
- ☐ Tetanus
- ☐ MMR
- ☐ Polio

ALLERGIES: List all allergies (foods, drugs, environment). ☐ None

______
______
______
______

CURRENT MEDICATIONS: List the following that you are currently taking: Prescription medications, over-the-counter (OTC) medications, vitamin supplements, and herbal supplements. ☐ None

Medication	Frequency

ACCIDENTS/ INJURIES: Describe all serious accidents, severe injuries, head injury, or fractrures. Include the date each occurred. ☐ None

Accident/Injury:	Date:

Copyright © 2008, 2004, 2000, 1995, 1990 by Saunders, an imprint of Elsevier Inc. All rights reserved.

C

FAMILY HISTORY

For each member of your family, follow the purple or blue line across the page and check boxes for:
1. Their present state of health
2. Any illnesses they have had

	Good Health	Poor Health	Deceased	If deceased, write in age and cause of death.	Allergies or Asthma	Diabetes	Heart Disease	Stroke	Cancer	High Blood Pressure	Glaucoma	Arthritis	Ulcer	Kidney Disease	Mental Health Problems	Alcohol/Drug Abuse	Obesity	High Cholesterol	Thyroid Disease
Father:																			
Mother:																			
Brothers/Sisters:																			

D

SOCIAL HISTORY

EDUCATION ______ High school ______ College ______ Post graduate

Occupation ______ Years ______

Previous occupations ______ Years ______

______ Years ______

Have you ever been exposed to any of the following in your environment?

☐ Excess dust (coal, lime, rock) ☐ Cleaning fluids/solvents ☐ Radiation ☐ Other toxic materials
☐ Sand ☐ Hair spray ☐ Insecticides
☐ Chemicals ☐ Smoke or auto exhaust fumes ☐ Paints

Please answer the follwing questions by placing an X in the box in front of the word Yes or No, except where you are asked for specific information. This information is obviously highly confidential and will be released to other health professionals or insurance carriers ONLY with your consent.

DIET:

Do you eat a good breakfast? ☐ Yes ☐ No
Do you snack between meals (soft drinks, chips, candy bars)? ☐ Yes ☐ No
Do you eat fresh fruits and vegetables each day? ☐ Yes ☐ No
Do you eat whole grain breads and cereals? ☐ Yes ☐ No
Is your diet high in fat content? ☐ Yes ☐ No
Is your diet high in cholesterol content? ☐ Yes ☐ No
Is your diet high in salt content? ☐ Yes ☐ No
Are you allergic to any foods? ☐ Yes ☐ No
How many glasses of water do you drink each day? ______
How would you describe your overall eating habits? ☐ Excellent ☐ Good ☐ Fair ☐ Poor

PERSONAL HISTORY:

Do you find it hard to make decisions? ☐ Yes ☐ No
Do you find it hard to concentrate or remember? ☐ Yes ☐ No
Do you feel depressed? ☐ Yes ☐ No
Do you have difficulty relaxing? ☐ Yes ☐ No
Do you have a tendency to worry a lot? ☐ Yes ☐ No
Have you gained or lost much weight recently? ☐ Yes ☐ No
Do you lose your temper often? ☐ Yes ☐ No
Are you disturbed by any work or family problems? ☐ Yes ☐ No
Are you having sexual difficulties? ☐ Yes ☐ No
Have you ever considered committing suicide? ☐ Yes ☐ No
Have you ever desired or sought psychiatric help? ☐ Yes ☐ No

EXERCISE:

Do you exercise on a regular basis? ☐ Yes ☐ No
Does your job require strenuous, sustained physical work? ☐ Yes ☐ No

SLEEP PATTERNS:

Do you seem to feel exhausted or fatigued most of the time? ☐ Yes ☐ No
Do you have difficulty either falling asleep or staying asleep? ☐ Yes ☐ No

USE OF TOBACCO/ALCOHOL/CAFFEINE/DRUGS: Amt:

How much do you smoke per day? ☐ Cigarettes __ ☐ Cigars/pipes __
☐ Don't smoke

Do you take two or more alcoholic drinks per day? ☐ Yes ☐ No
Do you drink six or more cups of coffee or tea per day? ☐ Yes ☐ No
Are you a regular user of sleeping pills, marijuana, tranquilizers, pain killers, etc? ☐ Yes ☐ No
Have you ever used heroin, cocaine, LSD, PCP, etc? ☐ Yes ☐ No

List any country outside the USA you have visited in the past six months? ______

When did you have your last physical examination? ______

Copyright © 2008, 2004, 2000, 1995, 1990 by Saunders, an imprint of Elsevier Inc. All rights reserved.

Patient's Name ______________________________

E

REVIEW OF SYSTEMS

HEAD AND NECK
____ Frequent headaches
____ Neck pain
____ Neck lumps or swelling

EYES
____ Wears glasses
____ Blurry vision
____ Eyesight worsening
____ Sees double
____ Sees halo
____ Eye pain or itching
____ Watering eyes
____ Eye trouble

EARS
____ Hearing difficulties
____ Earaches
____ Running ears
____ Buzzing in ears
____ Motion sickness

MOUTH
____ Dental problems
____ Swellings on gums or jaws
____ Sore tongue
____ Taste changes

NOSE AND THROAT
____ Congested nose
____ Running nose
____ Sneezing spells
____ Headcolds
____ Nose bleeds
____ Sore throat
____ Enlarged tonsils
____ Hoarse voice

RESPIRATORY
____ Wheezes or gasps
____ Coughing spells
____ Coughs up phlegm
____ Coughed up blood
____ Chest colds
____ Excessive sweating, night sweats

CARDIOVASCULAR
____ High blood pressure
____ Racing heart
____ Chest pains
____ Dizzy spells
____ Shortness of breath
____ Shortness of breath at night
____ More pillows to breathe
____ Swollen feet or ankles
____ Leg cramps
____ Heart murmur

DIGESTIVE
____ Heartburn
____ Bloated stomach
____ Belching
____ Stomach pains
____ Nausea
____ Vomited blood
____ Difficulty swallowing
____ Constipation
____ Loose bowels
____ Black stools
____ Grey stools
____ Pain in rectum
____ Rectal bleeding

URINARY
____ Night frequency
____ Day frequency
____ Wets pants or bed
____ Burning on urination
____ Brown, black, or bloody urine
____ Difficulty starting urine
____ Urgency

MALE GENITAL
____ Weak urine stream
____ Prostate trouble
____ Burning or discharge
____ Lumps on testicles
____ Painful testicles

FEMALE GENITAL
__/__/__ Last menstrual period
__/__/__ Last Pap test
____ Post-menopausal or hysterectomy
____ Noticed vaginal bleeding
____ Abnormal LMP
____ Heavy bleeding during periods
____ Bleeding between periods
____ Bleeding after intercourse
____ Recent vaginal itching/ discharge
____ No monthly breast exam
____ Lump or pain in breasts
____ Complications with birth control

OBSTETRIC HISTORY
____ Gravida
____ Para
____ Pre-term
____ Miscarriages
____ Still births
____ Has had an abortion

MUSCULOSKELETAL
____ Aching muscles
____ Swollen joints
____ Back or shoulder pains
____ Painful feet
____ Disability

SKIN
____ Skin problems
____ Itching or burning skin
____ Bleeds easily
____ Bruises easily

NEUROLOGICAL
____ Faintness
____ Numbness
____ Convulsions
____ Change in handwriting
____ Trembles

F

PROGRESS NOTES

Date	

Copyright © 2008, 2004, 2000, 1995, 1990 by Saunders, an imprint of Elsevier Inc. All rights reserved.

Procedure 1-1: Consent to Treatment. Complete the consent to treatment form (below) using a classmate as the patient.

(attach label or complete blanks)

First name: ______________ Last name: ______________

Date of Birth: ________ Month ________ Day ________ Year

Account Number: ______________________________

Procedure Consent Form

I, ____, hereby consent to have

Dr. ________________, perform ____.

I have been fully informed of the following by my physician:

1. The nature of my condition.
2. The nature and purpose of the procedure.
3. An explanation of risks involved with the procedure.
4. Alternative treatments or procedures available.
5. The likely results of the procedure.
6. The risks involved with declining or delaying the procedure.

My physician has offered to answer all questions concerning the proposed procedure.

I am aware that the practice of medicine and surgery is not an exact science, and I acknowledge that no guarantees have been made to me about the results of the procedure.

Patient ______________________________ Date ______________

(or guardian and relationship)

Witnessed ______________________________ Date ______________

Copyright © 2008, 2004, 2000, 1995, 1990 by Saunders, an imprint of Elsevier Inc. All rights reserved.

Procedure 1-2: Release of Medical Information. Complete the release of medical information form (below) using a classmate as the patient.

RELEASE OF MEDICAL INFORMATION

All information contained in the medical record is confidential and the release of information is closely controlled. A properly completed and signed authorization is required for the release of the following information.

PATIENT INFORMATION

Patient Name ____________________

Address ____________________ Social Security #____________

City ____________ State ______ ZIP ____________ Birthdate____/____/____

Phone (Home) ____________ Work ____________

RELEASE FROM:

Name ____________________

Address ____________________

City ____________ State ______ ZIP ________

RELEASE TO:

Name ____________________

Address ____________________

City ____________ State ______ ZIP ________

INFORMATION TO BE RELEASED:

1. GENERAL RELEASE:

___Entire Medical Record (excluding protected information)
___Hospital Records only (specify)____________
___Lab Results only (specify) ____________
___X-ray Reports only (specify) ____________
___Other Records (specify) ____________

2. INFORMATION PROTECTED BY STATE/FEDERAL LAW:
If indicated below, I hereby authorize the disclosure and release of information regarding:

___Drug Abuse Diagnosis/Treatment
___Alcoholism Diagnosis/Treatment
___Mental Health Diagnosis/Treatment
___Sexually Transmitted Disease

PURPOSE/NEED FOR INFORMATION:

___Taking records to another doctor
___Moving
___Legal purposes
___Insurance purposes
___Workman's Compensation
___Other/Explain:____________

METHOD OF RELEASE:

___ US Mail
___ Fax
___ Telephone
___ To Patient

PATIENT AUTHORIZATION TO RELEASE INFORMATION:

Authorization is valid for 60 days only from the date of my signature. I reserve the right to revoke this authorization at any time prior to 60 days (except for action that has already been taken) by notifying the medical office in writing.

I understand that my records are protected under HIPAA (Health Insurance Portability and Accountability Act) Standards for Privacy of Individually Identifiable Information (45 CFR Parts 160 and 164) unless otherwise permitted by federal law. Any information released or received shall not be further relayed to any other facility or person without my written authorization. I also understand that such information will not be given, sold, transferred or in any way relayed to any other person or party not specified above without my further written authorization.

I hereby grant authorization to release the information listed above. I certify that this request has been made voluntarily and that the information given above is accurate to the best of my knowledge.

____________________ ____________
Signature of Patient/Legally Responsible Party Date

____________________ ____________
Witness Signature Date

OFFICE USE ONLY

Information indicated above released on ____________
Date

Explanation of information released: ____________

____

Signature and credentials of individual releasing information: ____________

Procedure 1-3: Preparing a Medical Record. Prepare a medical record.

Procedure 1-4: Obtaining and Recording Patient Symptoms. Practice obtaining patient symptoms, by completing Taking Patient Symptoms: Supplemental Education for Chapter 1 (pages 44 to 51 in this study guide).

Copyright © 2008, 2004, 2000, 1995, 1990 by Saunders, an imprint of Elsevier Inc. All rights reserved.

Notes

Copyright © 2008, 2004, 2000, 1995, 1990 by Saunders, an imprint of Elsevier Inc. All rights reserved.

EVALUATION OF COMPETENCY

Procedure 1-1: Completion of a Consent to Treatment Form

Name: ______________________________ Date: ______________

Evaluated By: ______________________________ Score: ______________

Performance Objective

Outcome:	Complete a consent to treatment form.	
Conditions:	Given a consent to treatment form.	
Standards:	Time: 10 minutes	Student completed procedure in ____ minutes.
	Accuracy: Satisfactory score on the Performance Evaluation Checklist	

Performance Evaluation Checklist

Trial 1	Trial 2	Point Value	*Performance Standards*
		•	Typed or printed required information on the consent to treatment form.
		•	Confirmed that the physician discussed the procedure with the patient.
		▷	Explained why the procedure should be discussed with the patient before the form is signed.
		•	Greeted the patient and introduced yourself.
		•	Explained the purpose of the form to the patient.
		•	Gave the consent form to the patient to read.
		•	Asked if the patient had any questions.
		•	Asked the patient to sign the form.
		•	Witnessed the patient's signature and dated the form.
		▷	Explained what "witnessing a signature" means.
		•	Provided the patient with a copy of the completed form.
		*	Filed the original form in the patient's medical record.
		▷	Explained why the form must be filed in the medical record.
		*	Completed the procedure within 10 minutes.
			TOTALS

Copyright © 2008, 2004, 2000, 1995, 1990 by Saunders, an imprint of Elsevier Inc. All rights reserved.

Evaluation of Student Performance

EVALUATION CRITERIA			COMMENTS
Symbol	Category	Point Value	
*	Critical Step	16 points	
•	Essential Step	6 points	
▷	Theory Question	2 points	
Score calculation: 100 points – ____ points missed ____ Score Satisfactory score: 85 or above			

AAMA/CAAHEP Competency Achieved:

☑ III. C. 3. c. (1) a. Respond to and initiate written communications.

Copyright © 2008, 2004, 2000, 1995, 1990 by Saunders, an imprint of Elsevier Inc. All rights reserved.

EVALUATION OF COMPETENCY

Procedure 1-2: Release of Medical Information

Name: ______________________________ Date: ______________

Evaluated By: ______________________________ Score: ______________

Performance Objective

Outcome:	1. Assist a patient in the completion of a release of medical information form.
	2. Release medical information according to a completed release of information form.
Conditions:	Given a release of medical information form and the patient's medical record.
Standards:	Time: 15 minutes. Student completed procedure in ____ minutes.
	Accuracy: Satisfactory score on the Performance Evaluation Checklist.

Performance Evaluation Checklist

Trial 1	*Trial 2*	*Point Value*	*Performance Standards*
			COMPLETION OF A RELEASE FORM
		•	Greeted the patient.
		•	Introduced yourself and explained the purpose of the form to the patient.
		▷	Explained the procedure to follow if you do not recognize the patient.
		•	Provided the patient with a release form.
		•	Asked the patient to complete the form.
		•	Provided assistance if needed.
		•	Checked to make sure all information was completed.
		•	Asked the patient to sign the form.
		•	Witnessed the patient's signature and dated the form.
		•	Provided the patient with a copy of the completed form.
		•	Copied the medical information requested on the form.
		*	Released only the information requested
		•	Included a copy of the completed form with the medical information.
		•	Documented what information was released along with the date of release.
		•	Signed the document with your name and credentials.
		*	Filed the original document and the release form in the patient's medical record.
		▷	Explained the reason for filing the form.
		•	Sent the medical information according to the medical office policy.

Copyright © 2008, 2004, 2000, 1995, 1990 by Saunders, an imprint of Elsevier Inc. All rights reserved.

Trial 1	Trial 2	Point Value	*Performance Standards*
			MAILED OR FAXED REQUESTS
		•	Checked the expiration date on the release of medical information form.
		▷	Explained the procedure to follow if the form is expired.
		•	Verified the signature on the form.
		▷	Stated what to do if in doubt regarding the authenticity of the signature.
		•	Copied the information requested on the form.
		*	Released only the information requested.
		•	Documented what information was released along with the date of release.
		•	Signed the document with your name and credentials.
		•	Filed the original document and the release form in the patient's medical record.
		•	Sent the medical information according to the medical office policy.
		*	Completed the procedure within 15 minutes.
			TOTALS

Evaluation of Student Performance

EVALUATION CRITERIA			COMMENTS
Symbol	Category	Point Value	
*	Critical Step	16 points	
•	Essential Step	6 points	
▷	Theory Question	2 points	

Score calculation: 100 points
− ______ points missed
______ Score
Satisfactory score: 85 or above

AAMA/CAAHEP Competency Achieved:

☑ III. C. 3. c. (2) (a): Identify and respond to issues of confidentiality.

☑ III. C. 3. c. (2) (b): Perform within legal and ethical boundaries.

☑ III. C. 3. c. (2) (e): Demonstrate knowledge of federal and state health care legislation and regulations.

☑ III. C. 3. c. (3) (a): Explain general office policies.

Copyright © 2008, 2004, 2000, 1995, 1990 by Saunders, an imprint of Elsevier Inc. All rights reserved.

EVALUATION OF COMPETENCY

Procedure 1-3: Preparing a Medical Record

Name: ______________________________ Date: ______________

Evaluated By: ______________________________ Score: ______________

Performance Objective

Outcome:	Prepare a medical record.
Conditions:	Given the following: patient registration form, Notice of Privacy Practices and acknowledgment form, file folder, metal fasteners, name labels, alphabetic labels, miscellaneous chart labels, chart dividers, preprinted forms, and a two-hole punch.
Standards:	Time: 10 minutes Student completed procedure in ____ minutes.
	Accuracy: Satisfactory score on the Performance Evaluation Checklist.

Performance Evaluation Checklist

Trial 1	Trial 2	Point Value	*Performance Standards*
		•	Greeted the patient and introduced yourself.
		•	Identified the patient and verified that the patient was a new patient.
		•	Asked the patient to complete a patient registration form, read an NPP, and sign an acknowledgment form.
		•	Offered to answer questions.
		•	Checked the registration form for accuracy and legibility.
		•	Copied the patient's insurance card.
		▷	Stated the purpose of copying the card.
		•	Entered the data on the completed registration form into the computer.
		•	Assembled supplies needed to prepare the medical record.
			Typed the patient's full name on the name label
		•	The patient's name was in transposed order.
		•	The name was typed using correct spacing.
		•	The patient's name was spelled correctly.
		•	Attached appropriate color-coded labels to the side tab.
		•	Attached the labels using the indentations on the tab.
		•	Attached the name label immediately above the alphabetical label.
		•	Attached additional labels to the folder as required.
		•	Inserted chart dividers onto the metal fasteners.
		•	Placed the original registration form in front of the medical record.
		•	Placed the signed NPP acknowledgement form in the record.

Copyright © 2008, 2004, 2000, 1995, 1990 by Saunders, an imprint of Elsevier Inc. All rights reserved.

Trial 1	Trial 2	Point Value	Performance Standards
		●	Placed the insurance card (copy) in the appropriate section of the record.
		●	Labeled preprinted forms with required information.
		▷	Stated examples of preprinted forms included in the medical record.
		●	Punched holes into the forms if required.
		●	Inserted each form under its proper chart divider.
		●	Checked the medical record to make sure it was prepared properly.
		*	Completed the procedure within 10 minutes.
			TOTALS

Evaluation of Student Performance

EVALUATION CRITERIA			COMMENTS
Symbol	**Category**	**Point Value**	
*	Critical Step	16 points	
●	Essential Step	6 points	
▷	Theory Question	2 points	
Score calculation: 100 points – _____ points missed ____ Score Satisfactory score: 85 or above			

AAMA/CAAHEP Competency Achieved:

☑ III. C. 3. b. (4) (h): Maintain medication and immunization records.

☑ III. C. 3. c. (2) (c): Establish and maintain the medical record.

☑ III. C. 3. c. (2) (e): Demonstrate knowledge of federal and state health care legislation and regulations.

☑ III. C. 3. c. (4) (c): Utilize computer software to maintain office systems.

☑ III. C. 3. a. (1) (c): Organize a patient's medical record.

Copyright © 2008, 2004, 2000, 1995, 1990 by Saunders, an imprint of Elsevier Inc. All rights reserved.

EVALUATION OF COMPETENCY

Procedure 1-4: Obtaining and Recording Patient Symptoms

Name: ______________________________ Date: ____________

Evaluated By: ______________________________ Score: ____________

Performance Objective

Outcome:	Obtain and record patient symptoms.
Conditions:	Given the following: medical record of the patient to be interviewed and a black ink pen.
Standards:	Time: 10 minutes Student completed procedure in ____ minutes.
	Accuracy: Satisfactory score on the Performance Evaluation Checklist

Performance Evaluation Checklist

Trial 1	Trial 2	Point Value	*Performance Standards*
		•	Assembled equipment.
		•	Made sure the correct patient record was obtained.
		•	Went to the waiting room and asked the patient to come back.
		•	Escorted the patient to a quiet room.
		•	In a calm and friendly manner, greeted the patient and introduced yourself.
		•	Identified the patient by full name and date of birth.
		•	Asked the patient to be seated.
		•	Seated yourself facing the patient at a distance of 3 to 4 feet.
		▷	Explained the purpose of this seating arrangement.
			Used good communication skills
		•	Used the patient's name of choice.
		•	Demonstrated genuine interest and concern for the patient.
		•	Maintained appropriate eye contact.
		•	Used terminology the patient could understand.
		•	Listened carefully and attentively to the patient.
		•	Paid attention to the patient's nonverbal messages.
		•	Avoided judgmental comments.
		•	Avoided rushing the patient.
		•	Located the progress note sheet in the medical record.
		•	Charted the date, time and CC abbreviation
		•	Used an open-ended question to obtain the chief complaint.
		▷	Explained why an open-ended questions should be used.

Copyright © 2008, 2004, 2000, 1995, 1990 by Saunders, an imprint of Elsevier Inc. All rights reserved.

Trial 1	*Trial 2*	*Point Value*	*Performance Standards*
			Charted the chief complaint
		•	Limited the CC to one or two symptoms.
		•	Referred to a specific rather than a vague symptom.
		•	Charted concisely and briefly.
		•	Used the patient's own words as much as possible.
		•	Included the duration of the symptom.
		•	Avoided using names of diseases.
		•	Obtained additional information regarding the chief complaint using what, when and where questions.
		•	Thanked the patient and proceeded to the next step in the patient workup.
		•	Informed the patient that the physician will be in soon.
		•	Placed the medical record in the appropriate location for review by the physician.
		*	Completed the procedure within 10 minutes.
			TOTALS

CHART	
Date	

Copyright © 2008, 2004, 2000, 1995, 1990 by Saunders, an imprint of Elsevier Inc. All rights reserved.

Evaluation of Student Performance

EVALUATION CRITERIA			COMMENTS
Symbol	Category	Point Value	
*	Critical Step	16 points	
•	Essential Step	6 points	
▷	Theory Question	2 points	
Score calculation: 100 points – ______ points missed ____ Score Satisfactory score: 85 or above			

AAMA/CAAHEP Competency Achieved:

☑ III. C. 3. b. (4) (a): Perform telephone and in-person screening.

☑ III. C. 3. b. (4) (c) : Obtain and record patient history.

☑ III. C. 3. c. (1) (b): Recognize and respond to verbal communications.

☑ III. C. 3. c. (1) (c): Recognize and respond to nonverbal communications.

☑ III. C. 3. c. (1) (d): Demonstrate telephone techniques.

☑ III. C. 3. c. (2) (d): Document appropriately.

Copyright © 2008, 2004, 2000, 1995, 1990 by Saunders, an imprint of Elsevier Inc. All rights reserved.

TAKING PATIENT SYMPTOMS: SUPPLEMENTAL EDUCATION FOR CHAPTER 1

Taking patient symptoms is a frequent and important responsibility of the medical assistant. Because of this, the medical assistant must have a thorough knowledge of symptoms and related terminology. A **symptom** is defined as any change in the body or its functioning that indicates the presence of disease. The medical assistant will be able to observe **objective** symptoms presented by the patient, such as coughing, a rash, and swelling. On the other hand, the medical assistant must rely on information relayed by the patient in order to obtain data on **subjective** symptoms. Examples of subjective symptoms include pain, pruritus, and vertigo.

This section is designed as supplemental education for Chapter 1 (The Medical Record) in your textbook. Completion of the exercises in this section will assist you in recording patient symptoms effectively and thoroughly, which is essential to an accurate diagnosis by the physician.

Learning Objectives

After completing this chapter, you should be able to do the following:

1. Explain the purpose of analyzing a symptom.
2. State the seven basic types of information that must be obtained to analyze a symptom.
3. Analyze a symptom by using direct questions.

Analysis of a Symptom

Before a symptom can be analyzed, the **chief complaint** must first be identified. The chief complaint (CC) is the patient's reason for seeking care, or the symptom causing the patient the most trouble. An open-ended question should be used to elicit the chief complaint from the patient, and it should be charted following the charting guidelines presented in your textbook (pages 34 and 35). The next step is to analyze the chief complaint in detail from the time of its onset. The purpose of this is to provide a complete description of the current status of the chief complaint.

Analyzing the chief complaint requires a combination of good listening and writing skills. The medical assistant must also know what information should be recorded for each symptom as well as the questions to ask the patient to obtain this information. A list and explanation of the information required for each symptom, along with examples of questions to ask the patient, are presented below.

Type of Information Required

The following information is needed for each symptom to provide a full description of the current status of the chief complaint:

1. **Location of the Symptom**. This refers to the specific area of the body where the symptom is located. Locating the symptom is the first step in determining the cause of the patient's disease. The patient may refer to the location in general terms, for example, the head, arm, stomach, or back. It is important that the medical assistant be more specific than this, however, and determine the exact location using descriptions such as "occurs in the lower back" or "occurs under the sternum." Questions that assist in accomplishing this are as follows:

   - Where exactly does it hurt?
   - Can you show me where it hurts?
   - Do you feel it anywhere else?

2. **Quality of the Symptom**. The quality of the symptom includes a complete and concise description of the symptom. The medical assistant should use informative terms to describe the character of each symptom. For example, if the patient complains of pain, the character of the pain must be included. Terms that can be used to describe pain include:

   - Burning
   - Aching
   - Sharp
   - Dull
   - Throbbing
   - Cramplike
   - Squeezing

Copyright © 2008, 2004, 2000, 1995, 1990 by Saunders, an imprint of Elsevier Inc. All rights reserved.

If the patient has vomited, the medical assistant will need to indicate the color, odor, and consistency of the vomitus. If the patient has a cough, the medical assistant will need to indicate if it is productive or nonproductive and whether or not blood is present. Refer to the table of terms on pp. 50-51 of this manual, which will assist you in describing symptoms. Specific examples of questions that are helpful in determining the quality of the symptom are as follows:

- Describe it (the symptom) to me as fully as possible.
- What is it (the symptom) like?

3. **Severity of the Symptom**. The severity refers to the quantitative aspect of the symptom. It includes the following:

- Intensity of the symptom (e.g., mild, moderate, severe)
- Number (e.g., of convulsions, of nosebleeds)
- Volume (e.g., of vomitus, of blood, of mucus)
- Size or extent (e.g., of the rash, edema, lumps, or masses)

This information assists the physician in determining the extensiveness or seriousness of the illness. Questions to determine severity are often specific to that symptom. For example, if the patient has a productive cough, the medical assistant will need to determine how much phlegm is being coughed up (e.g., a teaspoon, half a cup). At first, this area may appear difficult. As you practice taking symptoms, however, you will learn what questions to ask the patient, and eventually it will become automatic. The examples at the end of this section as well as the student practice problems provide guidance in developing skill in this area. Some examples of general questions that can be used to determine the severity of a symptom are as follows:

- How bad is it (the symptom)?
- Does it (the symptom) limit your normal activities?

4. **Chronology and Timing of the Symptom**. Chronology and timing include a sequential account of the symptom up to the time the patient came to the medical office for treatment. This information is important in determining the duration of the symptom and change in it since it first occurred. Chronology and timing include the following four areas:

   a. **Date of Onset:** The date of onset of the symptom should be indicated, if possible, as a calendar date and clock time. Because of this, the patient may need some time to recall this information. Examples of questions that help obtain this information are as follows:

   - When did you experience this (the symptom) for the first time?
   - Exactly when did this begin?

   b. **Duration:** The duration of the symptom refers to how long the symptom lasts after it occurs, for example: 10 minutes, 2 hours, continuously. Examples of questions to obtain this information are as follows:

   - How long does it last after occurring?
   - For what length of time do you experience this symptom?

Copyright © 2008, 2004, 2000, 1995, 1990 by Saunders, an imprint of Elsevier Inc. All rights reserved.

c. **Frequency:** The frequency of the symptom refers to how often the symptom occurs, for example: twice a day, a single attack every 2 weeks. Examples of questions to obtain this information are as follows:

- How often does it occur?
- How often has the symptom recurred?

d. **Change over Time:** This area refers to any change in the symptom since it first occurred. A change in a symptom reflects the nature of the underlying disease, which, in turn, assists the physician in making a diagnosis. Examples of questions to obtain this information are as follows:

- Has the symptom changed since it first occurred?
- Is it (the symptom) getting better, worse, or staying the same?

5. **Manner of Onset**. The manner of onset refers to what the patient was doing when the symptom first occurred and exactly what was experienced by the patient when the symptom began. These data help provide information on the pathologic process responsible for the symptom. For example, the patient may have been lifting a heavy object before experiencing low back pain. As is evident, this information helps the physician in making an accurate diagnosis. Examples of questions that are helpful in determining the manner of onset are as follows:

- What exactly did you experience when it (the symptom) first occurred?
- What was the first thing you noticed?
- Did it (the symptom) come on suddenly or gradually?
- What were you doing when it (the symptom) began?
- Where were you when this happened?
- How were you feeling before it (the symptom) began?

6. **Modifying Factors**. Symptoms are often influenced by activities or physiological processes such as physical exercise, change in weather, bodily functions (e.g., bowel movements, eating, coughing), pregnancy, emotional states, and fatigue. Some activities may aggravate the symptom while others may alleviate it. These influences may help to determine what is causing the problem. For example, pain that becomes worse after the patient eats but is relieved after taking an antacid assists the physician in focusing on gastrointestinal disorders. Questions to assist in determining modifying factors are as follows:

- Does anything make it (the symptom) better?
- Does anything make it worse?
- What have you done to make it better?
- What did you do to help it?
- Are you taking any medication for it? Did it help?

7. **Associated Symptoms**. There is usually more than one symptom present with a disease process. Determining these additional symptoms gives the physician a complete picture of the illness. Examples of questions that help to identify the presence of additional symptoms are as follows:

- Are you having any other symptoms?
- What other problems have you noticed since you became ill?

Copyright © 2008, 2004, 2000, 1995, 1990 by Saunders, an imprint of Elsevier Inc. All rights reserved.

Examples

The following examples illustrate how to analyze a symptom. The chief complaint is listed first, followed by questions to ask the patient from the seven basic categories of information.

> ***Example:*** *Chief Complaint: Headaches that began 2 months ago.*

1. Using your finger, point to the location of the headache.
2. Describe the pain. Is it sharp, dull, throbbing?
3. Are you able to carry on normal activities when you have a headache?
4. Is it sometimes more severe than usual?
5. When exactly did your headaches begin?
6. How long does your headache last when it occurs?
7. How often do you get a headache?
8. Since your headaches began, have they gotten better or worse, or have they stayed the same?
9. What were you doing the first time you experienced a headache?
10. What was your health status before your headaches began?
11. Do you get a headache before, during, or after a particular activity, such as reading or watching TV?
12. Does anything make your headache better?
13. Are you taking any medication for your headache? Does it help?
14. Have you had any other problems since your headaches began, such as nausea, vomiting, dizziness, or problems with vision?

> ***Example:*** *Chief Complaint: The patient has been coughing for the past 3 days.*

1. Does it hurt when you cough? Where? Show me with one of your fingers.
2. What is the cough like?
3. Can you cough for me?
4. Do you bring up any phlegm when you cough? What color is it? Is blood present?
5. Describe the pain. Is it sharp, dull, squeezing?
6. Do you become exhausted when you cough?
7. How much phlegm do you bring up? A teaspoon? Half a cup?
8. How much blood is present in the phlegm?
9. When did your cough first begin?
10. Does it seem like an attack? How long does the attack last?
11. How often do you get a coughing attack?
12. Does your cough seem to be getting better or worse?
13. What was the first thing you noticed when you became ill?
14. How were you feeling before your symptoms began?
15. Is there anything that makes your cough better?
16. Is there anything that makes your cough worse?

Copyright © 2008, 2004, 2000, 1995, 1990 by Saunders, an imprint of Elsevier Inc. All rights reserved.

17. Do you cough more at night or during the day?
18. Are you taking any medication for it? Does it help?
19. Are you having any other problems?

PRACTICE PROBLEMS

In the space provided, indicate examples of direct questions to ask the patient to obtain the necessary information for the symptom(s) presented in the chief complaint.

Problem 1

Chief Complaint: Earache and fever for the past 2 days.

Questions:

Problem 2

Chief Complaint: Rash with itching that began 3 days ago.

Questions:

Copyright © 2008, 2004, 2000, 1995, 1990 by Saunders, an imprint of Elsevier Inc. All rights reserved.

Problem 3

Chief Complaint: Pain during urination that began yesterday.

Questions:

Problem 4

Chief Complaint: Low back pain for the past 3 months.

Questions:

Problem 5

Chief Complaint: Sore throat and fever for the past 24 hours.

Questions:

Copyright © 2008, 2004, 2000, 1995, 1990 by Saunders, an imprint of Elsevier Inc. All rights reserved.

Problem 6

Chief Complaint: Chest pain that occurred this morning.

Questions:

Terms for Describing Symptoms

PAIN
Burning, aching, sharp, dull, throbbing, cramping, squeezing
Radiating, transient, constant
Localized, superficial, deep

RESPIRATIONS
Rapid, irregular, shallow, deep, labored, gasping, noisy, wheezing
Apnea, dyspnea, orthopnea
Discomfort, pain, cyanosis, cough

COUGH
Nonproductive, productive
Persistent, dry, hacking, barking, spasmodic
Phlegm: color, consistency, presence or absence of blood
Exhausting or painful

CARDIOVASCULAR
Pain, palpitations
Sharp, radiating
Dyspnea, orthopnea
Cyanosis

GASTROINTESTINAL
Abdomen: flaccid, rigid, distended
Appetite: anorexia, intolerance to foods
Heartburn, pain after eating, belching, nausea, vomiting, flatulence, change in bowel habits, constipation, diarrhea, black stools

URINE/STOOL
Abnormality: color, odor, consistency, frequency
Contents: sediment, mucus, blood
Elimination: urgency, nocturia, pain, burning

SKIN
Rash: pruritus, red, swelling, distribution
Lesions: color, character, distribution
Pallor, flushing, jaundice, warm, dry, cold, clammy
Ecchymosis, petechiae, cyanosis, edema
Pruritus, sweating, change in color, bruises easily

Copyright © 2008, 2004, 2000, 1995, 1990 by Saunders, an imprint of Elsevier Inc. All rights reserved.

Ears
Pain, loss of hearing, tinnitus, vertigo
Discharge, infection

Eyes
Itching, burning, blurry vision, seeing double, photophobia
Discharge, watering, infection

Copyright © 2008, 2004, 2000, 1995, 1990 by Saunders, an imprint of Elsevier Inc. All rights reserved.

Notes

Copyright © 2008, 2004, 2000, 1995, 1990 by Saunders, an imprint of Elsevier Inc. All rights reserved.

2

Medical Asepsis and the OSHA Standard

CHAPTER ASSIGNMENTS

√ After Completing	Date Due	Textbook Page (s)	TEXTBOOK ASSIGNMENTS	Possible Points	Points You Earned
		49-82	Read Chapter 2: Medical Asepsis and the OSHA Standard		
		59 78	Read Case Study 1 Case Study 1 questions	5	
		65 78	Read Case Study 2 Case Study 2 questions	5	
		69 78	Read Case Study 3 Case Study 3 questions	5	
		79	Apply Your Knowledge questions	10	
			TOTAL POINTS		

√ After Completing	Date Due	Study Guide Page(s)	STUDY GUIDE ASSIGNMENTS (CTA: Critical Thinking Activity)	Possible Points	Points You Earned
		57	Pretest	10	
		58	Key Term Assessment	23	
		59-63	Evaluation of Learning questions	45	
		64	CTA A: Infection Process Cycle	5	
		64	CTA B: Handwashing	8	
		65	CTA C: Personal Protective Equipment: Gloves	8	
		65	CTA D: Personal Protective Equipment	30	
		65-66	CTA E: Discarding Medical Waste	20	
			CD Activity: Chapter 2 Discard It! (Record points earned)		

Copyright © 2008, 2004, 2000, 1995, 1990 by Saunders, an imprint of Elsevier Inc. All rights reserved.

√ After Completing	Date Due	Study Guide Page(s)	STUDY GUIDE ASSIGNMENTS (CTA: Critical Thinking Activity)	Possible Points	Points You Earned
		66	CTA F: Dear Gabby	10	
		67	CTA G: Crossword Puzzle	25	
		68	CTA H: Road to Recovery Game: OSHA Standard (Record points earned)		
			CD Activity: Chapter 2 Quiz Show (Record points earned)		
		57	Posttest	10	
			ADDITIONAL ASSIGNMENTS		
			TOTAL POINTS		

Copyright © 2008, 2004, 2000, 1995, 1990 by Saunders, an imprint of Elsevier Inc. All rights reserved.

√ When Assigned By Your Instructor	Study Guide Page(s)	Practices Required	LABORATORY ASSIGNMENTS (Procedure Number and Name)	*Score
	75	5	**Practice for Competency** 2-1: Handwashing Textbook reference: pp. 54-56	
	77-78		**Evaluation of Competency** 2-1: Handwashing	*
	75	4	**Practice for Competency** 2-2: Applying an Alcohol-Based Handrub Textbook reference: p. 57	
	79-80		**Evaluation of Competency** 2-2: Applying an Alcohol-Based Handrub	*
	75	5	**Practice for Competency** 2-3: Application and Removal of Clean Disposable Gloves Textbook reference: pp. 58-59	
	81-82		**Evaluation of Competency** 2-3: Application and Removal of Clean Disposable Gloves	*
			ADDITIONAL ASSIGNMENTS	

Copyright © 2008, 2004, 2000, 1995, 1990 by Saunders, an imprint of Elsevier Inc. All rights reserved.

Notes

Copyright © 2008, 2004, 2000, 1995, 1990 by Saunders, an imprint of Elsevier Inc. All rights reserved.

Name GRACE V. MAURICIO Date ___________

PRETEST

True or False

T 1. A microorganism is a tiny living plant or animal that cannot be seen with the naked eye.

F 2. A disease-producing microorganism is known as a nonpathogen.

T 3. Microorganisms grow best in an acidic environment.

T 4. Coughing and sneezing help force pathogens from the body.

F 5. An alcohol-based handrub should be used to sanitize hands that are visibly soiled.

T 6. OSHA stands for Occupational Safety and Health Administration.

T 7. A biohazard warning label must be fluorescent orange or orange-red in color.

F 8. Prescription eyeglasses are acceptable eye protection when handling blood.

_____ 9. Hepatitis B is an infection of the liver caused by a virus.

_____ 10. Many people do not develop symptoms when they first become infected with HIV.

POSTTEST

True or False

T 1. Bacteria and viruses are examples of microorganisms.

F 2. An anaerobe can exist only in the presence of oxygen. (w/o)

T 3. The optimum growth temperature is the temperature at which a microorganism grows the best.

T 4. Medical asepsis are practices which help keep an area free from infection.

F 5. Resident flora are picked up in the course of daily activities and are usually pathogenic.

_____ 6. The purpose of the OSHA Standard is to prevent exposure of employees to bloodborne pathogens.

_____ 7. OSHA requires the Exposure Control Plan to be updated annually.

_____ 8. An engineering control is a physical or mechanical device used to remove health hazards from the workplace.

_____ 9. A reagent strip that has been used to test urine is an example of regulated medical waste.

_____ 10. The most common means of transmitting hepatitis C is through sexual intercourse.

Copyright © 2008, 2004, 2000, 1995, 1990 by Saunders, an imprint of Elsevier Inc. All rights reserved.

KEY TERM ASSESSMENT

Directions: Match each medical term with its definition.

__C__ 1. Aerobe
__Q__ 2. Anaerobe
__U__ 3. Antiseptic
__E__ 4. Asepsis
_____ 5. Bloodborne pathogens
__N__ 6. Cilia
__R__ 7. Contaminate
_____ 8. Exposure incident
__V__ 9. Hand hygiene
_____ 10. Infection
__P__ 11. Microorganism
__G__ 12. Nonintact skin
__O__ 13. Nonpathogen
_____ 14. Occupational exposure
_____ 15. Opportunistic infection
__H__ 16. Optimum growth temperature
__A__ 17. Pathogen
__I__ 18. pH
_____ 19. Post-exposure prophylaxis
_____ 20. Regulated medical waste
__S__ 21. Reservoir host
__F__ 22. Susceptible
__B__ 23. Transient flora

A. A disease-producing microorganism
B. Microorganisms that reside on the superficial skin layers and are picked up in the course of daily activities
C. A microorganism that needs oxygen in order to live and grow
D. Reasonably anticipated skin, eye, mucous membrane, or parenteral contact with bloodborne pathogens or other potentially infectious materials that may result from the performance of an employee's duties
E. Free from infection or pathogens
F. Easily affected; lacking resistance
G. Skin that has a break in the surface
H. The temperature at which an organism grows best 98.6°F
I. The degree to which a solution is acidic or basic
J. A specific eye, mouth, other mucous membrane, nonintact skin, or parenteral contact with blood or other potentially infectious materials that results from an employee's duties
K. Pathogenic microorganisms capable of causing disease that are present in human blood
L. The condition in which the body, or part of it, is invaded by a pathogen
M. Any waste containing infectious material that may pose a threat to health and safety
N. Slender hairlike processes
O. A microorganism that does not normally produce disease
P. A microscopic plant or animal
Q. A microorganism that grows best in the absence of oxygen
R. To soil or to make impure
S. The organism that becomes infected by a pathogen and also serves as a source of transfer of pathogens to others
T. An infection resulting from a defective immune system that cannot defend the body from pathogens normally found in the environment
U. An agent that kills microorganisms or inhibits their growth
V. The process of cleaning or sanitizing the hands
W. Treatment administered to an individual after exposure to an infectious disease to prevent the disease

Copyright © 2008, 2004, 2000, 1995, 1990 by Saunders, an imprint of Elsevier Inc. All rights reserved.

EVALUATION OF LEARNING

Directions: Fill in each blank with the correct answer.

1. List four examples of types of microorganisms.

bacteria, viruses, protozoa, fungi, and animal parasites

2. Define medical asepsis.

medical asepsis means that an object or area is clean and free from infection.

3. What type of microorganisms are still present on an object that is medically aseptic?

RESIDENT FLORA

4. What is the name given to the organism that uses organic or living substances for food?

HETEROTROPHS

5. Why do most microorganisms prefer a neutral pH?

If the environment of the microorganisms becomes too acidic or too basic, they die.

6. List five examples of how microorganisms can enter the body.

1. OPEN WOUNDS 3. NOSE 5. EYES
2. MOUTH 4. THROAT

7. List three examples of how a microorganism can be transmitted from one person to another.

1.

8. List four examples of factors that would make a host more susceptible to the entrance of a pathogen.

1. POOR HEALTH 3. POOR NUTRITION
2. POOR HYGIENE 4. STRESS

9. List five protective devices of the body that prevent the entrance of microorganisms.

1. SKIN 4. COUGHING + SNEEZING
2. MUCOUS MEMBRANES 5. TEARS + SWEAT
3. MUCUS + CILIA

10. What is the difference between resident flora and transient flora?

Copyright © 2008, 2004, 2000, 1995, 1990 by Saunders, an imprint of Elsevier Inc. All rights reserved.

11. List three examples of when handwashing should be performed in the medical office.

12. How does antiseptic handwashing sanitize the hands?

13. List three examples of when an alcohol-based handrub may be used to sanitize the hands.

14. What are the advantages and disadvantages of alcohol-based handrubs?

15. List six medical aseptic practices the medical assistant should follow in the medical office.

16. What does OSHA stand for, and what is its purpose?

17. What is the purpose of the OSHA Occupational Exposure to Bloodborne Pathogens Standard?

18. Who must follow the OSHA Standard? List examples.

19. What is the purpose of the Needlestick Safety and Prevention Act?

Copyright © 2008, 2004, 2000, 1995, 1990 by Saunders, an imprint of Elsevier Inc. All rights reserved.

20. List five examples of other potentially infectious materials (OPIM).

21. List examples of nonintact skin.

22. What is the purpose of the exposure control plan (ECP)?

23. List three examples of items to which a biohazard warning label must be attached.

24. What is the purpose of a Sharps Injury Log? What type of offices must maintain this log?

25. Define an engineering control and list three examples of engineering controls.

26. What is a safer medical device?

27. What should be done before and after gloves are applied?

Wash hands with soap and water.

28. List six guidelines that must be followed when using personal protective equipment.

29. What procedure should be followed when a sharps container located in an examining room becomes full? Explain the reason for your answer.

Copyright © 2008, 2004, 2000, 1995, 1990 by Saunders, an imprint of Elsevier Inc. All rights reserved.

30. Explain how to prepare regulated medical waste for pickup by a medical waste service.

31. How should regulated medical waste be stored while waiting pickup by the medical waste service? Explain why.

32. What information is included on a regulated medical waste tracking form?

33. List four guidelines that must be followed with respect to biohazard sharps containers.

34. What is the most likely means of contracting hepatitis B in the health care setting?

35. What side effects may occur following the administration of a hepatitis B vaccine?

36. What post-exposure prophylaxis (PEP) is recommended for an unvaccinated individual who has been exposed to hepatitis B?

37. What are the symptoms of acute viral hepatitis B in individuals who have symptoms?

38. Why is chronic viral hepatitis B considered such a serious condition?

Copyright © 2008, 2004, 2000, 1995, 1990 by Saunders, an imprint of Elsevier Inc. All rights reserved.

39. Why is chronic hepatitis C known as "an epidemic that occurred in the past?"

40. What are the symptoms of acute HIV infection?

41. Explain what occurs during the asymptomatic period and the symptomatic period of the AIDS infection cycle.

42. What are the characteristics of full-blown AIDS?

43. How is HIV transmitted? How is it *not* transmitted?

44. List five AIDS-defining conditions.

45. What is the CDC's definition of AIDS?

Copyright © 2008, 2004, 2000, 1995, 1990 by Saunders, an imprint of Elsevier Inc. All rights reserved.

CRITICAL THINKING ACTIVITIES

A. INFECTION PROCESS CYCLE

Carefully review the Infection Process Cycle and the requirements for growth needed by microorganisms. Create an environment in a medical office that would function to interrupt the Infection Process Cycle and discourage the growth of pathogens.

B. HANDWASHING

Using the principles outlined in the handwashing procedure, explain what might happen under the following circumstances:

1. The medical assistant's uniform touches the sink during the handwashing procedure.
2. The hands are not held lower than the elbows during the handwashing procedure.
3. Friction is not used to wash the hands.
4. Water is splashed on the medical assistant's uniform during the handwashing procedure.
5. The medical assistant continually uses water that is too cold to wash hands.
6. The medical assistant turns off the running water with his or her bare hands.
7. The medical assistant does not clean his or her fingernails daily.
8. The medical assistant's skin becomes chapped.

Copyright © 2008, 2004, 2000, 1995, 1990 by Saunders, an imprint of Elsevier Inc. All rights reserved.

C. PERSONAL PROTECTIVE EQUIPMENT: GLOVES

In which of the following situations does OSHA require the use of clean disposable gloves?

_____ 1. Performing a urinalysis on a urine specimen that contains blood

_____ 2. Sanitizing operating scissors for sterilization

_____ 3. Performing a finger puncture

_____ 4. Performing a vision screening test on a school-aged child

_____ 5. Cleaning up a blood spill on a laboratory work table

_____ 6. Drawing blood from an elderly patient

_____ 7. Measuring the weight of a college student

_____ 8. Testing a blood specimen for glucose

D. PERSONAL PROTECTIVE EQUIPMENT

Create a collage of items or articles that *can* and *cannot* be used as PPE following these guidelines:

1. Using items cut from a magazine, colored pencils, and markers, create a collage of items that are designated as personal protective equipment by OSHA.
2. On the reverse side of the sheet, create a collage of items or articles that are *not* permitted to be used as personal protective equipment.
3. In the classroom, choose a partner and trade sheets. For each PPE item: state examples of the procedures or tasks which may require its use. For each item that is not PPE: explain why it should not be used as PPE.

Examples of PPE

____

____

____

____

Not examples of PPE

____

____

____

____

E. DISCARDING MEDICAL WASTE

Indicate where each of the following (used) items should be discarded using these abbreviations:
RWC: regular waste container
BSC: biohazard sharps container
BB: biohazard bag waste container

_____ 1. Urine testing strip

_____ 2. Lancet

_____ 3. Gloves with blood on them

_____ 4. Blood tube

_____ 5. Tongue depressor

_____ 6. Razor blade

_____ 7. Capillary pipet

_____ 8. Dressing saturated with blood

Copyright © 2008, 2004, 2000, 1995, 1990 by Saunders, an imprint of Elsevier Inc. All rights reserved.

_____ 9. Patient drape

_____ 10. An empty urine container

_____ 11. Sutures caked with blood

_____ 12. Thermometer probe cover

_____ 13. Patient gown

_____ 14. Disposable diaper

_____ 15. Dressing saturated with a purulent discharge

_____ 16. Clean disposable gloves

_____ 17. Disposable vaginal speculum

_____ 18. An outdated vaccine

_____ 19. Syringe and needle

_____ 20. Examining-table paper

F. DEAR GABBY

Gabby is away on vacation and wants you to fill in for her. In the space provided, respond to the following letter using the knowledge you have acquired in this chapter.

Dear Gabby:

I am writing to you because I am very concerned about my younger sister "Tuesday." For the past 2 weeks, Tuesday has been extremely tired and does not feel like eating. She also vomits several times a day and says that her joints ache. Tuesday is 26 years old and a single mother with two small children. Tuesday has been dating "Alex" for the past 4 months. It is well-known around town that Alex sometimes injects himself with illegal drugs and I think there's a chance that Tuesday is also using drugs.

I told Tuesday that she needs to see her doctor right away, but she will not listen to me. She says it just seems like a prolonged case of the flu and it will probably go away soon. I did an Internet search of her symptoms and it sounds to me like she has hepatitis C.

Gabby, am I just being overprotective of my sister, or should I insist that she see her doctor?

Wanting to Know in Wyoming

____

____

____

____

____

____

____

____

____

____

Copyright © 2008, 2004, 2000, 1995, 1990 by Saunders, an imprint of Elsevier Inc. All rights reserved.

G. CROSSWORD PUZZLE

Medical Asepsis and the OSHA Standard

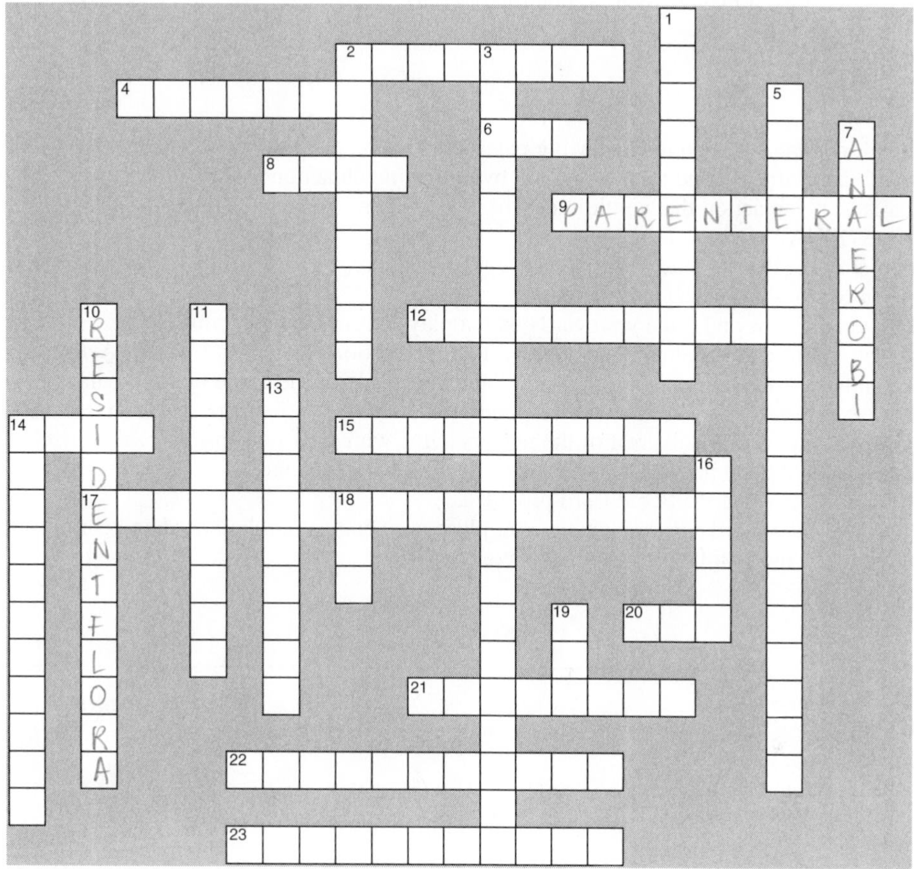

Directions: Complete the crossword puzzle using the clues provided below.

ACROSS

2 MO that causes disease
4 Acute viral hepatitis B symptom
6 After exposure, may prevent disease
8 Vaginal secretions (ex)
9 Piercing of the skin barrier
12 #1 aseptic practice
14 Hepatitis B passive immunizing agent
15 #1 chronic viral disease in U.S.
17 Health hazard eliminator
20 Protector of public health
21 Example of an MO
22 Lacking resistance
23 HBV serious complication

DOWN

1 Found in antimicrobial soap
2 Shortly before or after birth
3 AIDS-defining condition
5 Way to prevent an NSI
7 Grows best without oxygen
10 Normally live on the skin
11 Can live dry for 1 week
13 Body invasion by a pathogen
14 Eats "live stuff"
16 HIV screening test
18 Discard in a biohazard container
19 Scrubs are not this

Copyright © 2008, 2004, 2000, 1995, 1990 by Saunders, an imprint of Elsevier Inc. All rights reserved.

H. ROAD TO RECOVERY GAME

Object: The object of the game is to lead your "patient" to recovery by correctly determining if a response to a situation in the medical office meets the OSHA BBP Standard or violates the OSHA Standard.

Needed: **Road to Recovery** game board (located at the end of this manual)
A token for each player (such as a button or coin)
Dice (1)
Game cards
Score card

Directions:

1. Cut out the situation game cards on the following pages.
2. On the reverse of each card respond to the situation by indicating an action that could be taken. For approximately half of your cards, state an action that would **meet** the OSHA Standard; for the other half, state an action that would **violate** the OSHA Standard.
3. Get into a group of two. (Please note: This is an exception to the regular **Road to Recovery** directions which specify a group of four.)
4. Get into your playing groups and trade your cards with a player from another group.
5. Place one complete set of cards on the game board with the Situations facing up (and the Actions facing down).
6. Play **Road to Recovery** following the directions on the reverse side of the game board. A player should pick up a card and read the Situation and the Action and respond by indicating whether the action **meets** the OSHA Standard or **violates** the OSHA Standard. If the rest of the players agree with your response, award yourself 5 points. If a question arises as to the correct answer, consult your instructor for assistance.
7. Keep track of your points using the Score Card provided.
8. After completing one set of cards on the game board, place a second set on the board and continue playing the game. Continue playing until all the sets of cards have been used.

ROAD TO RECOVERY
SCORE CARD

Name: ______________________________

Recording Points:
Using the Game Card Points box, cross off a number each time you answer a game card correctly (starting with 5 and continuing in sequence). Your Total Game Card Points will be equal to the last number you crossed off. Record this number in the space provided (1). Record any extra points you were awarded during the game (2) and any points that were deducted (3). To determine your total points, add (1) and (2) together and deduct (3). Record this number in the Total Points Earned space provided. Compare your score with the other player and determine where you placed. Place a check mark next to the level of recovery your patient attained.

Game Card Points:

5	75	145
10	80	150
15	85	155
20	90	160
25	95	165
30	100	170
35	105	175
40	110	180
45	115	185
50	120	190
55	125	195
60	130	200
65	135	205
70	140	210

Calculation of Points:

(1) Total Game Card Points: ________

(2) Additional Points Awarded: ________

(3) Deducted Points: ________

TOTAL POINTS EARNED: ________

LEVEL OF RECOVERY:

Patient's Name: ______________________

☐ First Place: **Fully Recovered**

☐ Second Place: **Almost Recovered**

Copyright © 2008, 2004, 2000, 1995, 1990 by Saunders, an imprint of Elsevier Inc. All rights reserved.

SITUATION: You just gave an injection to a patient and after withdrawing the needle, you notice that there is no sharps container in the room.

SITUATION: A part-time clinical medical assistant was just hired. She is not immunized against hepatitis B.

SITUATION: You go into an examining room and notice that the biohazard sharps container in that room is completely full.

SITUATION: You are getting ready to apply gloves and notice that you have a cut on your finger.

SITUATION: A clinical medical assistant who has worked at the office for 5 years changes her mind and decides she wants the hepatitis B vaccine.

SITUATION: You are performing laboratory testing. You accidentally drop a blood tube, and it breaks.

SITUATION: You accidentally get some blood on your bare hands while removing your gloves.

SITUATION: You are wearing a protective lab coat over your scrubs. While performing a laboratory test, some blood splashes onto your lab coat, but does not penetrate through to your scrubs.

SITUATION: You are wearing a protective laboratory coat over your scrubs, and you are getting ready to leave for the day.

ACTION:	ACTION:	ACTION:
ACTION:	ACTION:	ACTION:
ACTION:	ACTION:	ACTION:

SITUATION: You remove your gloves after giving an injection to a patient and accidentally discard them into the biohazard sharps container.

SITUATION: A new clinical medical assistant was just hired at the medical office, and she is allergic to latex gloves.

SITUATION: During an office meeting, a co-worker suggests an idea to save money by emptying full sharps containers into a biohazard bag so that the containers can be reused.

SITUATION: You are separating serum from whole blood, and you accidentally spill some of the serum on the counter top.

SITUATION: You have just drawn blood from a patient, and you accidentally stick yourself with the needle.

SITUATION: A new employee wants to know where she should eat her lunch.

SITUATION: By mistake, you throw a reusable tourniquet into the sharps container after drawing a patient's blood.

SITUATION: Your office only has one refrigerator and blood tubes need to be stored in it, but the staff would like to put their lunches in it.

SITUATION: You are applying a pair of disposable gloves, and one of the gloves tears while you are pulling it on.

ACTION:	ACTION:	ACTION:
ACTION:	ACTION:	ACTION:
ACTION:	ACTION:	ACTION:

SITUATION: You are removing a stopper from a tube of blood so that you can transfer the serum to another tube. A small amount of serum accidentally spatters into your eye.

SITUATION: You have just been assigned the responsibility of performing all required venipunctures in your office. You notice that the sharps container is located on the opposite side of the room to the blood drawing chair.

SITUATION: A technician is coming to your office today to repair your blood chemistry analyzer.

SITUATION: A new employee has been hired who has already had the hepatitis B vaccination series.

SITUATION: Utility gloves are used and reused in your office for the sanitization of medical instruments.

SITUATION: Your office has run out of biohazard bags used to transport specimens to the lab and you notice that an employee is using plastic bags as a substitute.

SITUATION: A medical assisting extern student does not wear gloves to recap a needle after drawing medication into a syringe to give an injection to a patient.

SITUATION: You accidentially close (and lock in place) the lid of a sharps container that is only half full.

SITUATION: You notice that after an externship student performs an allergy injection, she lays the used needle and syringe on the counter. She then discards it in the sharps container after applying a Band aid to the patient's finger.

ACTION:	ACTION:	ACTION:
ACTION:	ACTION:	ACTION:
ACTION:	ACTION:	ACTION:

PRACTICE FOR COMPETENCY

Medical Asepsis

Procedure 2-1: Handwashing. Perform the handwashing procedure. List five medically aseptic steps that must be followed during this procedure.

Medically Aseptic Steps to Follow during Handwashing

1. ____
____
2. ____
____
3. ____
____
4. ____
____
5. ____
____

Procedure 2-2: Alcohol-based Handrub. Apply an alcohol-based handrub. Practice applying both a gel and a foam handrub. List the brand name(s) of the handrubs you applied and list the ingredients contained in them.

Procedure 2-3: Clean Disposable Gloves. Apply and remove clean disposable gloves. What size gloves fit you the best?

____
____

Copyright © 2008, 2004, 2000, 1995, 1990 by Saunders, an imprint of Elsevier Inc. All rights reserved.

Notes

Copyright © 2008, 2004, 2000, 1995, 1990 by Saunders, an imprint of Elsevier Inc. All rights reserved.

EVALUATION OF COMPETENCY

Procedure 2-1: Handwashing

Name: ______________________________ Date: ____________

Evaluated By: ______________________________ Score: ____________

Performance Objective

Outcome: Perform handwashing.

Conditions: Using a sink.

Given liquid soap or bar soap and paper towels.

Standards: Time: 5 minutes. Student completed procedure in ____ minutes.

Accuracy: Satisfactory score on the Performance Evaluation Checklist.

Performance Evaluation Checklist

Trial 1	*Trial 2*	*Point Value*	*Performance Standards*
		•	Removed watch or pushed it up on the forearm.
		•	Removed rings.
		▷	Stated the reason for removing rings.
		•	Stood at sink with clothing away from edge of sink.
		•	Turned on faucets with paper towel.
		▷	Explained the reason for turning on faucets with paper towel.
		•	Adjusted the water to a warm temperature.
		•	Discarded towel into trash can.
		•	Wet hands and forearms with water.
		•	Held hands lower than elbows at all times.
		▷	Explained why the hands should be held lower than elbows.
		•	Did not touch the inside of sink with hands.
		•	Applied soap to hands.
		•	Washed palms and backs of hands with 10 circular motions and friction.
		▷	Explained why circular motions and friction are needed to wash hands.
		•	Washed fingers with 10 circular motions.
		•	Washed fingers while interlaced using friction and circular motions.
		•	Rinsed well (keeping hands lower than elbows).
		•	Washed wrists and forearms using friction and circular motions.
		•	Cleaned fingernails using manicure stick.

Copyright © 2008, 2004, 2000, 1995, 1990 by Saunders, an imprint of Elsevier Inc. All rights reserved.

Trial 1	Trial 2	Point Value	Performance Standards
		•	Rinsed arms and hands.
		•	Repeated handwashing procedure (if necessary).
		•	Dried hands gently and thoroughly.
		▷	Stated the reason for drying hands gently and completely.
		•	Turned off faucets using paper towel.
		•	Did not touch sink area with bare hands.
		▷	Explained the reason for not touching sink area with bare hands.
		*	Completed the procedure within 5 minutes.
			TOTALS

Evaluation of Student Performance

EVALUATION CRITERIA			COMMENTS
Symbol	Category	Point Value	
*	Critical Step	16 points	
•	Essential Step	6 points	
▷	Theory Question	2 points	
Score calculation: 100 points – ______ points missed ____ Score Satisfactory score: 85 or above			

AAMA/CAAHEP Competency Achieved:

☑ III. C. 3. b. (1) (a): Perform handwashing.

☑ III. C. 3. b. (1) (e): Practice Standard Precautions.

Copyright © 2008, 2004, 2000, 1995, 1990 by Saunders, an imprint of Elsevier Inc. All rights reserved.

EVALUATION OF COMPETENCY

Procedure 2-2: Applying an Alcohol-Based Handrub

Name: ______________________________ Date: ____________

Evaluated By: ______________________________ Score: ____________

Performance Objective

Outcome: Apply an alcohol-based handrub.

Conditions: Given an alcohol-based handrub.

Standards: Time: 2 minutes. Student completed procedure in ____ minutes.

Accuracy: Satisfactory score on the Performance Evaluation Checklist.

Performance Evaluation Checklist

Trial 1	Trial 2	Point Value	*Performance Standards*
		•	Inspected the hands to make sure they are not visibly soiled.
		▷	Stated the procedure to follow if the hands are visibly soiled.
		•	Removed watch or pushed it up on the forearm.
		•	Removed rings.
			Applied the alcohol-based handrub to the palm of one hand as follows:
		•	***Gel or lotion:*** Applied an amount of gel or lotion approximately equal to the size of a dime.
		•	***Foam:*** Applied an amount of foam approximately equal to the size of a walnut.
		▷	Explained why it is important not to use more than the recommended amount of handrub.
		•	Thoroughly spread the handrub over the surface of both hands up to ½ inch above the wrist.
		•	Spread the handrub around and under the fingernails.
		▷	Explained why it is important to cover the entire surface of the hands.
		•	Rubbed the hands together until they are dry.
		•	Did not touch anything until the hands were dry.
		*	Completed the procedure within 2 minutes.
			TOTALS

Copyright © 2008, 2004, 2000, 1995, 1990 by Saunders, an imprint of Elsevier Inc. All rights reserved.

Evaluation of Student Performance

EVALUATION CRITERIA			COMMENTS
Symbol	Category	Point Value	
✶	Critical Step	16 points	
●	Essential Step	6 points	
▷	Theory Question	2 points	
Score calculation: 100 points – ______ points missed ____ Score Satisfactory score: 85 or above			

AAMA/CAAHEP Competency Achieved:

☑ III. C. 3. b. (1) (e): Practice Standard Precautions.

Copyright © 2008, 2004, 2000, 1995, 1990 by Saunders, an imprint of Elsevier Inc. All rights reserved.

EVALUATION OF COMPETENCY

Procedure 2-3: Application and Removal of Clean Disposable Gloves

Name: ______________________________ Date: ______________

Evaluated By: ______________________________ Score: ______________

Performance Objective

Outcome: Apply and remove clean disposable gloves.

Conditions: Given the appropriate sized clean disposable gloves.

Standards: Time: 5 minutes. Student completed procedure in ____ minutes.

Accuracy: Satisfactory score on the Performance Evaluation Checklist.

Performance Evaluation Checklist

Trial 1	Trial 2	Point Value	*Performance Standards*
			Application of Clean Gloves
		•	Removed all rings.
		▷	Stated why rings should be removed.
		•	Sanitized the hands.
		•	Chose the appropriate sized gloves.
		▷	Explained what can happen if the gloves are too small or too large.
		•	Applied the gloves.
		•	Adjusted the gloves so that they fit comfortably.
		•	Inspected the gloves for tears.
		▷	Stated the procedure to follow if a glove is torn.
			Removal of Clean Gloves
		•	Grasped the outside of the left glove 1 to 2 inches from the top with the gloved right hand.
		•	Slowly pulled left glove off the hand.
		•	Pulled the left glove free and scrunched it into a ball with the gloved right hand.
		•	Placed the index and middle fingers of the left hand on the inside of the right glove.
		•	Did not allow the clean hand to touch outside of the glove.
		•	Pulled the glove off the right hand enclosing the balled-up left glove.
		•	Discarded both gloves in an appropriate waste container.

Copyright © 2008, 2004, 2000, 1995, 1990 by Saunders, an imprint of Elsevier Inc. All rights reserved.

		▷	Stated when gloves should be discarded in a biohazardous waste container.
		•	Sanitized the hands.
		*	Completed the procedure in 5 minutes.
			TOTALS

Evaluation of Student Performance

EVALUATION CRITERIA			COMMENTS
Symbol	Category	Point Value	
*	Critical Step	16 points	
•	Essential Step	6 points	
▷	Theory Question	2 points	
Score calculation: 100 points – ______ points missed ____ Score Satisfactory score: 85 or above			

AAMA/CAAHEP Competency Achieved:

☑ III. C. 3. b. (1) (e): Practice Standard Precautions.

Copyright © 2008, 2004, 2000, 1995, 1990 by Saunders, an imprint of Elsevier Inc. All rights reserved.

3

Sterilization and Disinfection

CHAPTER ASSIGNMENTS

√ After Completing	Date Due	Textbook Page(s)	TEXTBOOK ASSIGNMENTS	Possible Points	Points You Earned
		83-116	Read Chapter 3: Sterilization and Disinfection		
		86 113	Read Case Study 1 Case Study 1 questions	5	
		96 113	Read Case Study 2 Case Study 2 questions	5	
		101 113	Read Case Study 3 Case Study 3 questions	5	
		114	Apply Your Knowledge questions	10	
			TOTAL POINTS		

√ After Completing	Date Due	Study Guide Page(s)	STUDY GUIDE ASSIGNMENTS (CTA: Critical Thinking Activity))	Possible Points	Points You Earned
		87	Pretest	10	
		88	Key Term Assessment	16	
		89-91	Evaluation of Learning questions	31	
		92-93	CTA A: Material Safety Data Sheet	17	
		93-94	CTA B: Obtaining a Material Data Safety Sheet	10	
		94	CTA C: Sanitization	8	
		95	CTA D: Storage of a Chemical Disinfectant	4	
		95-96	CTA E: Sterilization	10	
		98	CTA F: What Comes Next? Game (Record points earned)		
			CD Activity: Chapter 3 What Happens Now? (Record points earned)		

Copyright © 2008, 2004, 2000, 1995, 1990 by Saunders, an imprint of Elsevier Inc. All rights reserved.

√ After Completing	Date Due	Study Guide Page(s)	STUDY GUIDE ASSIGNMENTS (CTA: Critical Thinking Activity))	Possible Points	Points You Earned
			CD Activity: Chapter 3 Quiz Show (Record points earned)		
		87	Posttest	10	
			ADDITIONAL ASSIGNMENTS		
			TOTAL POINTS		

Copyright © 2008, 2004, 2000, 1995, 1990 by Saunders, an imprint of Elsevier Inc. All rights reserved.

√ When Assigned By Your Instructor	Study Guide Page(s)	Practices Required	LABORATORY ASSIGNMENTS (Procedure Number and Name)	*Score
	101	3	DVD **Practice for Competency** 3-1: Sanitization of Instruments Textbook reference: pp. 91-95	
	103-105		**Evaluation of Competency** 3-1: Sanitization of Instruments	*
	101	3	**Practice for Competency** 3-2: Chemical Disinfection of Articles Textbook reference: pp. 97-99	
	107-108		**Evaluation of Competency** 3-2: Chemical Disinfection of Articles	*
	101	Paper: 3 Muslin: 3	DVD **Practice for Competency** 3-3: Wrapping Instruments Using Paper or Muslin Textbook reference: pp. 103-105	
	109-110		**Evaluation of Competency** 3-3: Wrapping Instruments Using Paper or Muslin	*
	101	3	**Practice for Competency** 3-4: Wrapping Instruments Using a Pouch Textbook reference: pp. 105-106	
	111-112		**Evaluation of Competency** 3-4: Wrapping Instruments Using a Pouch	
	101	3	DVD **Practice for Competency** 3-5: Sterilizing Articles in the Autoclave Textbook reference: pp. 110-112	
	113-114		**Evaluation of Competency** 3-5: Sterilizing Articles in the Autoclave	*
			ADDITIONAL ASSIGNMENTS	

Copyright © 2008, 2004, 2000, 1995, 1990 by Saunders, an imprint of Elsevier Inc. All rights reserved.

Notes

Copyright © 2008, 2004, 2000, 1995, 1990 by Saunders, an imprint of Elsevier Inc. All rights reserved.

Name ______________________________ Date ______________

PRETEST

True or False

_____ 1. A bacterial spore consists of a hard, thick-walled capsule that can resist adverse conditions.

_____ 2. The purpose of sanitization is to remove all microorganisms and spores from a contaminated article.

_____ 3. According to OSHA, gloves do not need to be worn during the sanitization process.

_____ 4. Glutaraldehyde (Cidex) is a high-level disinfectant.

_____ 5. OSHA recommends a 10%-bleach solution be used to decontaminate blood spills.

_____ 6. Sterilization is the process of destroying all forms of microbial life except for bacterial spores.

_____ 7. Autoclave tape indicates whether or not an autoclaved item is sterile.

_____ 8. The wrapper used to autoclave articles should prevent contaminants from getting in during handling and storage.

_____ 9. Tap water should be used in the autoclave.

_____ 10. The inside of the autoclave should be wiped every day with a damp cloth.

POSTTEST

True or False

_____ 1. The agent used to destroy microorganisms on an article depends on the size of the article.

_____ 2. The purpose of the Hazard Communications Standard is to make sure that employees do not use hazardous chemicals in the workplace.

_____ 3. The Hazard Communications Standard requires that the label of a hazardous chemical include information on how to store and handle the chemical.

_____ 4. Stethoscopes must be decontaminated using a high-level disinfectant.

_____ 5. Protective eyewear must be worn when working with isopropyl alcohol.

_____ 6. The shelf life of a disinfectant indicates how long a disinfectant retains its effectiveness.

_____ 7. The best means of determining the effectives of the sterilization process are biologic indicators.

_____ 8. The proper time for sterilizing an article in the autoclave depends on what is being autoclaved.

_____ 9. A pack that has been in the storage cupboard for 4 weeks should be resterilized.

_____ 10. Ethylene oxide gas is used by medical manufactureres to sterilize disposable items.

Copyright © 2008, 2004, 2000, 1995, 1990 by Saunders, an imprint of Elsevier Inc. All rights reserved.

KEY TERM ASSESSMENT

Directions: Match each medical term with its definition.

_____ 1. Antiseptic

_____ 2. Autoclave

_____ 3. Contaminate

_____ 4. Critical item

_____ 5. Decontamination

_____ 6. Detergent

_____ 7. Disinfectant

_____ 8. Incubate

_____ 9. Load

_____ 10. Material safety data sheet

_____ 11. Noncritical item

_____ 12. Sanitization

_____ 13. Semicritical item

_____ 14. Spore

_____ 15. Sterilization

_____ 16. Thermolabile

A. To provide proper conditions for growth and development
B. To soil, stain, or pollute; to make impure
C. Easily affected or changed by heat
D. A substance that inhibits disease-producing microorganisms but not their spores (usually applied to living tissues)
E. An item that comes in contact with intact skin but not mucous membranes
F. A hard, thick-walled capsule formed by some bacteria that contains only the essential parts of the protoplasm of the bacterial cell
G. An item that comes in contact with sterile tissue or the vascular system
H. An apparatus for the sterilization of materials, using steam under pressure
I. An agent that cleanses by emulsifying dirt and oil
J. An item that comes in contact with nonintact skin or intact mucous membranes
K. The articles that are being sterilized
L. An agent used to destroy pathogenic microorganisms but not necessarily their spores (usually applied to inanimate objects)
M. A sheet that provides information regarding a chemical and its hazards, and measures to take to avoid injury and illness when handling the chemical
N. A process to remove organic matter from an article and to lower the number of microorganisms to a safe level as determined by public health requirements
O. The process of destroying all forms of microbial life, including bacterial spores
P. The use of physical or chemical means to destroy bloodborne pathogens on an item so that it is no longer capable of transmitting disease, making it safe to handle

Copyright © 2008, 2004, 2000, 1995, 1990 by Saunders, an imprint of Elsevier Inc. All rights reserved.

EVALUATION OF LEARNING

Directions: Fill in each blank with the correct answer.

1. How does one determine what type of physical or chemical agent to use to destroy microorganisms on an article?

2. List two diseases that are caused by bacteria that produce spores.

3. What is the purpose of the Hazard Communication Standard?

4. List four examples of hazardous chemicals that may be used in the medical office.

5. What information must be included on a hazardous chemical label as required by the Hazard Communication Standard?

6. List and describe the information that must be included in a Material Safety Data Sheet.

7. What is the purpose of sanitizing an article?

8. What is the advantage of using the ultrasound method to clean instruments?

9. Why should gloves be worn during the sanitization procedure?

Copyright © 2008, 2004, 2000, 1995, 1990 by Saunders, an imprint of Elsevier Inc. All rights reserved.

10. What is the definition of high-level disinfection?

11. List one example of an item that requires high-level disinfection. List one example of a high-level disinfectant.

12. List two examples of items that can be disinfected through intermediate-level disinfection. List one example of an intermediate-level disinfectant.

13. List two examples of items that are disinfected by low-level disinfection.

14. What disinfectant does OSHA recommend for the decontamination of blood spills?

15. Why is it important to remove all organic matter from an article before it is disinfected?

16. Explain the difference between the shelf life and use life of a chemical disinfectant.

17. What is the purpose of the pressure used in the autoclaving process?

18. Why is it important that all air be removed from the autoclave during the sterilization process?

19. What are the most common temperature and pressure used to sterilize materials with the autoclave?

20. What information does the CDC recommend be recorded in an autoclave log regarding each cycle?

Copyright © 2008, 2004, 2000, 1995, 1990 by Saunders, an imprint of Elsevier Inc. All rights reserved.

21. What is the function of a sterilization indicator?

22. What is the purpose of wrapping articles to be autoclaved?

23. List two properties of a good wrapper for use in autoclaving.

24. List three examples of wrapping material used for the autoclave and identify an advantage of each type.

25. Why is more time needed to autoclave a large minor office surgery pack?

26. What is "event-related sterility"?

27. Describe the care an autoclave should receive on a daily basis.

28. Why is a longer exposure period needed to ensure sterilization when using the dry heat oven?

29. What effect does moist heat have on instruments with sharp cutting edges?

30. How does the medical manufacturing industry use ethylene oxide gas sterilization?

31. What guidelines must be followed when using cold sterilization?

Copyright © 2008, 2004, 2000, 1995, 1990 by Saunders, an imprint of Elsevier Inc. All rights reserved.

CRITICAL THINKING ACTIVITIES

A. MATERIAL SAFETY DATA SHEET

Refer to the Material Safety Data Sheet in the text (Figure 3-2) and answer the following questions.

1. When was this MSDS last revised? ______
2. Is glutaraldehyde soluble in water? ______
3. Describe the appearance and odor of glutaraldehyde.
______
4. What is the pH of glutaraldehyde? ______
5. Is glutaraldehyde flammable? ______
6. Is glutaraldehyde stable? ______
7. What conditions should be avoided with glutaraldehyde? ______
8. How can glutaraldehyde enter the body?
______
______
9. What symptoms occur if glutaraldehyde does the following?
   a. Comes in contact with the skin ______
   b. Is splashed into the eyes ______
   c. Is inhaled ______
   d. Is ingested ______
10. What preexisting conditions can an individual possess that can be aggravated by glutaraldehyde?
______
11. Does glutaraldehyde cause cancer? ______
12. What are the emergency and first aid procedures for glutaraldehyde for the following?
   a. Skin
   ______
   ______
   b. Eyes
   ______
   ______
   c. Inhalation
   ______
   ______
   d. Ingestion
   ______
   ______
13. What should be done if glutaraldehyde is spilled?
______
______
______

Copyright © 2008, 2004, 2000, 1995, 1990 by Saunders, an imprint of Elsevier Inc. All rights reserved.

14. What is the disposal method for glutaraldehyde?

____

15. How should glutaraldehyde be stored?

____

16. What type of ventilation is needed when working with glutaraldehyde?

____

17. What skin and eye protection should be taken with glutaraldehyde?

____

B. OBTAINING A MATERIAL SAFETY DATA SHEET

Obtain an MSDS for one of the following hazardous chemicals and answer the questions below. Internet sites for obtaining an MSDS are listed below:

www.msdssearch.com
www.hazard.com/msds

- Cidex
- MetriCide
- Cidex OPA
- Cavicide
- Wavicide
- Biozide
- Sporox II
- Vesphene
- Envirocide
- Clorox bleach

1. What is the chemical name of this hazardous chemical? _______________
2. What is the trade or brand name of this chemical? _______________
3. Who manufactures this chemical? _______________
4. What number would you call if an emergency occurred with this chemical?

   ____

5. What type of symptoms occur if this chemical does the following?
   a. Comes in contact with the skin _______________
   b. Is splashed into the eyes _______________
   c. Is inhaled _______________
   d. Is ingested _______________
6. What are the emergency and first aid procedures for this chemical?

   ____

7. What should be done if this chemical is spilled?

   ____

Copyright © 2008, 2004, 2000, 1995, 1990 by Saunders, an imprint of Elsevier Inc. All rights reserved.

8. What is the disposal method for this chemical?

____

____

9. How should this chemical be stored?

____

____

10. What type of protection should be taken when working with this chemical?

____

____

C. SANITIZATION

For each of the following situations involving sanitization, write C if the technique is correct and I if the technique is incorrect. If the situation is correct, state the principle underlying the technique. If the situation is incorrect, explain what might happen if the technique was performed in the incorrect manner.

_____ 1. A contaminated surgical instrument is left in the examination room.

____

____

_____ 2. The medical assistant does not wear gloves when sanitizing surgical instruments.

____

____

_____ 3. The medical assistant piles instruments while preparing them for sanitization.

____

____

_____ 4. The medical assistant forgets to read the material safety data sheet before decontaminating some surgical instruments in Cidex.

____

____

_____ 5. The medical assistant uses laundry detergent to sanitize surgical instruments.

____

____

_____ 6. Dried blood is not completely cleansed from hemostatic forceps before they are sterilized in the autoclave.

____

____

_____ 7. The medical assistant checks all instruments for proper working condition before sterilizing them.

____

____

_____ 8. The medical assistant lubricates hemostatic forceps with a steam-penetrable lubricant before sterilizing them.

____

____

Copyright © 2008, 2004, 2000, 1995, 1990 by Saunders, an imprint of Elsevier Inc. All rights reserved.

D. STORAGE OF A CHEMICAL DISINFECTANT

You have just received a 0.5 gallon container of Cidex Plus. You look at the label on the container and note the following:

- Expiration date: 8/7/09
- Use life: 28 days
- Reuse life: 28 days

Based on this information, answer the following questions.

1. If the Cidex Plus is left unopened on the shelf, when would it expire and need to be discarded?
____
2. You open and activate the Cidex Plus on 9/1/08. What date should you write on the container?
____
3. You next fill a disinfectant container with the Cidex Plus and disinfect some articles in it. On what date would the Cidex Plus be unusable and need to be disposed?
____
4. On what date would you need to discard the rest of the container of Cidex Plus if it is not used?
____

E. STERILIZATION

For each of the following situations involving sterilization of articles in the autoclave, write C if the technique is correct, and I if the technique is incorrect. If the situation is correct, state the principle underlying the technique. If the situation is incorrect, explain what might happen if the technique was performed in the incorrect manner.

_____ 1. The medical assistant opens a hemostat before placing it in a sterilization pouch.
____
____

_____ 2. Tap water is used to fill the water reservoir of the autoclave.
____
____

_____ 3. When loading the autoclave, the medical assistant places glass jars in an upright position.
____
____

_____ 4. The medical assistant places 4 sterilization pouches on top of each other in the autoclave.
____
____

_____ 5. The medical assistant places small packs to be sterilized approximately 1 to 3 inches apart in the autoclave.
____
____

_____ 6. Spore strips are placed in the autoclave where steam will penetrate them most easily.
____
____

_____ 7. The medical assistant begins timing the load in the autoclave after the proper temperature of 250°F has been reached.
____
____

Copyright © 2008, 2004, 2000, 1995, 1990 by Saunders, an imprint of Elsevier Inc. All rights reserved.

_____ 8. The medical assistant removes the load from the autoclave while it is still wet.

____

____

_____ 9. The medical assistant notices a tear in one of the wrappers while removing articles from the autoclave. He or she rewraps and resterilizes the article.

____

____

_____ 10. The medical assistant notices that a sterilized wrapped article stored on the storage shelf has opened up. He or she retapes the pack and places it back on the storage shelf.

____

____

Copyright © 2008, 2004, 2000, 1995, 1990 by Saunders, an imprint of Elsevier Inc. All rights reserved.

Notes

Copyright © 2008, 2004, 2000, 1995, 1990 by Saunders, an imprint of Elsevier Inc. All rights reserved.

F. WHAT COMES NEXT? GAME

Object: The object of the game is to achieve sterilization of an article by determining the correct sequence of events in the sanitization and sterilization procedure.

Directions:

1. Cut out the game cards on the following page.
2. Make your cards unique by coloring and decorating them.
3. Review the sequence of steps in the sanitization and sterilization procedures.
4. Get into a group of three students.
5. Hold your game cards with the steps facing you.
6. Each player places the first step in the sanitization/sterilization procedure face down on the table.
7. When all players have placed a card on the table, turn the cards over.
8. Award yourself 5 points if you have correctly determined the proper step in the sequence. If you have a question regarding the correct answer, consult your instructor.
9. In turn, each player can earn an additional 5 points by stating a fact about that step in the procedure. For example, if the step is "Apply Gloves," a fact about this step would be that both clean gloves and utility gloves must be worn during the sanitization procedure.
10. Keep track of your points on the Score Card provided.
11. Keep the cards in their proper sequence on the table and continue the game until all of the game cards have been used.

WHAT COMES NEXT?
SCORE CARD

Name: ______________________________

Recording Points:
Cross off a number each time you properly sequence a game card (starting with 5 and continuing in sequence). Cross off another number if you are able to state a fact about the step in the procedure. Your total points will be equal to the last number you crossed off. Record this number in the space provided and check the level that you achieved.

Game Card Points:	
5	75
10	80
15	85
20	90
25	95
30	100
35	105
40	110
45	115
50	120
55	125
60	130
65	135
70	140

TOTAL POINTS: _______

LEVEL:

- ☐ 100 to 120 points: **Sterile**—You got rid of all MOs and spores!
- ☐ 80 to 100 points: **Aseptic**—You got rid of the pathogenic MOs.
- ☐ 60 to 80 points: **Contaminated**—Your article is still contaminated.

Copyright © 2008, 2004, 2000, 1995, 1990 by Saunders, an imprint of Elsevier Inc. All rights reserved.

Read MSDS	Apply gloves	Rinse contaminated instruments	Decontaminate instruments
Clean instruments manually	Thoroughly rinse instruments	Dry instruments	Check working order and lubricate instruments
Wrap instruments	Load the autoclave	Operate the autoclave	Store instruments

What comes next?	What comes next?	What comes next?	What comes next?
What comes next?	What comes next?	What comes next?	What comes next?
What comes next?	What comes next?	What comes next?	What comes next?

PRACTICE FOR COMPETENCY

Sterilization and Disinfection

Procedure 3-1: Sanitizing Instruments. Sanitize instruments. In the space provided, indicate the following:

A. Name of the disinfectant ______________________________

B. Name of the instrument cleaner ______________________________

C. Names of instruments sanitized ______________________________

____

____

Procedure 3-2: Chemical Disinfection of Articles. Chemically disinfect contaminated articles. In the space provided, indicate the following:

A. Name of the disinfectant ______________________________

B. Names of articles disinfected ______________________________

____

____

Procedures 3-3 and 3-4: Wrapping Articles for the Autoclave. Wrap articles for autoclaving. In the space provided, list the information you indicated on the label of each pack which includes the contents of the pack, the date, and your initials.

Information indicated on the label of the wrapped article:

____

____

____

____

____

____

____

____

Procedure 3-5: Sterilizing Articles in the Autoclave. Sterilize articles in the autoclave. In the space provided, indicate the articles you sterilized.

____

____

____

____

Copyright © 2008, 2004, 2000, 1995, 1990 by Saunders, an imprint of Elsevier Inc. All rights reserved.

Notes

Copyright © 2008, 2004, 2000, 1995, 1990 by Saunders, an imprint of Elsevier Inc. All rights reserved.

EVALUATION OF COMPETENCY

Procedure 3-1: Sanitization of Instruments

Name: ______________________________ Date: ______________

Evaluated By: ______________________________ Score: ______________

Performance Objective

Outcome: Sanitize instruments.

Conditions: Given the following: disposable gloves, utility gloves, contaminated instruments, chemical disinfectant and MSDS, disinfectant container, cleaning solution and MSDS, basin, nylon brush, wire brush, paper towels, cloth towel, and instrument lubricant.

Standards: Time: 10 minutes. Student completed procedure in ____ minutes.

Accuracy: Satisfactory score on the Performance Evaluation Checklist.

Performance Evaluation Checklist

Trial 1	Trial 2	Point Value	*Performance Standards*
		•	Reviewed the MSDS for hazardous chemicals being used.
		•	Applied gloves.
		•	Transported the contaminated instruments to the cleaning area.
		•	Applied heavy-duty utility gloves over the disposable gloves.
		▷	Stated the purpose of the utility gloves.
		•	Separated sharp instruments and delicate instruments from other instruments.
		▷	Explained why instruments should be separated.
		•	Immediately rinsed the instruments thoroughly under warm running water.
		▷	Stated why the instruments should be rinsed immediately.
			Decontaminated the Instruments
		•	Checked the expiration date of the chemical disinfectant.
		▷	Explained why an expired disinfectant should not be used.
		•	Observed all personal safety precautions listed on the label.
		•	Followed label directions for proper mixing and use of the disinfectant.
		•	Labeled the disinfecting container with the name of the disinfectant and the reuse expiration date.
		•	Poured the disinfectant into the labeled container.
		•	Completely submerged the articles in the disinfectant.
		•	Covered the disinfectant container.
		▷	Stated the reason for covering the container.
		•	Disinfected the articles for 10 minutes.
		▷	Explained the reason for decontaminating the instruments.

Copyright © 2008, 2004, 2000, 1995, 1990 by Saunders, an imprint of Elsevier Inc. All rights reserved.

Trial 1	Trial 2	Point Value	*Performance Standards*
			Cleaned the Instruments: Manual Method
		•	Checked the expiration date of the cleaning agent.
		•	Observed all personal safety precautions.
		•	Followed label directions for proper use and mixing of the cleaning agent.
		•	Removed articles from disinfectant and placed them in the cleaning solution.
		•	Cleaned the surface of the instruments with a nylon brush.
		•	Cleaned grooves, crevices, or serrations with a wire brush.
		•	Removed stains using commercial stain remover.
		•	Scrubbed the instruments until they were visibly clean.
		▷	Explained why all organic matter must be removed.
			Cleaned the Instruments: Ultrasound Method
		•	Prepared the cleaning solution in the ultrasonic cleaner.
		•	Observed all personal safety precautions listed on label.
		•	Removed the articles from the disinfectant.
		•	Separated instruments of dissimilar metals.
		•	Properly placed the instruments in the ultrasonic cleaner.
		•	Positioned hinged instruments in an open position.
		▷	Stated why hinged instruments must be in an open position.
		•	Ensured that sharp instruments did not touch other instruments.
		•	Checked to make sure all instruments were fully submerged.
		•	Placed the lid on the ultrasonic cleaner.
		•	Turned on the ultrasonic cleaner.
		•	Cleaned the instruments for the length of time recommended by the manufacturer.
		•	Removed the instruments from the machine.
		•	Rinsed each instrument thoroughly with warm water for 20 to 30 seconds.
		▷	Explained why instruments should be rinsed thoroughly.
		•	Dried each instrument with a paper towel.
		•	Placed instrument on a towel for additional drying.
		▷	Stated the reason for drying the instruments.
		•	Checked each instrument for defects and proper working condition.
		•	Lubricated hinged instruments in an open position.
		•	Opened and closed the instrument to distribute the lubricant.
		•	Placed the lubricated instrument on a towel to drain.
		▷	Stated the reason for lubricating instruments.
		•	Disposed of the cleaning solution according to the manufacturer's instructions.

Copyright © 2008, 2004, 2000, 1995, 1990 by Saunders, an imprint of Elsevier Inc. All rights reserved.

Trial 1	Trial 2	Point Value	*Performance Standards*
		•	Removed both sets of gloves.
		•	Sanitized hands.
		•	Wrapped the instruments.
		•	Sterilized the instruments in the autoclave.
		*	Completed the procedure within 10 minutes.
			TOTALS

Evaluation of Student Performance

EVALUATION CRITERIA			COMMENTS
Symbol	Category	Point Value	
*	Critical Step	16 points	
•	Essential Step	6 points	
▷	Theory Question	2 points	
Score calculation: 100 points – ______ points missed ____ Score Satisfactory score: 85 or above			

AAMA/CAAHEP Competency Achieved:

☑ III. C. 3. b. (1) (c): Perform sterilization techniques.

Copyright © 2008, 2004, 2000, 1995, 1990 by Saunders, an imprint of Elsevier Inc. All rights reserved.

Notes

Copyright © 2008, 2004, 2000, 1995, 1990 by Saunders, an imprint of Elsevier Inc. All rights reserved.

EVALUATION OF COMPETENCY

Procedure 3-2: Chemical Disinfection of Articles

Name: ______________________________ Date: ______________

Evaluated By: ______________________________ Score: ______________

Performance Objective

Outcome: Chemically disinfect articles.

Conditions: Given the following: disposable gloves, utility gloves, contaminated articles, chemical disinfectant and MSDS, disinfectant container, and paper towels.

Standards: Time: 10 minutes. Student completed procedure in ____ minutes.

Accuracy: Satisfactory score on the Performance Evaluation Checklist.

Performance Evaluation Checklist

Trial 1	*Trial 2*	*Point Value*	*Performance Standards*
		•	Applied gloves and sanitized the articles.
		•	Reviewed the MSDS for the chemical disinfectant.
		▷	Described what information is included on an MSDS.
		•	Checked the expiration date of the disinfectant.
		▷	Explained why an expired disinfectant should not be used.
		•	Observed all personal safety precautions listed on the container label.
		•	Followed the directions on the label for proper use and reuse of the disinfectant.
		•	Completely immersed articles in the chemical disinfectant.
		•	Covered disinfectant container.
		▷	Stated the reason for covering the container.
		•	Disinfected articles for the proper length of time as indicated on the label of the container.
		•	Rinsed the articles thoroughly.
		▷	Stated the reason for rinsing the articles.
		•	Dried the articles.
		•	Properly disposed of the disinfectant.
		▷	Stated the purpose of proper disposal.
		•	Removed gloves.
		•	Sanitized hands.
		•	Properly stored the articles.
		*	Completed the procedure within 10 minutes.
			TOTALS

Copyright © 2008, 2004, 2000, 1995, 1990 by Saunders, an imprint of Elsevier Inc. All rights reserved.

Evaluation of Student Performance

EVALUATION CRITERIA			COMMENTS
Symbol	**Category**	**Point Value**	
✶	Critical Step	16 points	
●	Essential Step	6 points	
▷	Theory Question	2 points	
Score calculation: 100 points – ____ points missed ____ Score Satisfactory score: 85 or above			

AAMA/CAAHEP Competency Achieved:

☑ III. C. 3. b. (1) (c): Perform sterilization techniques.

Copyright © 2008, 2004, 2000, 1995, 1990 by Saunders, an imprint of Elsevier Inc. All rights reserved.

EVALUATION OF COMPETENCY

Procedure 3-3: Wrapping Instruments Using Paper or Muslin

Name: ______________________________ Date: ______________

Evaluated By: ______________________________ Score: ______________

Performance Objective

Outcome: Wrap an instrument for autoclaving.

Conditions: Given the following: sanitized instrument, wrapping material, sterilization indicator strip, autoclave tape, and a permanent marker.

Standards: Time: 5 minutes. Student completed procedure in ____ minutes.

Accuracy: Satisfactory score on the Performance Evaluation Checklist.

Performance Evaluation Checklist

Trial 1	*Trial 2*	*Point Value*	*Performance Standards*
		•	Sanitized hands.
		•	Assembled equipment.
		•	Selected the appropriate-sized wrapping material.
		•	Checked the expiration date on the sterilization indicator box.
		▷	Stated why outdated strips should not be used.
		•	Placed wrapping material on clean, flat surface.
		•	Turned the wrap in a diagonal position.
		•	Placed instrument in the center of wrapping material.
		•	Placed instruments with movable joints in an open position.
		▷	Stated why instruments with movable joints must be placed in an open position.
		•	Placed a sterilization indicator in the center of the pack.
		•	Folded wrapping material up from the bottom and doubled back a small corner.
		•	Folded over one edge of wrapping material and doubled back the corner.
		•	Folded over the other edge of wrapping material and doubled back the corner.
		•	Folded the pack up from the bottom and secured with autoclave tape.
		•	Ensured that the pack was firm enough for handling, but loose enough to permit proper circulation of steam.
		▷	Stated why instruments are wrapped for autoclaving.
		•	Labeled and dated the pack. Included your initials.
		▷	Stated the purpose of dating the pack.
		*	Completed the procedure within 5 minutes.
			TOTALS

Copyright © 2008, 2004, 2000, 1995, 1990 by Saunders, an imprint of Elsevier Inc. All rights reserved.

Evaluation of Student Performance

EVALUATION CRITERIA			COMMENTS
Symbol	Category	Point Value	
✶	Critical Step	16 points	
•	Essential Step	6 points	
▷	Theory Question	2 points	
Score calculation: 100 points – ______ points missed ____ Score Satisfactory score: 85 or above			

AAMA/CAAHEP Competency Achieved:

☑ III. C. 3. b. (1) (b): Wrap items for autoclaving.

Copyright © 2008, 2004, 2000, 1995, 1990 by Saunders, an imprint of Elsevier Inc. All rights reserved.

EVALUATION OF COMPETENCY

Procedure 3-4: Wrapping Instruments Using a Pouch

Name: ______________________________ Date: ______________

Evaluated By: ______________________________ Score: ______________

Performance Objective

Outcome: Wrap an instrument for autoclaving.

Conditions: Given the following: sanitized instrument, sterilization pouch, and a permanent marker.

Standards: Time: 5 minutes. Student completed procedure in ____ minutes.

Accuracy: Satisfactory score on the Performance Evaluation Checklist.

Performance Evaluation Checklist

Trial 1	*Trial 2*	*Point Value*	*Performance Standards*
		•	Sanitized hands.
		•	Assembled equipment.
		•	Selected the appropriate-sized pouch.
		•	Placed the pouch on a clean, flat surface.
		•	Labeled and dated the pack. Included your initials.
		•	Inserted the instrument into the open end of the pouch.
		•	Sealed the pouch.
		•	Sterilized the pack in the autoclave.
		▷	Stated how long the pack is sterile once it has been autoclaved.
		*	Completed the procedure within 5 minutes.
			TOTALS

Copyright © 2008, 2004, 2000, 1995, 1990 by Saunders, an imprint of Elsevier Inc. All rights reserved.

Evaluation of Student Performance

EVALUATION CRITERIA			COMMENTS
Symbol	Category	Point Value	
✶	Critical Step	16 points	
●	Essential Step	6 points	
▷	Theory Question	2 points	
Score calculation: 100 points – ______ points missed ____ Score Satisfactory score: 85 or above			

AAMA/CAAHEP Competency Achieved:

☑ III. C. 3. b. (1) (b): Wrap items for autoclaving.

Copyright © 2008, 2004, 2000, 1995, 1990 by Saunders, an imprint of Elsevier Inc. All rights reserved.

EVALUATION OF COMPETENCY

Procedure 3-5: Sterilizing Articles in the Autoclave

Name: ______________________________ Date: ______________

Evaluated By: ______________________________ Score: ______________

Performance Objective

Outcome:	Sterilize a load of contaminated articles in the autoclave.
Conditions:	Using an autoclave.
	Given the following: autoclave operating manual, distilled water, wrapped articles, and heat-resistant gloves.
Standards:	Time: 10 minutes. Student completed procedure in ____ minutes.
	Accuracy: Satisfactory score on the Performance Evaluation Checklist.

Performance Evaluation Checklist

Trial 1	Trial 2	Point Value	*Performance Standards*
		•	Assembled equipment.
		•	Checked the water level in the autoclave.
		•	Properly loaded the autoclave.
			Manually Operated the Autoclave
		•	Determined the sterilizing time for the type of articles being autoclaved.
		•	Turned on the autoclave.
		•	Filled the chamber with water.
		•	Closed and latched the door.
		•	Set the timing control.
		▷	Stated when the timer should be set.
		•	Vented the chamber of steam.
		•	Dried the load.
		▷	Stated the reason for drying the load.
			Automatically Operated the Autoclave
		•	Closed and latched the door.
		•	Turned on the autoclave.
		•	Determined the sterilization program.
		•	Pressed the appropriate program button.
		•	Pressed the start button.

Copyright © 2008, 2004, 2000, 1995, 1990 by Saunders, an imprint of Elsevier Inc. All rights reserved.

Trial 1	Trial 2	Point Value	Performance Standards
		▷	Stated the purpose of each control or indicator on the autoclave.
		•	Turned off the autoclave.
		•	Removed the load with heat-resistant gloves.
		▷	Stated the reason for using heat-resistant gloves.
		•	Inspected the packs as they were removed for damage.
		▷	Explained what should be done if a pack is torn.
		•	Checked the sterilization indicators on the outside of the packs.
		•	Recorded information in the autoclave log.
		•	Stored the articles in a clean dust-proof area.
		•	Placed the most recently sterilized packs behind previously sterilized packs.
		•	Maintained appropriate daily care of the autoclave.
		▷	Described the care the autoclave should receive each day.
		*	Completed the procedure within 10 minutes.
			TOTALS

Evaluation of Student Performance

EVALUATION CRITERIA			COMMENTS
Symbol	Category	Point Value	
*	Critical Step	16 points	
•	Essential Step	6 points	
▷	Theory Question	2 points	
Score calculation: 100 points – ____ points missed ____ Score Satisfactory score: 85 or above			

AAMA/CAAHEP Competency Achieved:

☑ III. C. 3. b. (1) (b): Perform sterilization techniques.

Copyright © 2008, 2004, 2000, 1995, 1990 by Saunders, an imprint of Elsevier Inc. All rights reserved.

4

Vital Signs

CHAPTER ASSIGNMENTS

√ After Completing	Date Due	Textbook Page(s)	TEXTBOOK ASSIGNMENTS	Possible Points	Points You Earned
		117-168	Read Chapter 4: Vital Signs		
		138 163	Read Case Study 1 Case Study 1 questions	5	
		141 163	Read Case Study 2 Case Study 2 questions	5	
		146 164	Read Case Study 3 Case Study 3 questions	5	
		164-165	Apply Your Knowledge questions	10	
			TOTAL POINTS		
√ After Completing	**Date Due**	**Study Guide Page(s)**	**STUDY GUIDE ASSIGNMENTS (CTA: Critical Thinking Activity)**	**Possible Points**	**Points You Earned**
		119	Pretest	10	
		120-121	Key Term Assessment	55	
		122-130	Evaluation of Learning questions	88	
		130-131	CTA A: Measurement of Body Temperature	18	
		132	CTA B: Alterations in Body Temperature	5	
		132	CTA C: Pulse Sites	6	
			CD Activity: Chapter 4 Where's the Beat? (Record points earned)		
		132-133	CTA D: Pulse and Respiratory Rates	3	
		133-134	CTA E: Pulse Oximetry	18	
		134	CTA F: Blood Pressure Measurement	6	

Copyright © 2008, 2004, 2000, 1995, 1990 by Saunders, an imprint of Elsevier Inc. All rights reserved.

√ After Completing	Date Due	Study Guide Page(s)	STUDY GUIDE ASSIGNMENTS (CTA: Critical Thinking Activity)	Possible Points	Points You Earned
		135	CTA G: Proper BP Cuff Selection	12	
		135	CTA H: Reading Blood Pressure Values	24	
			CD Activity: Chapter 4 Under Pressure (Record points earned)		
		136	CTA I: Interpreting Blood Pressure Readings	10	
		136	CTA J: Hypertension	20	
		138	CTA K: Crossword Puzzle	30	
		139-140	CTA L: Go To! Game (Record points earned)		
		143	CTA M: Road to Recovery Game: Vital Signs Terminology (Team Players) (Record points earned)		
			CD Activity: Chapter 4: Road to Recovery Game Vital Signs Terminology (Individual Player) (Record points earned)		
			CD Activity: Chapter 4 Animations	20	
		119	Posttest	10	
			ADDITIONAL ASSIGNMENTS		
			TOTAL POINTS		

Copyright © 2008, 2004, 2000, 1995, 1990 by Saunders, an imprint of Elsevier Inc. All rights reserved.

√ When Assigned By Your Instructor	Study Guide Page(s)	Practices Required	LABORATORY ASSIGNMENTS	*Score
	153	5	**Practice for Competency** 4-1: Measuring Oral Body Temperature—Electronic Thermometer Textbook reference: pp. 128-129	
	159-160		**Evaluation of Competency** 4-1: Measuring Oral Body Temperature—Electronic Thermometer	*
	153	3	**Practice for Competency** 4-2: Measuring Axillary Body Temperature— Electronic Thermometer Textbook reference: p. 130	
	161-162		**Evaluation of Competency** 4-2: Measuring Axillary Body Temperature— Electronic Thermometer	*
	153	3	**Practice for Competency** 4-3: Measuring Rectal Body Temperature— Electronic Thermometer Textbook reference: pp. 131-132	
	163-164		**Evaluation of Competency** 4-3: Measuring Rectal Body Temperature— Electronic Thermometer	*
	153	5	**Practice for Competency** 4-4: Measuring Aural Body Temperature— Tympanic Membrane Thermometer Textbook reference: pp. 132-134	
	165-166		**Evaluation of Competency** 4-4: Measuring Aural Body Temperature— Tympanic Membrane Thermometer	*
	153	5	**Practice for Competency** 4-5: Measuring Temporal Body Temperature Textbook reference: pp. 135-136	
	167-168	5	**Evaluation of Competency** 4-5: Measuring Temporal Body Temperature	*
	155	10	**Practice for Competency** 4-6: Measuring Pulse and Respiration Textbook reference: pp. 147-148	

Copyright © 2008, 2004, 2000, 1995, 1990 by Saunders, an imprint of Elsevier Inc. All rights reserved.

√ When Assigned By Your Instructor	Study Guide Page(s)	Practices Required	LABORATORY ASSIGNMENTS	*Score
	169-170		**Evaluation of Competency** 4-6: Measuring Pulse and Respiration	*
	155	5	**Practice for Competency** 4-7: Measuring Apical Pulse Textbook reference: p. 149	
	171-172		**Evaluation of Competency** 4-7: Measuring Apical Pulse	*
	155	5	**Practice for Competency** 4-8: Performing Pulse Oximetry Textbook reference: pp. 150-151	
	173-175		**Evaluation of Competency** 4-8: Performing Pulse Oximetry	*
	157	10	**Practice for Competency** 4-9: Measuring Blood Pressure Textbook reference: pp. 159-162	
	177-179		**Evaluation of Competency** 4-9: Measuring Blood Pressure	*
			ADDITIONAL ASSIGNMENTS	

Copyright © 2008, 2004, 2000, 1995, 1990 by Saunders, an imprint of Elsevier Inc. All rights reserved.

Name ______________________________ Date ______________

PRETEST

True or False

_____ 1. The heat-regulating center of the body is the medulla.

_____ 2. A vague sense of body discomfort, weakness, and fatigue that often marks the onset of a disease is known as the blahs.

_____ 3. If an axillary temperature of 100° F was taken orally, it would register as 101° F.

_____ 4. If the lens of a tympanic membrane thermometer is dirty, the reading may be falsely low.

_____ 5. Chemical thermometers should be stored in the freezer.

_____ 6. The femoral pulse site can be used to assess circulation to the foot.

_____ 7. The term used to describe an irregularity in the heart's rhythm is dysrhythmia.

_____ 8. Pulse oximetry provides the physician with information on the amount of oxygen being delivered to the tissues.

_____ 9. Blood pressure measures the contraction and relaxation of the heart.

_____10. When taking blood pressure, the stethoscope is placed over the brachial artery.

POSTTEST

True or False

_____ 1. A temperature of 100° F is classified as a low-grade fever.

_____ 2. The rectal site should not be used to take the temperature of a newborn.

_____ 3. A tympanic membrane thermometer should not be used to measure temperature on a patient who has a normal amount of cerumen in the ear.

_____ 4. A temporal artery temperature reading is the same as an oral reading.

_____ 5. Excessive pressure should not be applied when measuring a pulse because it could obstruct the pulse.

_____ 6. A child has a faster pulse rate than an adult.

_____ 7. The normal respiratory rate of an adult ranges between 10 and 18 respirations per minute.

_____ 8. The term used to describe a bluish discoloration of the skin due to a lack of oxygen is hypoxia.

_____ 9. The oxygen saturation level of a healthy individual falls between 85% to 90%.

_____10. When measuring blood pressure, the patient's arm should be positioned above the level of the heart.

Copyright © 2008, 2004, 2000, 1995, 1990 by Saunders, an imprint of Elsevier Inc. All rights reserved.

KEY TERM ASSESSMENT

Temperature

Directions: Match each medical term with its definition.

_______ 1. Afebrile

_______ 2. Antipyretic

_______ 3. Axilla

_______ 4. Celsius scale

_______ 5. Conduction

_______ 6. Convection

_______ 7. Crisis

_______ 8. Disinfectant

_______ 9. Fahrenheit scale

_______ 10. Febrile

_______ 11. Fever

_______ 12. Frenulum linguae

_______ 13. Hyperpyrexia

_______ 14. Hypothermia

_______ 15. Malaise

_______ 16. Radiation

A. An extremely high fever
B. An agent used to destroy disease-producing microorganisms but not necessarily their spores (usually applied to inanimate objects)
C. A body temperature that is below normal
D. The armpit
E. The transfer of energy, such as heat, through air currents
F. A body temperature that is above normal (pyrexia)
G. An agent that reduces fever
H. A temperature scale on which the freezing point of water is 32° and the boiling point of water is 212°
I. The transfer of energy, such as heat, in the form of waves
J. A temperature scale on which the freezing point of water is 0° and the boiling point is 100°
K. The midline fold that connects the undersurface of the tongue with the floor of the mouth
L. Pertaining to fever
M. The transfer of energy, from one object to another
N. A sudden falling of an elevated body temperature to normal
O. Without fever; the body temperature is normal
P. A vague sense of body discomfort, weakness, and fatigue often marking the onset of a disease and continuing through the course of the illness

Pulse

Directions: Match each medical term with its definition.

_______ 1. Antecubital space

_______ 2. Aorta

_______ 3. Bounding pulse

_______ 4. Bradycardia

_______ 5. Dysrhythmia

_______ 6. Intercostal

_______ 7. Pulse rhythm

_______ 8. Pulse volume

_______ 9. Tachycardia

_______ 10. Thready pulse

A. Between the ribs
B. A pulse with an increased volume that feels very strong and full
C. The strength of the heartbeat
D. The space located at the front of the elbow
E. An abnormally fast heart rate (over 100 beats per minute)
F. The major trunk of the arterial system of the body
G. The time interval between heartbeats
H. A pulse with a decreased volume that feels weak and thin
I. An irregular rhythm
J. An abnormally slow heart rate (below 60 beats per minute)

Copyright © 2008, 2004, 2000, 1995, 1990 by Saunders, an imprint of Elsevier Inc. All rights reserved.

Respiration and Pulse Oximetry

Directions: Match each medical term with its definition.

_______ 1. Alveolus

_______ 2. Apnea

_______ 3. Bradypnea

_______ 4. Cyanosis

_______ 5. Dyspnea

_______ 6. Eupnea

_______ 7. Exhalation

_______ 8. Hyperpnea

_______ 9. Hyperventilation

_______ 10. Hypopnea

_______ 11. Hypoxemia

_______ 12. Hypoxia

_______ 13. Inhalation

_______ 14. Orthopnea

_______ 15. Pulse oximeter

_______ 16. Pulse oximetry

_______ 17. SaO_2

_______ 18. SpO_2

_______ 19. Tachypnea

A. The act of breathing out
B. A reduction in the oxygen supply to the tissues of the body
C. A decrease in the oxygen saturation of the blood. May lead to hypoxia
D. The temporary cessation of breathing
E. An abnormal increase in the respiratory rate of more than 20 respirations per minute
F. A computerized device consisting of a probe and monitor used to measure the oxygen saturation of arterial blood
G. An abnormal decrease in the rate and depth of respiration
H. A thin-walled air sac of the lungs in which the exchange of oxygen and carbon dioxide takes place
I. The use of a pulse oximeter to measure the oxygen saturation of arterial blood
J. The act of breathing in
K. A bluish discoloration of the skin and mucous membranes first observed in the nailbeds and lips
L. Abbreviation for the percentage of hemoglobin that is saturated with oxygen in arterial blood
M. The condition in which breathing is easier when an individual is in a standing or sitting position
N. Shortness of breath or difficulty in breathing
O. Abbreviation for the percentage of hemoglobin that is saturated with oxygen in arterial blood as measured by a pulse oximeter
P. Normal respiration
Q. An abnormally fast and deep type of breathing usually associated with acute anxiety conditions
R. An abnormal decrease in the respiratory rate of less than 10 respirations per minute
S. An abnormal increase in the rate and depth of respiration

Blood Pressure

Directions: Match each medical term with its definition.

_______ 1. Diastole

_______ 2. Diastolic pressure

_______ 3. Hypertension

_______ 4. Hypotension

_______ 5. Meniscus

_______ 6. Pulse pressure

_______ 7. Sphygmomanometer

_______ 8. Stethoscope

_______ 9. Systole

_______ 10. Systolic pressure

A. The curved surface on a column of liquid in a tube
B. High blood pressure
C. The point of maximum pressure on the arterial walls
D. The phase in the cardiac cycle in which the heart relaxes between contractions
E. An instrument for measuring arterial blood pressure
F. The point of lesser pressure on the arterial walls
G. Low blood pressure
H. The phase in the cardiac cycle in which the ventricles contract, sending blood out of the heart and into the aorta and pulmonary aorta
I. An instrument for amplifying and hearing sounds produced by the body
J. The difference between the systolic and diastolic pressures

Copyright © 2008, 2004, 2000, 1995, 1990 by Saunders, an imprint of Elsevier Inc. All rights reserved.

EVALUATION OF LEARNING

Temperature

Directions: Fill in each blank with the correct answer.

1. Define a vital sign.

___

___

___

2. What are the four vital signs?

___

___

___

___

3. What general guidelines should be followed when measuring vital signs?

___

___

___

___

4. List four ways in which heat is produced in the body.

___

___

___

___

5. List four ways in which heat is lost from the body.

___

___

___

___

6. What is the normal body temperature range?

___

7. What is a fever?

___

___

8. How do diurnal variations affect body temperature?

___

___

9. How does vigorous physical exercise affect body temperature?

___

Copyright © 2008, 2004, 2000, 1995, 1990 by Saunders, an imprint of Elsevier Inc. All rights reserved.

10. How do emotional states affect the body temperature?

11. What symptoms occur with a fever?

12. Describe the following fever patterns:
    a. Continuous fever
    b. Intermittent fever
    c. Remittent fever

13. What is the subsiding stage of a fever?

14. What four sites are used for taking body temperature?

15. List three instances in which the axillary site for taking body temperature would be preferred over the oral site.

16. Why does the rectal method for taking body temperature provide a very accurate temperature measurement?

17. When might the rectal method be used to take body temperature?

18. When might the aural method be used to take body temperature?

19. How does a temperature taken through the rectal and axillary method compare (in terms of degrees) with a temperature taken through the oral method?

Copyright © 2008, 2004, 2000, 1995, 1990 by Saunders, an imprint of Elsevier Inc. All rights reserved.

20. List and describe the four types of themometers available for taking body temperature.

21. Describe the advantages of a tympanic membrane thermometer.

22. What is the purpose of using a probe cover with an electronic thermometer?

23. Explain how a tympanic membrane thermometer measures body temperature.

24. Explain how to clean the lens of a tympanic membrane thermometer.

25. List two reasons why the temporal artery is a good site to measure body temperature.

26. How does the temperature obtained through the temporal site compare with oral, rectal, and axillary body temperature?

27. List four factors that can result in a falsely low temperature reading when using the temporal artery thermometer.

28. Where should a chemical thermometer be stored? Explain why.

Pulse

Directions: Fill in each blank with the correct answer.

1. What causes the pulse to occur?

Copyright © 2008, 2004, 2000, 1995, 1990 by Saunders, an imprint of Elsevier Inc. All rights reserved.

2. What is the unit of measurement for pulse rate?

____

3. How does physical activity affect the pulse rate?

____

4. What is the most common site for taking the pulse?

____

5. List two reasons for taking the pulse at the apical pulse site.

____

____

6. Where is the apex of the heart located?

____

____

7. When is the brachial artery used as a pulse site?

____

8. When is the carotid artery used as a pulse site?

____

9. When is the femoral artery used as a pulse site?

____

10. What two pulse sites can be used to assess circulation to the foot?

____

11. List two reasons for measuring the pulse rate.

____

____

12. State the normal range for a pulse rate for an adult.

____

13. What is the normal pulse range for the following age groups:
    a. Newborn ______________________________
    b. Toddler ______________________________
    c. Preschooler ______________________________
    d. School-age ______________________________
    e. Adult after age 60 ______________________________

14. What is the normal pulse range for a well-trained athlete?

____

Copyright © 2008, 2004, 2000, 1995, 1990 by Saunders, an imprint of Elsevier Inc. All rights reserved.

15. What may cause tachycardia?

____

16. If the rhythm and volume of a patient's pulse are normal, the medical assistant would record it as:

____

Respiration

Directions: Fill in each blank with the correct answer.

1. What is the purpose of respiration?

____

____

2. What is the purpose of inhalation?

____

____

3. What is the purpose of exhalation?

____

____

4. What is included in one complete respiration?

____

____

5. The exchange of oxygen and carbon dioxide between the body cells and blood is known as

____

6. What is the name of the control center for involuntary respiration?

____

7. Why must respiration be taken without the patient's awareness?

____

8. What is the normal respiratory rate (range) for a normal adult?

____

9. List two factors that will increase the respiratory rate.

____

____

10. Describe a normal rhythm for respiration.

____

____

11. What are two conditions in which hyperventilation may occur?

____

Copyright © 2008, 2004, 2000, 1995, 1990 by Saunders, an imprint of Elsevier Inc. All rights reserved.

12. What type of patient might experience hypopnea?

13. Where is cyanosis first observed?

14. What might cause cyanosis to occur?

15. What are two conditions in which dyspnea may occur?

16. Describe the character of normal breath sounds.

17. Describe the character of the following abnormal breath sounds:
    a. Crackles
    b. Rhonchi
    c. Wheezes

Pulse Oximetry

Directions: Fill in each blank with the correct answer.

1. What is the purpose of pulse oximetry?

2. What is the function of hemoglobin?

3. What is the oxygen saturation level of a healthy individual?

4. What might occur if the oxygen saturation level falls between 85% and 90%?

Copyright © 2008, 2004, 2000, 1995, 1990 by Saunders, an imprint of Elsevier Inc. All rights reserved.

5. List three patient conditions that can cause a decreased SpO_2 value.

____

____

____

6. When might pulse oximetry be used for the short-term continuous montioring of a patient?

____

____

7. What is the purpose of the pulse oximeter post test (POST)?

____

____

8. What type of site must be used for applying a pulse oximeter probe?

____

____

9. How can dark fingernail polish cause a falsely low SpO_2 reading?

____

____

10. How can patient movement cause an inaccurate SpO_2 reading?

____

____

11. What type of patients may make it difficult to properly align the oximeter probe?

____

____

12. List three conditions that can cause poor peripheral blood flow.

____

____

13. Why must a reusable oximeter probe be free of all dirt and grime before it is used?

____

____

Blood Pressure

Directions: Fill in each blank with the correct answer.

1. What does blood pressure measure?

____

____

2. Why is the diastolic pressure lower than the systolic pressure?

____

____

____

Copyright © 2008, 2004, 2000, 1995, 1990 by Saunders, an imprint of Elsevier Inc. All rights reserved.

3. What is considered normal blood pressure for an adult?

____

4. State the blood pressure range for each of the following:

   a. Prehypertension: _______________

   b. Hypertension, stage 1: _______________

   c. Hypertension, stage 2: _______________

5. Why should blood pressure readings always be interpreted using the patient's baseline blood pressure?

____

____

6. How does age affect blood pressure?

____

7. How do diurnal variations affect the blood pressure?

____

____

8. What are the two types of stethoscope chest pieces and the use of each?

____

____

____

____

9. What are the parts of a sphygmomanometer?

____

____

10. List the two types of sphygmomanometers.

____

11. List the three different cuff sizes and give examples of when each would be employed.

____

____

____

12. Explain how to determine the proper cuff size for a patient.

____

____

13. What may occur if blood pressure is taken using a cuff that is too small or too large?

____

____

Copyright © 2008, 2004, 2000, 1995, 1990 by Saunders, an imprint of Elsevier Inc. All rights reserved.

14. List the five phases included in the Korotkoff sounds and describe what type of sound is heard during each phase.

____

____

____

____

____

CRITICAL THINKING ACTIVITIES

A. MEASUREMENT OF BODY TEMPERATURE

For each of the following situations involving the measurement of body temperature, write C if the technique is correct and I if the technique is incorrect. If the situation is correct, state the principle underlying the technique. If the situation is incorrect, explain what might happen if the technique were performed in the incorrect manner.

Electronic Thermometer

____ 1. The medical assistant takes a patient's oral temperature immediately after the patient has consumed a cup of coffee.

____

____

____ 2. The medical assistant instructs the patient not to talk while his or her oral temperature is being measured.

____

____

____ 3. The medical assistant forgets to lubricate the rectal probe before taking a patient's rectal temperature.

____

____

____ 4. An axillary temperature reading is recorded as follows: 102.2° F.

____

____

____ 5. The medical assistant discards a used rectal probe in a regular waste container.

____

____

____ 6. The medical assistant's bare fingers accidentally touch a used oral probe cover while discarding it.

____

____

Tympanic Membrane Thermometer

____ 1. A tympanic membrane thermometer is used to take the temperature of a patient with impacted cerumen.

____

____

____ 2. A thermometer with a dirty probe lens is used to take the patient's temperature.

____

____

Copyright © 2008, 2004, 2000, 1995, 1990 by Saunders, an imprint of Elsevier Inc. All rights reserved.

____ 3. The ear canal is straightened before taking a patient's aural temperature.

____ 4. The medical assistant does not seal the opening of the ear canal with the probe when taking aural temperature.

____ 5. The probe is positioned toward the opposite temple when taking aural temperature.

____ 6. The medical assistant waits 30 seconds before taking the patient's temperature in the same ear.

Temporal Artery Thermometer

____ 1. The medical assistant checks to make sure the proble lens is clean and intact before using a temporal artery thermometer.

____ 2. The medical assistant brushes hair away from the patient's forehead before measuring the patient's temperature.

____ 3. The medical assistant slides the temporal artery probe across the patient's forehead while continually depressing the scan button.

____ 4. The medical assistant quickly scans the patient's forehead during temporal artery temperature measurement.

____ 5. After scanning the forehead, the medical assistant records the patient's temporal artery temperature reading.

____ 6. The medical assistant cleans the temporal artery thermometer by immersing it in warm, sudsy water.

Copyright © 2008, 2004, 2000, 1995, 1990 by Saunders, an imprint of Elsevier Inc. All rights reserved.

B. ALTERATIONS IN BODY TEMPERATURE

Label the diagram below with the terms that describe the body temperature alteration.

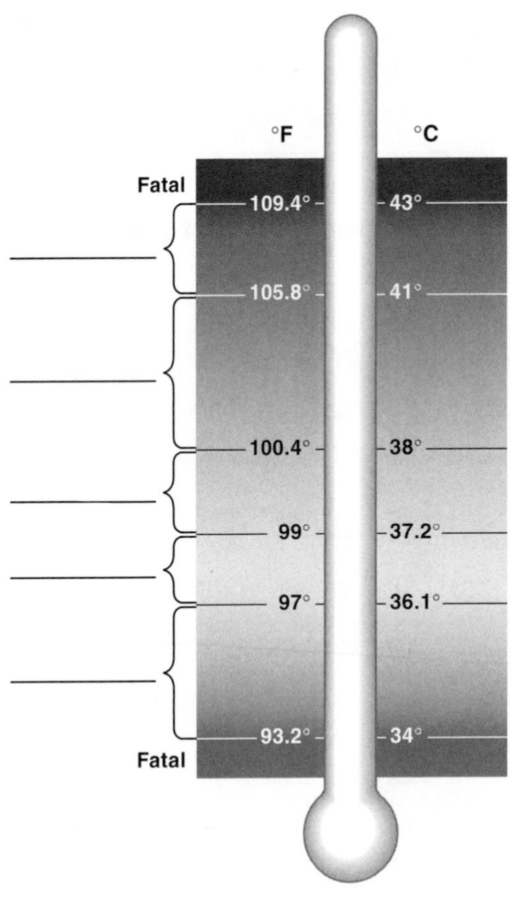

C. PULSE SITES

Locate the pulse at the following sites and record the pulse rates below:

1. Brachial pulse ____________________
2. Temporal pulse ____________________
3. Carotid pulse ____________________
4. Femoral pulse ____________________
5. Popliteal pulse ____________________
6. Dorsalis pedis pulse ____________________

D. PULSE AND RESPIRATORY RATES

Take the pulse and respiration of a person before and after vigorous exercise. Record results below:

1. Before vigorous exercise

____

____

2. After vigorous exercise

____

____

Copyright © 2008, 2004, 2000, 1995, 1990 by Saunders, an imprint of Elsevier Inc. All rights reserved.

3. Compare the results and explain how exercise affects the pulse and respiratory rates.

E. PULSE OXIMETRY

Your physician asks you to measure the oxygen saturation level of the patients listed below. For each situation, answer the following questions:

a. What would you do in each situation to prevent an inaccurate pulse oximetry reading?

b. What occurs with each of these situations and how does it affect the SpO_2 reading?

1. Kelly Collins, a patient with chronic bronchitis, is wearing navy blue nail polish.

2. Melvin Hosey has Parkinson's disease and is having difficulty controlling tremors in his hands.

3. Scott Kimes, a patient with emphysema, frequently experiences periods of prolonged coughing.

4. Nicole Lowe has returned to the office for a recheck of her viral pneumonia. You are getting ready to measure her oxygen saturation and notice that bright sunlight is coming through the window where she is seated and shining on her hand.

5. Rebecca Bensie, a patient on oxygen therapy, is morbidly obese, and you are having trouble properly aligning the oximeter probe on her finger.

6. Doug Habbershaw, a patient with peripheral vascular disease, has come to the office for a health check-up.

7. Emily Lacey has come to the office because she has been experiencing dyspnea. Her hands are very cold, and it is interfering with the pulse oximetry procedure.

8. Susan Boone, a patient with asthma, is wearing artificial fingernails.

Copyright © 2008, 2004, 2000, 1995, 1990 by Saunders, an imprint of Elsevier Inc. All rights reserved.

9. Frank Stewart, a patient with congestive heart failure, is at the office to have a mole removed from his back. There are bright overhead lights in the room, and they cannot be turned off because the physician needs to have good lighting to perform the surgery.

____

____

10. Wanda Weaver is having a sebaceous cyst removed from her chest and has been sedated for the procedure. You have applied an automatic blood pressure cuff to her right arm. The physician asks you to apply an oximeter probe to continuously monitor her oxygen saturation level during the procedure.

____

____

11. Which control, indicator, or display is involved when the following occurs:
    a. The oximeter is searching for a pulse ______________________________
    b. The oximeter can't find a pulse ______________________________
    c. The oximeter is portraying the strength of the pulse ______________________________
    d. The pulse is audibly broadcasted by a beeping sound ______________________________
    e. The oximeter displays the oxygen saturation level ______________________________
    f. The oximeter displays the pulse rate ______________________________
    g. The battery is low ______________________________
    h. You turn the oximeter off ______________________________

F. BLOOD PRESSURE MEASUREMENT

Using the principles outlined in the Procedure for Measuring Blood Pressure, explain what happens under the following circumstances:

1. The blood pressure is taken on a patient who has just undergone vigorous physical exercise.

____

2. The blood pressure is taken on a patient with tight sleeves.

____

____

3. An adult cuff is used to measure blood pressure on a young child.

____

____

4. The rubber bladder is not centered over the brachial artery.

____

____

5. The cuff is placed ½ inch above the bend in the elbows.

____

____

6. The manometer is viewed from a distance of 4 feet.

____

____

Copyright © 2008, 2004, 2000, 1995, 1990 by Saunders, an imprint of Elsevier Inc. All rights reserved.

G. PROPER BP CUFF SELECTION

Listed below are the measurements of the arm circumference (in cm) of different patients. Using Table 4-9 on page 155 of your textbook, indicate what size blood pressure cuff (child, small adult, adult, large adult, or adult thigh) should be used with each of these patients.

1. 47 cm ______________________
2. 20 cm ______________________
3. 32 cm ______________________
4. 16 cm ______________________
5. 38 cm ______________________
6. 27 cm ______________________
7. 52 cm ______________________
8. 24 cm ______________________

Measure the arm circumference of four classmates and record the values below. Next to each value, indicate what size blood pressure cuff should be used with each of these individuals.

1. ______________________
2. ______________________
3. ______________________
4. ______________________

H. READING BLOOD PRESSURE VALUES

Read and record the following blood pressure measurements in the space provided.

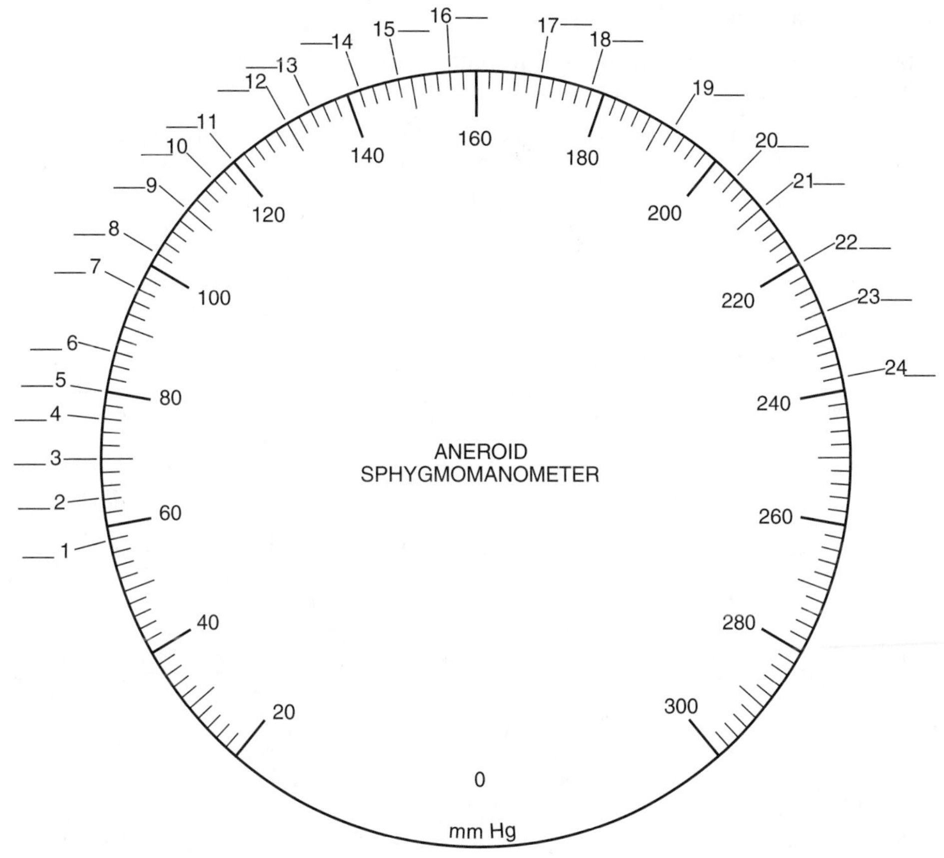

Copyright © 2008, 2004, 2000, 1995, 1990 by Saunders, an imprint of Elsevier Inc. All rights reserved.

I. INTERPRETING BLOOD PRESSURE READINGS

Classify each of the following blood pressure readings into its appropriate category. The readings are based on the average of two or more properly measured, seated blood pressure readings taken at each of two or more visits.

Normal
Prehypertension
Hypertension: Stage 1
Hypertension: Stage 2

1. 90/66 ________________________
2. 126/76 ________________________
3. 146/88 ________________________
4. 120/88 ________________________
5. 120/80 ________________________
6. 158/102 ________________________
7. 134/82 ________________________
8. 180/106 ________________________
9. 104/60 ________________________
10. 148/94 ________________________

J. HYPERTENSION

Create a profile of an individual who is at risk for developing hypertension following these guidelines:

1. Using colored pencils, crayons, or markers, draw a figure of an individual exhibiting risk factors for hypertension. Be as creative as possible.
2. Do not use any text in your drawing other than to label items you have drawn in your picture (e.g., cigarettes). A picture is worth a thousand words!
3. Include at least six risk factors for hypertension in your drawing. The Hypertension Patient Teaching Box in your textbook (page 154 can be used as a reference source).
4. In the classroom, choose a partner and trade drawings. Identify the risk factors for hypertension in your partner's drawing. Discuss with your partner what this person could do to lower his or her chances of developing hypertension.

Copyright © 2008, 2004, 2000, 1995, 1990 by Saunders, an imprint of Elsevier Inc. All rights reserved.

AT RISK FOR HYPERTENSION

K. CROSSWORD PUZZLE
Vital Signs

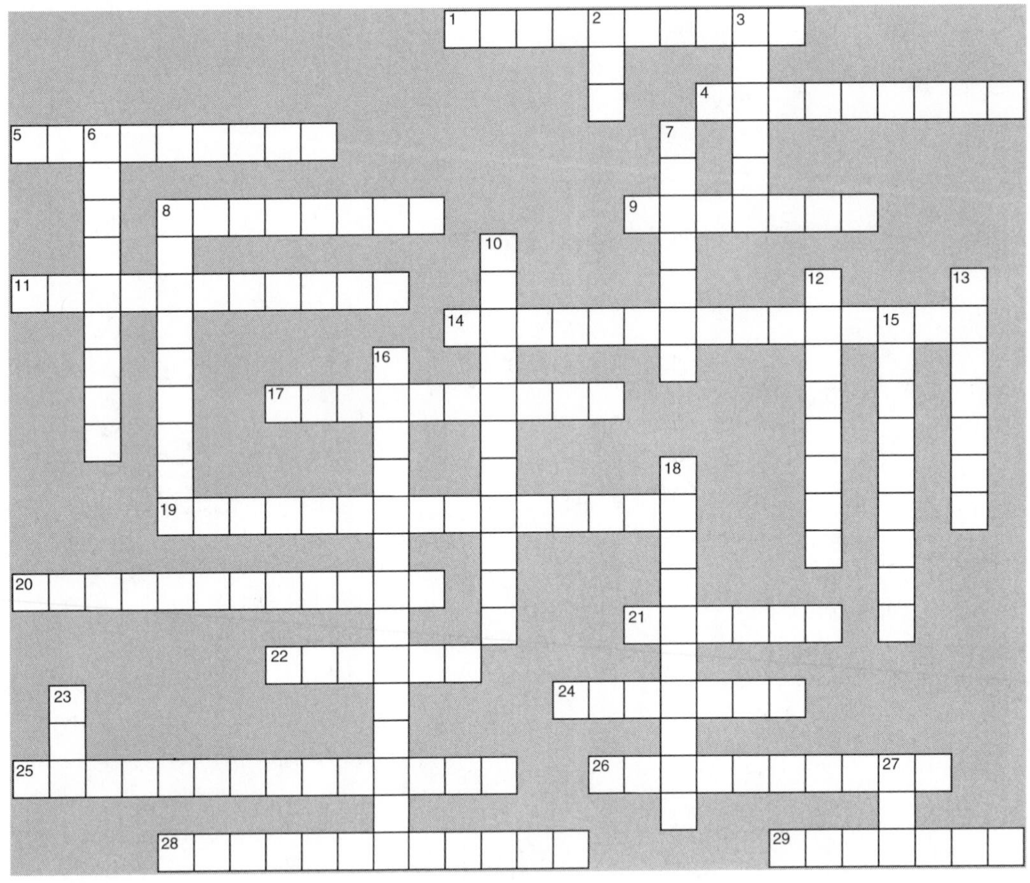

Directions: Complete the crossword puzzle using the clues presented below. All of your answers can be found in either a "box" or a "table" in your textbook.

ACROSS
1 Diaphragm or bell
4 Angled stethoscope earpieces
5 BP sounds
8 Has an S-shape
9 European temp measurement
11 Fever reducer
14 Fever increases this by 7%
17 U.S. temp measurement
19 Lowers pulse rate over time
20 Above 140/90
21 High BP might cause this
22 2400 mg or less per day
24 Asthma breath sounds
25 Center BP cuff over this
26 Risk factor for high BP
28 Cools body
29 Cracked earpieces can cause this

DOWN
2 Pulse range for exercising
3 Body temperature increaser
6 Fever that occurs with the flu
7 Invented the stethoscope
8 COPD example
10 Profuse perspiration
12 Do this after aerobic exercise
13 Leading cause of COPD
15 Fever causer
16 Drug to help COPD
18 BP position for patient's arm
23 220 minus your age
27 Good cholesterol

Copyright © 2008, 2004, 2000, 1995, 1990 by Saunders, an imprint of Elsevier Inc. All rights reserved.

Notes

Copyright © 2008, 2004, 2000, 1995, 1990 by Saunders, an imprint of Elsevier Inc. All rights reserved.

L. GO TO! GAME

Object: The object of **GO TO!** is to demonstrate your knowledge of locating pulse sites and answering questions relating to the vital signs.

Needed: **GO TO!** Gameboard (located in this chapter)
Completed Evaluation of Learning questions from this chapter
A small token for each player (such as a small button)
Dice (2)
Score Card

Directions:

1. Complete and review the Vital Signs Evaluation of Learning questions in your Study Guide.
2. Get into a group of four players.
3. Each player will select one of the four vital signs question sections (temperature, pulse, respiration, or blood pressure). The player will then tear that page out of the manual.
4. In turn, each player rolls the dice and GOES TO the pulse site indicated on the game board. (If a player rolls an 11, he or she loses a turn and the next player rolls the dice.)
5. If the player:
   A. *Goes to the correct pulse site*, he or she asks for a question from a vital signs category (other than his or her own category). Example: "Blood pressure."
   B. *Does not go to the correct pulse site,* the player is not permitted to request a question and must wait until his or her next turn to earn points.
6. The player with the category selected reads a question from his or her page of questions.
7. If the player answers the question correctly, he or she is awarded 5 points. If the player does not answer the question correctly, no points are awarded.
8. If you have any questions regarding the correct pulse site or answer to a question, consult your instructor for assistance.
9. Keep track of your points using the Score Card provided.
10. Once all of the questions from a category have been used, that category is deleted as a possible selection.
11. Continue until all of the Evaluation of Learning questions have been answered.
12. Calculate your points and determine the Knowledge Level you attained.

GO TO!
SCORE CARD

Name: ______________________________

Recording Points:
Cross off a number each time you answer a question correctly (starting with 5 and continuing in sequence). Your points will be equal to the last number you crossed off. Record this number in the space provided and determine the Knowledge Level you attained.

Points:	
5	75
10	80
15	85
20	90
25	95
30	100
35	105
40	110
45	115
50	120
55	125
60	130
65	135
70	140

TOTAL POINTS: _______

LEVEL OF KNOWLEDGE:

☐ 75 points and above: **Sheer genius**
☐ 55 to 70 points: **Shows great promise**
☐ 35 to 50 points: **Time to study**
☐ Below 35 points: **Brain freeze**

Copyright © 2008, 2004, 2000, 1995, 1990 by Saunders, an imprint of Elsevier Inc. All rights reserved.

GO TO!

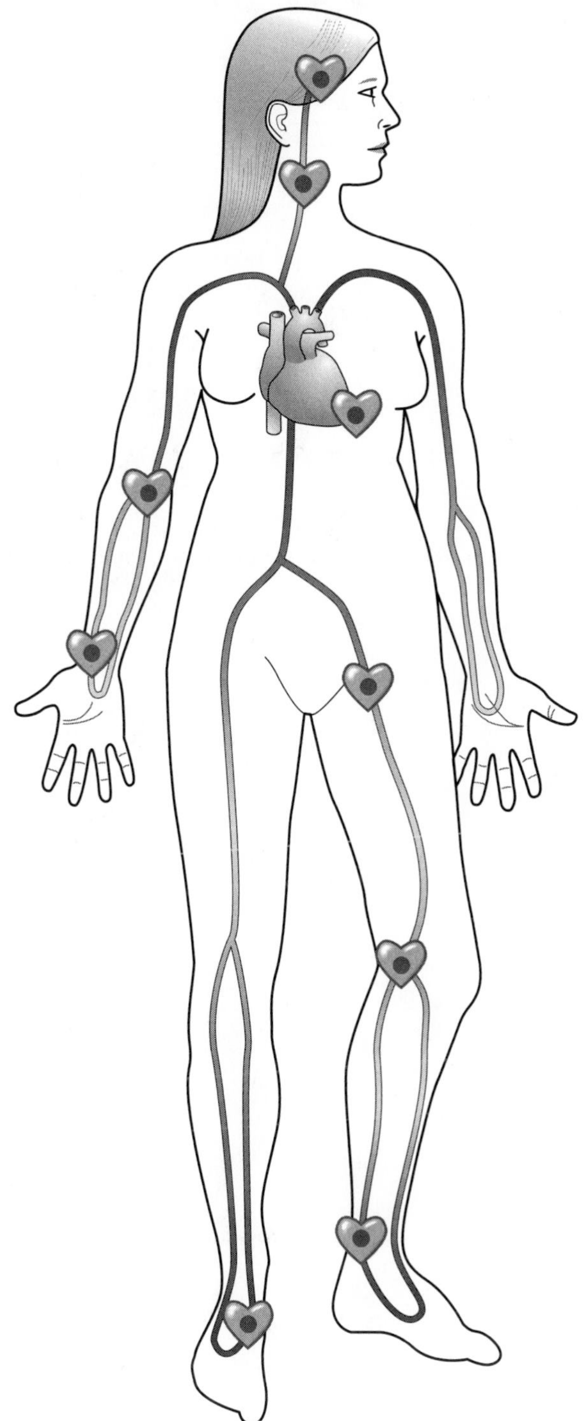

PULSE SITES	
Dice throws:	
Value	Go to
2	Radial
3	Apical
4	Brachial
5	Temporal
6	Carotid
7	Femoral
8	Popliteal
9	Dorsalis pedis
10	Posterior tibial
11	Dysrhythmia detected *Lose this turn*
12	Pulse is regular and strong Go wherever you want *Bonus of 5 points*

Copyright © 2008, 2004, 2000, 1995, 1990 by Saunders, an imprint of Elsevier Inc. All rights reserved.

M. ROAD TO RECOVERY GAME

Object: The object of the game is to lead your "patient" to recovery by correctly providing the definition to medical terms relating to vital signs.

Needed: **Road to Recovery** game board (located at the end of this manual)
Game cards
A token for each player (such as a button or coin)
Dice (1)
Score Card

Directions

1. Cut out the terminology game cards on the following pages.
2. Study the terms and definitions in preparation for the game.
3. Place one complete set of terms on the game board with the definitions facing up (and the medical terms facing down).
4. Play **Road to Recovery** following the directions on the reverse side of the game board.
5. Keep track of your points using the Score Card provided.
6. If time permits, place the set of cards on the game board again with the medical terms face-up and the definitions face-down and continue playing the game until all the cards have been used.

ROAD TO RECOVERY
SCORE CARD

Name: ________________________________

Recording Points:
Using the Game Card Points box, cross off a number each time you answer a game card correctly (starting with 5 and continuing in sequence). Your total game card points will be equal to the last number you crossed off. Record this number in the space provided (1). Record any extra points you were awarded during the game (2), and any points that were deducted (3). To determine your total points, add (1) and (2) together and deduct (3). Record this number in the Total Points Earned space provided. Compare your score with the other players and determine where you placed. Place a checkmark next to the level of recovery your patient attained.

Game Card Points:			
5	75	145	215
10	80	150	220
15	85	155	225
20	90	160	230
25	95	165	235
30	100	170	240
35	105	175	245
40	110	180	250
45	115	185	255
50	120	190	260
55	125	195	265
60	130	200	270
65	135	205	275
70	140	210	280

Calculation of Points:

(1) Total Game Card Points: ________

(2) Additional Points Awarded: ________

(3) Deducted Points: ________

TOTAL POINTS EARNED: ________

LEVEL OF RECOVERY:

Patient's Name: ____________________

☐ First Place: **Fully Recovered**
☐ Second Place: **Almost Recovered**
☐ Third Place: **Still Recovering**
☐ Fourth Place: **Gasping for Air**

Copyright © 2008, 2004, 2000, 1995, 1990 by Saunders, an imprint of Elsevier Inc. All rights reserved.

Notes

Copyright © 2008, 2004, 2000, 1995, 1990 by Saunders, an imprint of Elsevier Inc. All rights reserved.

Adventitious sounds	Afebrile	Alveolus	Antecubital space
Antipyretic	Aorta	Apnea	Axilla
Bounding pulse	Bradycardia	Bradypnea	Celsius scale
Conduction	Convection	Crisis	Cyanosis

The space located at the front of the elbow	A thin-walled air sac of the lungs in which the exchange of oxygen and carbon dioxide takes place	Without fever; the body temperature is normal	Abnormal breath sounds
The armpit	The temporary cessation of breathing	The major trunk of the arterial system of the body	An agent that reduces fever
A temperature scale on which the freezing point of water is 0° and the boiling point of water is 100°	An abnormal decrease in the respiratory rate of less than 10 respirations per minute	An abnormally slow heart rate (less than 60 beats per minute)	A pulse with an increased volume that feels very strong and full
A bluish discoloration of the skin and mucous membranes	A sudden falling of an elevated body temperature to normal	The transfer of energy through air currents	The transfer of energy from one object to another by direct contact.

Diastole	Diastolic pressure	Disinfectant	Dyspnea
Dysrhythmia	Eupnea	Exhalation	Fahrenheit scale
Febrile	Fever	Frenulum linguae	Hyperpnea
Hyperpyrexia	Hypertension	Hyperventilation	Hypopnea

Shortness of breath or difficulty breathing	An agent used to destroy disease-producing microorganisms but not necessarily their spores (usually applied to inanimate objects)	The point of lesser pressure on the arterial wall	The phase in the cardiac cycle in which the heart relaxes between contractions
A temperature scale on which the freezing point of water is 32° and the boiling point of water is 212°	The act of breathing out	Normal respiration (16 to 20 resp/min)	An irregular rhythm
An abnormal increase in the rate and depth of respiration	The midline fold that connects the undersurface of the tongue with the floor of the mouth	A body temperature that is above normal (synonym for pyrexia)	Pertaining to fever
An abnormal decrease in the rate and depth of respiration	An abnormally fast and deep type of breathing usually associated with acute anxiety conditions	High blood pressure	An extremely high fever

Hypotension	**Hypothermia**	**Hypoxemia**	**Hypoxia**
Inhalation	**Intercostal**	**Korotkoff sounds**	**Malaise**
Manometer	**Meniscus**	**Orthopnea**	**Pulse deficit**
Pulse oximeter	**Pulse oximetry**	**Pulse pressure**	**Pulse rhythm**

A reduction in the oxygen supply to the tissues of the body	A decrease in the oxygen saturation of the blood. May lead to hypoxia	A body temperature that is below normal	Low blood pressure
A vague sense of body discomfort, weakness, and fatigue	Sounds heard during the measurement of blood pressure that are used to determine the systolic and diastolic blood pressure reading	Between the ribs	The act of breathing in
A condition in which the radial pulse rate is less than the apical pulse rate	The condition in which breathing is easier in a standing or sitting position	The curved surface on a column of liquid in a tube	An instrument for measuring pressure
The time interval between heart beats	The difference between the systolic and diastolic pressures	The use of a pulse oximeter to measure the oxygen saturation of arterial blood	A computerized device consisting of a probe and monitor used to measure the oxygen saturation of arterial blood

Pulse volume	Pyrexia	Radiation	SaO_2
Sphygmomanometer	SpO_2	Stethoscope	Systole
Systolic pressure	Tachycardia	Tachypnea	Thready pulse

Abbreviation for the percentage of hemoglobin that is saturated with oxygen in arterial blood

The transfer of energy in the form of waves

A body temperature that is above normal (synonym for fever)

The strength of the heart beat

The phase in the cardiac cycle in which the ventricles contract

An instrument for amplifying and hearing sounds produced by the body

Abbreviation for the percentage of hemoglobin that is saturated with oxygen in arterial blood as measured by a pulse oximeter

An instrument for measuring arterial blood pressure

A pulse with a decreased volume that feels weak and thin

An abnormal increase in the respiratory rate of more than 20 respirations per minute

An abnormally fast heart rate (over 100 beats per minute)

The point of maximum pressure on the arterial walls

PRACTICE FOR COMPETENCY

Measuring Body Temperature

Measure body temperature with each of the following types of thermometers and record results in the chart provided.

Procedures 4-1, 4-2, and 4-3: Electronic Thermometer (Oral, Axillary, and Rectal)

Procedure 4-4: Tympanic Membrane Thermometer (Aural)

Procedure 4-5: Temporal Artery Thermometer

CHART	
Date	

Copyright © 2008, 2004, 2000, 1995, 1990 by Saunders, an imprint of Elsevier Inc. All rights reserved.

CHART	
Date	

Copyright © 2008, 2004, 2000, 1995, 1990 by Saunders, an imprint of Elsevier Inc. All rights reserved.

PRACTICE FOR COMPETENCY

Measuring Pulse, Respiration, and Oxygen Saturation

Procedure 4-6: Pulse and Respiration. Measure the radial pulse and respiration. Describe the rhythm and volume of the pulse. Describe the rhythm and depth of the respirations. Record the results in the chart provided.

Procedure 4-7: Apical Pulse. Measure apical pulse. Describe the rhythm and volume of the pulse. Record the results in the chart provided.

Procedure 4-8: Pulse Oximetry. Measure the oxgygen saturation level and record the results in the chart provided.

CHART	
Date	

Copyright © 2008, 2004, 2000, 1995, 1990 by Saunders, an imprint of Elsevier Inc. All rights reserved.

CHART	
Date	

Copyright © 2008, 2004, 2000, 1995, 1990 by Saunders, an imprint of Elsevier Inc. All rights reserved.

PRACTICE FOR COMPETENCY

Measuring Blood Pressure

Procedure 4-9: Blood Pressure. Measure blood pressure. Record results in the chart provided.

Chart	
Date	

Copyright © 2008, 2004, 2000, 1995, 1990 by Saunders, an imprint of Elsevier Inc. All rights reserved.

CHART

Date	

Copyright © 2008, 2004, 2000, 1995, 1990 by Saunders, an imprint of Elsevier Inc. All rights reserved.

EVALUATION OF COMPETENCY

Procedure 4-1: Measuring Oral Body Temperature—Electronic Thermometer

Name: ______________________________ Date: ______________

Evaluated By: ______________________________ Score: ______________

Performance Objective

Outcome:	Measure oral body temperature.
Conditions:	Given the following: electronic thermometer and oral probe, probe cover, and a waste container.
Standards:	Time: 5 minutes. Student completed procedure in ____ minutes.
	Accuracy: Satisfactory score on the Performance Evaluation Checklist.

Performance Evaluation Checklist

Trial 1	Trial 2	Point Value	*Performance Standards*
		•	Sanitized hands.
		•	Assembled equipment.
		•	Removed thermometer from its storage base.
		•	Attached oral probe to thermometer unit.
		•	Inserted probe into the thermometer.
		•	Greeted the patient and introduced yourself.
		•	Identified the patient and explained the procedure.
		•	Asked the patient if he/she has ingested hot or cold beverages.
		▷	Explained what to do if the patient has recently ingested a hot or cold beverage.
		•	Removed probe from the thermometer.
		▷	Explained what occurs when probe is removed from the thermometer.
		•	Attached probe cover to probe.
		▷	Stated the purpose of the probe cover.
		•	Correctly inserted the probe in patient's mouth.
		•	Instructed the patient to keep the mouth closed.
		▷	Explained why the mouth should be kept closed.
		•	Held probe in place until an audible tone was heard.
		•	Noted patient's temperature reading on display screen.
		•	Removed probe from patient's mouth.
		•	Discarded probe cover in a regular waste container.
		•	Did not allow fingers to come in contact with cover.

Copyright © 2008, 2004, 2000, 1995, 1990 by Saunders, an imprint of Elsevier Inc. All rights reserved.

Trial 1	Trial 2	Point Value	*Performance Standards*
		●	Returned probe to the thermometer unit.
		▷	Stated what occurs when probe is returned to the thermometer.
		●	Returned the thermometer unit to its storage base.
		●	Sanitized hands.
		●	Charted the results correctly.
		*	The temperature recording was identical to the reading on the display screen.
		▷	Stated the normal body temperature range for an adult (97° to 99° F).
		*	Completed the procedure within 5 minutes.
			TOTALS

CHART	
Date	

Evaluation of Student Performance

EVALUATION CRITERIA			COMMENTS
Symbol	Category	Point Value	
*	Critical Step	16 points	
●	Essential Step	6 points	
▷	Theory Question	2 points	

Score calculation: 100 points
– ______ points missed
____ Score
Satisfactory score: 85 or above

AAMA/CAAHEP Competency Achieved:

☑ III. C. 3. b. (4) (b): Obtain vital signs.

Copyright © 2008, 2004, 2000, 1995, 1990 by Saunders, an imprint of Elsevier Inc. All rights reserved.

EVALUATION OF COMPETENCY

Procedure 4-2: Measuring Axillary Body Temperature—Electronic Thermometer

Name: ______________________________ Date: ______________

Evaluated By: ______________________________ Score: ______________

Performance Objective

Outcome:	Measure axillary body temperature.
Conditions:	Given the following: electronic thermometer and oral probe, probe cover, and a waste container.
Standards:	Time: 5 minutes. Student completed procedure in ____ minutes.
	Accuracy: Satisfactory score on the Performance Evaluation Checklist.

Performance Evaluation Checklist

Trial 1	*Trial 2*	*Point Value*	*Performance Standards*
		•	Sanitized hands.
		•	Assembled equipment.
		•	Removed thermometer from its storage base.
		•	Attached oral probe to thermometer unit.
		•	Inserted probe into the thermometer.
		•	Greeted the patient and introduced yourself.
		•	Identified the patient and explained the procedure.
		•	Removed clothing from patient's shoulder and arm.
		•	Made sure that the axilla was dry.
		•	Removed probe from the thermometer.
		•	Attached probe cover to probe.
		•	Placed probe in the center of the patient's axilla.
		•	Ensured that the arm was held close to the body.
		▷	Explained why the arm must be held close to the body.
		•	Held probe in place until an audible tone was heard.
		•	Removed probe from patient's axilla.
		•	Noted patient's temperature reading on display screen.
		•	Discarded probe cover in a regular waste container.
		•	Did not allow fingers to come in contact with cover.
		•	Returned probe to the thermometer unit.
		•	Returned the thermometer unit to its storage base.

Copyright © 2008, 2004, 2000, 1995, 1990 by Saunders, an imprint of Elsevier Inc. All rights reserved.

Trial 1	Trial 2	Point Value	*Performance Standards*
		•	Sanitized hands.
		•	Charted the results correctly.
		✶	The temperature recording was identical to the reading on the display screen.
		✶	Completed the procedure within 5 minutes.
			TOTALS

CHART	
Date	

Evaluation of Student Performance

EVALUATION CRITERIA			COMMENTS
Symbol	Category	Point Value	
✶	Critical Step	16 points	
•	Essential Step	6 points	
▷	Theory Question	2 points	
Score calculation: 100 points – ______ points missed ______ Score Satisfactory score: 85 or above			

AAMA/CAAHEP Competency Achieved:

☑ III. C. 3. b. (4) (b): Obtain vital signs.

Copyright © 2008, 2004, 2000, 1995, 1990 by Saunders, an imprint of Elsevier Inc. All rights reserved.

EVALUATION OF COMPETENCY

Procedure 4-3: Measuring Rectal Body Temperature—Electronic Thermometer

Name: ______________________________ Date: ______________

Evaluated By: ______________________________ Score: ______________

Performance Objective

Outcome: Measure rectal body temperature.

Conditions: Given the following: electronic thermometer, rectal probe, probe cover, lubricant, disposable gloves, tissues, and a waste container.

Standards: Time: 5 minutes. Student completed procedure in ____ minutes.

Accuracy: Satisfactory score on the Performance Evaluation Checklist.

Performance Evaluation Checklist

Trial 1	*Trial 2*	*Point Value*	*Performance Standards*
		•	Sanitized hands.
		•	Assembled equipment.
		•	Removed thermometer from its storage base.
		•	Attached rectal probe to thermometer unit.
		•	Inserted probe into the thermometer.
		•	Greeted the patient and introduced yourself.
		•	Identified the patient and explained the procedure.
		•	Applied gloves.
		▷	Stated the reason for applying gloves.
		•	Positioned and draped the patient.
		▷	Explained how to position an adult and an infant.
		•	Removed probe from the thermometer.
		•	Attached probe cover to probe.
		•	Applied lubricant up to a level of 1 inch.
		▷	Stated the purpose of the lubricant.
		•	Instructed patient to lie still.
		•	Separated the buttocks and properly inserted the thermometer.
		▷	Stated how far the thermometer should be inserted for adults, children, and infants.
		•	Held probe in place until an audible tone was heard.
		•	Removed the probe in the same direction as it was inserted.

Copyright © 2008, 2004, 2000, 1995, 1990 by Saunders, an imprint of Elsevier Inc. All rights reserved.

Trial 1	Trial 2	Point Value	Performance Standards
		•	Noted patient's temperature reading on display screen.
		•	Discarded probe cover in a regular waste container.
		▷	Explained why the cover can be discarded in a regular waste container.
		•	Returned probe to the thermometer unit.
		•	Returned the thermometer unit to its storage base.
		•	Wiped the anal area with tissues.
		•	Removed gloves and sanitized hands.
		•	Charted the results correctly.
		✶	The temperature recording was identical to the reading on the display screen.
		✶	Completed the procedure within 5 minutes.
			TOTALS

CHART	
Date	

Evaluation of Student Performance

EVALUATION CRITERIA			COMMENTS
Symbol	Category	Point Value	
✶	Critical Step	16 points	
•	Essential Step	6 points	
▷	Theory Question	2 points	

Score calculation: 100 points
– ______ points missed
____ Score

Satisfactory score: 85 or above

AAMA/CAAHEP Competency Achieved:

☑ III. C. 3. b. (4) (b): Obtain vital signs.

Copyright © 2008, 2004, 2000, 1995, 1990 by Saunders, an imprint of Elsevier Inc. All rights reserved.

EVALUATION OF COMPETENCY

Procedure 4-4: Measuring Aural Body Temperature—Tympanic Membrane Thermometer

Name: ______________________________ Date: ______________

Evaluated By: ______________________________ Score: ______________

Performance Objective

Outcome:	Measure aural body temperature.
Conditions:	Given the following: tympanic membrane thermometer, probe cover, and a waste container.
Standards:	Time: 5 minutes. Student completed procedure in ____ minutes.
	Accuracy: Satisfactory score on the Performance Evaluation Checklist.

Performance Evaluation Checklist

Trial 1	Trial 2	Point Value	*Performance Standards*
		•	Sanitized hands.
		•	Assembled equipment.
		•	Greeted the patient and introduced yourself.
		•	Identified the patient and explained the procedure.
		•	Removed thermometer from its storage base.
		•	Checked to make sure the probe lens was clean and intact.
		▷	Stated what might occur if the lens was dirty.
		•	Placed a cover on the probe.
		▷	Explained the purpose of the probe cover.
		•	Observed the screen to determine if the thermometer is ready to use.
		•	Held the thermometer in the dominant hand.
		•	Straightened the patient's ear canal with the nondominant hand.
		▷	Explained the purpose of straightening the ear canal.
		•	Inserted the probe into the patient's ear canal and sealed the opening without causing the patient discomfort.
		•	Pointed the tip of the probe toward the opposite temple.
		▷	Stated the reason for pointing the probe toward the opposite temple.
		•	Asked the patient to remain still.
		•	Depressed the activation button for 1 full second or until an audible tone is heard.
		•	Removed the thermometer from the ear canal and noted the patient's temperature on the display screen.
		▷	Stated what should be done if the temperature seems too low.

Copyright © 2008, 2004, 2000, 1995, 1990 by Saunders, an imprint of Elsevier Inc. All rights reserved.

Trial 1	Trial 2	Point Value	Performance Standards
		•	Disposed of the probe cover in a waste container.
		•	Replaced the thermometer in its storage base.
		▷	Explained the reason for storing the thermometer in its base.
		•	Sanitized hands.
		•	Charted the results correctly.
		*	The temperature recording was identical to the reading on the display screen.
		*	Completed the procedure within 5 minutes.
			TOTALS

CHART	
Date	

Evaluation of Student Performance

EVALUATION CRITERIA			COMMENTS
Symbol	Category	Point Value	
*	Critical Step	16 points	
•	Essential Step	6 points	
▷	Theory Question	2 points	
Score calculation: 100 points – ____ points missed ____ Score Satisfactory score: 85 or above			

AAMA/CAAHEP Competency Achieved:

☑ III. C. 3. b. (4) (b): Obtain vital signs.

Copyright © 2008, 2004, 2000, 1995, 1990 by Saunders, an imprint of Elsevier Inc. All rights reserved.

EVALUATION OF COMPETENCY

Procedure 4-5: Measuring Temporal Body Temperature

Name: ______________________________ Date: ______________

Evaluated By: ______________________________ Score: ______________

Performance Objective

Outcome: Measure temporal body temperature.

Conditions: Given the following: temporal artery thermometer, disposable probe cover, antiseptic wipe, waste container.

Standards: Time: 5 minutes. Student completed procedure in ____ minutes.

Accuracy: Satisfactory score on the Performance Evaluation Checklist.

Performance Evaluation Checklist

Trial 1	*Trial 2*	*Point Value*	*Performance Standards*
		•	Sanitized the hands and assembled equipment.
		•	Greeted the patient and introduced yourself.
		•	Identified the patient and explained the procedure.
		•	Checked to make sure the probe lens is clean and intact.
		▷	Stated why the lens should be clean.
		•	Placed a disposable cover onto the probe or cleaned the probe with an antiseptic wipe and allowed it to dry.
		•	Selected an appropriate site.
		•	Brushed away any hair that is covering the scanning sites.
		▷	Explained why hair must be brushed away.
		•	Held the thermometer in the dominant hand with the thumb on the scan button.
		•	Gently positioned the probe of the thermometer on the center of the patient's forehead.
		•	Depressed the scan button and kept it depressed for the entire measurement.
		▷	Stated why the scan button must be continually depressed.
		•	Slowly and gently slid the probe straight across the forehead midway between the eyebrow and the upper hairline.
		•	Continued until the hairline was reached making sure to keep the probe flush against the forehead.
		•	Keeping the button depressed, lifted the probe from the forehead and placed it behind the earlobe for 1 to 2 seconds.
		▷	Stated why the probe is placed behind the earlobe.

Copyright © 2008, 2004, 2000, 1995, 1990 by Saunders, an imprint of Elsevier Inc. All rights reserved.

Trial 1	Trial 2	Point Value	Performance Standards
		•	Released the scan button and noted the temperature on the display screen.
		•	Disposed of the probe cover in a regular waste container.
		•	Wiped the probe with an antiseptic wipe and allowed it to dry.
		•	Sanitized hands.
		•	Charted the results correctly.
		*	The temperature recording was identical to the reading on the display screen.
		•	Stored the thermometer in a clean, dry area.
		*	Completed the procedure within 5 minutes.
			TOTALS

CHART	
Date	

Evaluation of Student Performance

EVALUATION CRITERIA			COMMENTS
Symbol	Category	Point Value	
*	Critical Step	16 points	
•	Essential Step	6 points	
▷	Theory Question	2 points	
Score calculation: 100 points – ______ points missed ____ Score Satisfactory score: 85 or above			

AAMA/CAAHEP Competency Achieved:

☑ III. C. 3. b. (4) (b): Obtain vital signs.

Copyright © 2008, 2004, 2000, 1995, 1990 by Saunders, an imprint of Elsevier Inc. All rights reserved.

EVALUATION OF COMPETENCY

Procedure 4-6: Measuring Pulse and Respiration

Name: ______________________________ Date: ______________

Evaluated By: ______________________________ Score: ______________

Performance Objective

Outcome:	Measure radial pulse and respiration.
Conditions:	Using a watch with a second hand.
Standards:	Time: 5 minutes. Student completed procedure in ____ minutes.
	Accuracy: Satisfactory score on the Performance Evaluation Checklist.

Performance Evaluation Checklist

Trial 1	*Trial 2*	*Point Value*	*Performance Standards*
		•	Sanitized hands.
		•	Greeted the patient and introduced yourself.
		•	Identified the patient and explained the procedure.
		•	Observed patient for any signs that might affect the pulse rate or respiratory rate.
		▷	Stated two factors that would increase the pulse rate.
		•	Positioned the patient in a comfortable position.
		•	Placed three middle fingertips over the radial pulse site.
		▷	Explained why the pulse should not be taken with the thumb.
		•	Applied moderate, gentle pressure until the pulse was felt.
		▷	Stated what will occur if too much pressure is applied over the radial artery.
		•	Counted the pulse for 30 seconds and made a mental note of the number.
		•	Determined the rhythm and volume of the pulse.
		▷	Stated when the pulse should be measured for a full minute.
		•	Continued to hold the fingers on the patient's wrist.
		▷	Explained why respirations should be taken without the patient's awareness.
		•	Observed the rise and fall of patient's chest.
		•	Counted the number of respirations for 30 seconds and made a mental note of the number.
		▷	Stated what makes up one respiration.
		•	Determined the rhythm and depth of the respirations.
		•	Observed the patient's color.

Copyright © 2008, 2004, 2000, 1995, 1990 by Saunders, an imprint of Elsevier Inc. All rights reserved.

Trial 1	Trial 2	Point Value	*Performance Standards*
		•	Sanitized hands.
		•	Multiplied the pulse and respiration values by 2.
		•	Charted the results correctly.
		*	The pulse rate was within ±2 beats of the evaluator's reading.
		*	The respiratory rate was within 1 respiration of the evaluator's measurement.
		▷	Stated the normal adult range for the pulse rate (60 to 100 bpm).
		▷	Stated the normal adult range for the respiratory rate (12 to 20 respirations/minute).
		*	Completed the procedure within 5 minutes.
			TOTALS

CHART	
Date	

Evaluation of Student Performance

EVALUATION CRITERIA			COMMENTS
Symbol	Category	Point Value	
*	Critical Step	16 points	
•	Essential Step	6 points	
▷	Theory Question	2 points	
Score calculation: 100 points – ______ points missed ____ Score Satisfactory score: 85 or above			

AAMA/CAAHEP Competency Achieved:

☑ III. C. 3. b. (4) (b): Obtain vital signs.

Copyright © 2008, 2004, 2000, 1995, 1990 by Saunders, an imprint of Elsevier Inc. All rights reserved.

EVALUATION OF COMPETENCY

Procedure 4-7: Measuring Apical Pulse

Name: ______________________________ Date: ____________

Evaluated By: ______________________________ Score: ____________

Performance Objective

Outcome:	Measure apical pulse.
Conditions:	Given the following: stethoscope and antiseptic wipe.
	Using a watch with a second hand.
Standards:	Time: 5 minutes. Student completed procedure in ____ minutes.
	Accuracy: Satisfactory score on the Performance Evaluation Checklist.

Performance Evaluation Checklist

Trial 1	*Trial 2*	*Point Value*	*Performance Standards*
		•	Sanitized hands.
		•	Greeted the patient and introduced yourself.
		•	Identified the patient and explained the procedure.
		•	Observed the patient for any signs that might affect the pulse rate.
		•	Assembled equipment.
		•	Rotated the chest piece to the bell position.
		•	Cleaned earpieces and chest piece with antiseptic wipe.
		▷	Stated the reason for cleaning stethoscope with an antiseptic.
		•	Positioned patient.
		•	Asked the patient to unbutton or remove his/her shirt.
		•	Warmed chest piece of the stethoscope.
		▷	Explained the reason for warming chest piece.
		•	Inserted earpieces of stethoscope in a forward position in the ears.
		▷	Explained why the earpieces must be directed forward.
		•	Placed the chest piece over the apex of the heart.
		▷	Described the location of the apex of the heart.
		•	Counted the number of heartbeats for 30 seconds and multiplied by 2.
		*	The reading was within ±2 beats of the evaluator's reading.
		•	Sanitized hands.

Copyright © 2008, 2004, 2000, 1995, 1990 by Saunders, an imprint of Elsevier Inc. All rights reserved.

		•	Charted the results correctly.
		•	Cleaned earpieces and chest piece with an antiseptic wipe.
		✶	Completed the procedure within 5 minutes.
			TOTALS

CHART	
Date	

Evaluation of Student Performance

EVALUATION CRITERIA			COMMENTS
Symbol	Category	Point Value	
✶	Critical Step	16 points	
•	Essential Step	6 points	
▷	Theory Question	2 points	
Score calculation: 100 points – ______ points missed ____ Score Satisfactory score: 85 or above			

AAMA/CAAHEP Competency Achieved:

☑ III. C. 3. b. (4) (b): Obtain vital signs.

Copyright © 2008, 2004, 2000, 1995, 1990 by Saunders, an imprint of Elsevier Inc. All rights reserved.

EVALUATION OF COMPETENCY

Procedure 4-8: Performing Pulse Oximetry

Name: ______________________________ Date: ____________

Evaluated By: ______________________________ Score: ____________

Performance Objective

Outcome: Perform pulse oximetry.

Conditions: Given the following: handheld pulse oximeter, reusable finger probe, and an antiseptic wipe.

Standards: Time: 5 minutes. Student completed procedure in ____ minutes.

Accuracy: Satisfactory score on the Performance Evaluation Checklist.

Performance Evaluation Checklist

Trial 1	*Trial 2*	*Point Value*	*Performance Standards*
		•	Sanitized hands and assembled equipment.
		•	Ensured the probe opened and closed smoothly and that the windows were clean.
		•	Disinfected the probe windows and platforms and allowed them to dry.
		▷	Stated the purpose of disinfecting the probe windows.
		•	If necessary, connected the probe to the cable.
		•	Connected the cable to the monitor.
		•	Did not lift or carry the monitor by the cable.
		•	Greeted the patient and introduced yourself.
		•	Identified the patient and explained the procedure.
		•	Seated the patient in a chair with the lower arm supported and the palm facing down.
		▷	Explained why the arm should be supported.
		•	Selected an appropriate finger to apply the probe.
		•	Observed the patient's finger to make sure it is free of dark fingernail polish or an artificial nail.
		•	Checked to make sure the patient's fingertip is clean.
		•	Checked to make sure the patient's finger is not cold.
		▷	Explained what to do if the patient's finger is cold
		•	Made sure that ambient light will not interfere with the measurement.
		▷	Explained why ambient light should be avoided.
		•	Positioned the probe securely on the fingertip.
		•	Allowed the cable to lay across the back of the hand and parallel to the arm of the patient.

Copyright © 2008, 2004, 2000, 1995, 1990 by Saunders, an imprint of Elsevier Inc. All rights reserved.

Trial 1	Trial 2	Point Value	*Performance Standards*
		•	Instructed the patient to remain still and to breathe normally.
		▷	Stated why the patient must remain still.
		•	Turned on the pulse oximeter.
		•	Waited while the oximeter went through its power-on self test (POST).
		▷	Explained what to do if the oximeter fails the POST.
		•	Allowed several seconds for the oximeter to detect the pulse and calculate the oxygen saturation.
		•	Ensured that the pulse strength indicator fluctuates with each pulsation and that the pulse signal is strong.
		▷	Stated what should be done if the oximeter is unable to locate a pulse.
		•	Left the probe in place until the oximeter displayed a reading.
		•	Noted the oxygen saturation value and pulse rate.
		*	The reading was identical to the evaluator's reading.
		▷	Stated the normal oxygen saturation level of a healthy adult (95% to 99%).
		•	Removed the probe from the patient's finger and turned off the oximeter.
		•	Sanitized hands.
		•	Charted the results correctly.
		•	Disconnected the cable from the monitor.
		•	Disinfected the probe with an antiseptic wipe.
		•	Properly stored the monitor in a clean dry area.
		*	Completed the procedure within 5 minutes.
			TOTALS

CHART	
Date	

Copyright © 2008, 2004, 2000, 1995, 1990 by Saunders, an imprint of Elsevier Inc. All rights reserved.

Evaluation of Student Performance

EVALUATION CRITERIA			COMMENTS
Symbol	Category	Point Value	
*	Critical Step	16 points	
•	Essential Step	6 points	
▷	Theory Question	2 points	
Score calculation: 100 points – ______ points missed ____ Score Satisfactory score: 85 or above			

AAMA/CAAHEP Competency Achieved:

☑ III. C. 3. b. (4) (b): Obtain vital signs.

Copyright © 2008, 2004, 2000, 1995, 1990 by Saunders, an imprint of Elsevier Inc. All rights reserved.

Notes

Copyright © 2008, 2004, 2000, 1995, 1990 by Saunders, an imprint of Elsevier Inc. All rights reserved.

EVALUATION OF COMPETENCY

Procedure 4-9: Measuring Blood Pressure

Name: ______________________________ Date: ______________

Evaluated By: ______________________________ Score: ______________

Performance Objective

Outcome: Measure blood pressure.

Conditions: Given the following: stethoscope, sphygmomanometer, and an antiseptic wipe.

Standards: Time: 5 minutes. Student completed procedure in ____ minutes.

Accuracy: Satisfactory score on the Performance Evaluation Checklist.

Performance Evaluation Checklist

Trial 1	*Trial 2*	*Point Value*	*Performance Standards*
		•	Sanitized hands.
		•	Assembled equipment.
		•	Rotated the chest piece to the diaphragm position.
		•	Cleaned earpieces and chest piece of stethoscope with an antiseptic wipe.
		•	Greeted the patient and introduced yourself.
		•	Identified the patient and explained the procedure.
		•	Observed patient for any signs that might influence the blood pressure reading.
		▷	Listed signs that would influence the blood pressure reading.
		•	Determined how high to pump the cuff (palpated systolic pressure or checking the patient's chart).
		•	Positioned patient in a sitting position.
		•	Made sure that the patient's arm was uncovered.
		•	Explained why blood pressure should not be taken over clothing.
		•	Positioned patient's arm at heart level with the palm facing up.
		•	Selected the proper cuff size.
		▷	Explained how to determine the proper cuff size.
		•	Located the brachial pulse with the fingertips.
		▷	Stated the location of the brachial pulse.
		•	Centered bladder over the brachial pulse site.
		▷	Explained why the bladder should be centered over the brachial pulse site.
		•	Placed cuff on patient's arm 1 to 2 inches above bend in elbow.
		•	Wrapped cuff smoothly and snugly around patient's arm and secured it.

Copyright © 2008, 2004, 2000, 1995, 1990 by Saunders, an imprint of Elsevier Inc. All rights reserved.

Trial 1	Trial 2	Point Value	*Performance Standards*
		•	Positioned self and/or manometer for direct viewing and at a distance of no more than 3 feet.
		•	Inserted earpieces of stethoscope in a forward position in the ears.
		•	Located the brachial pulse again.
		▷	Stated the purpose of locating the brachial pulse again.
		•	Placed diaphragm of the stethoscope over the brachial pulse site to make a tight seal.
		▷	Explained why there should be good contact of the chest piece with the skin.
		•	Made sure chest piece was not touching cuff.
		▷	Explained why the chest piece should not touch the cuff.
		•	Closed valve on bulb by turning thumbscrew to the right.
		•	Rapidly pumped air into cuff up to a level of 20 to 30 mm Hg above the palpated or previously measured systolic pressure.
		•	Released pressure at a moderate, steady rate by turning thumbscrew to the left.
		•	Heard and noted the first clear tapping sound (systolic pressure).
		•	Continued to deflate the cuff for another 10 mm/Hg.
		•	Heard and noted the point on the scale at which the sounds ceased (diastolic pressure).
		•	Quickly and completely deflated cuff to zero and removed earpieces from ears.
		▷	Stated how long one should wait before taking the blood pressure again on the same arm.
		•	Carefully removed cuff from patient's arm.
		•	Sanitized hands.
		•	Charted the results correctly.
		*	The reading was within ±2 mm of mercury of the evaluator's reading.
		▷	Stated the normal blood pressure for an adult (Less than 120/80).
		•	Cleaned earpieces and chest piece with an antiseptic wipe.
		*	Completed the procedure within 5 minutes.
			TOTALS

CHART	
Date	

Copyright © 2008, 2004, 2000, 1995, 1990 by Saunders, an imprint of Elsevier Inc. All rights reserved.

EVALUATION CRITERIA			COMMENTS
Symbol	Category	Point Value	
✶	Critical Step	16 points	
●	Essential Step	6 points	
▷	Theory Question	2 points	
Score calculation: 100 points – ____ points missed ____ Score Satisfactory score: 85 or above			

AAMA/CAAHEP Competency Achieved:

☑ III. C. 3. b. (4) (b): Obtain vital signs.

Copyright © 2008, 2004, 2000, 1995, 1990 by Saunders, an imprint of Elsevier Inc. All rights reserved.

Notes

Copyright © 2008, 2004, 2000, 1995, 1990 by Saunders, an imprint of Elsevier Inc. All rights reserved.

5

The Physical Examination

CHAPTER ASSIGNMENTS

√ After Completing	Date Due	Textbook Page(s)	TEXTBOOK ASSIGNMENTS	Possible Points	Points You Earned
		169-203	Read Chapter 5: The Physical Examination		
		174 200	Read Case Study 1 Case Study 1 questions	5	
		174 200	Read Case Study 2 Case Study 2 questions	5	
		191 200	Read Case Study 3 Case Study 3 questions	5	
		201	Apply Your Knowledge questions	10	
			TOTAL POINTS		

√ After Completing	Date Due	Study Guide Page(s)	STUDY GUIDE ASSIGNMENTS (CTA: Critical Thinking Activity)	Possible Points	Points You Earned
		185	Pretest	10	
		186	Key Term Assessment	16	
		187-188	Evaluation of Learning questions	20	
		189	CTA A: Reading Weight Measurements	15	
			CD Activity: Chapter 5 By the Pound (Record points earned)		
		190	CTA B: Reading Height Measurements	11	
			CD Activity: Chapter 5 Feet and Inches (Record points earned)		
		191	CTA C: Calculating BMI	2	
		191	CTA D: Dear Gabby	10	

Copyright © 2008, 2004, 2000, 1995, 1990 by Saunders, an imprint of Elsevier Inc. All rights reserved.

√ After Completing	Date Due	Study Guide Page(s)	STUDY GUIDE ASSIGNMENTS (CTA: Critical Thinking Activity)	Possible Points	Points You Earned
		191-192	CTA E: Patient Positions	10	
			CD Activity: Chapter 5 Let's Get Physical (Record points earned)		
		192	CTA F: Examination Techniques	10	
		192	CTA G: Otoscope	4	
		193	CTA H: Crossword Puzzle	25	
		185	Posttest	10	
			ADDITIONAL ASSIGNMENTS		
			TOTAL POINTS		

Copyright © 2008, 2004, 2000, 1995, 1990 by Saunders, an imprint of Elsevier Inc. All rights reserved.

√ When Assigned By Your Instructor	Study Guide Page(s)	Practices Required	LABORATORY ASSIGNMENTS (Procedure Number and Name)	*Score
	195	5	**Practice for Competency** 5-1: Measuring Weight and Height Textbook reference: pp. 180-181	
	197-199		**Evaluation of Competency** 5-1: Measuring Weight and Height	*
	195	3	**Practice for Competency** 5-2: Sitting Position Textbook reference: pp. 182-183	
	201-202		**Evaluation of Competency** 5-2: Sitting Position	*
	195	3	**Practice for Competency** 5-3: Supine Position Textbook reference: pp. 183-184	
	203-204		**Evaluation of Competency** 5-3: Supine Position	*
	195	3	**Practice for Competency** 5-4: Prone Position Textbook reference: pp. 184-185	
	205-206		**Evaluation of Competency** 5-4: Prone Position	*
	195	3	**Practice for Competency** 5-5: Dorsal Recumbent Position Textbook reference: pp. 185-186	
	207-208		**Evaluation of Competency** 5-5: Dorsal Recumbent Position	*
	195	3	**Practice for Competency** 5-6: Lithotomy Position Textbook reference: pp. 186-187	
	209-210		**Evaluation of Competency** 5-6: Lithotomy Position	*
	195	3	**Practice for Competency** 5-7: Sims Position Textbook reference: pp. 188	
	211-212		**Evaluation of Competency** 5-7: Sims Position	*
	195	3	**Practice for Competency** 5-8: Knee-Chest Position Textbook reference: pp. 189	
	213-214		**Evaluation of Competency** 5-8: Knee-Chest Position	*

Copyright © 2008, 2004, 2000, 1995, 1990 by Saunders, an imprint of Elsevier Inc. All rights reserved.

√ When Assigned By Your Instructor	Study Guide Page(s)	Practices Required	LABORATORY ASSIGNMENTS (Procedure Number and Name)	*Score
	195	3	DVD **Practice for Competency** 5-9: Fowler's Position Textbook reference: p. 190	
	215-216		**Evaluation of Competency** 5-9: Fowler's Position	*
	195	3	DVD **Practice for Competency** 5-10: Assisting with the Physical Examination Textbook reference: pp. 197-199	
	217-219		**Evaluation of Competency** 5-10: Assisting with the Physical Examination	*
			ADDITIONAL ASSIGNMENTS	

Copyright © 2008, 2004, 2000, 1995, 1990 by Saunders, an imprint of Elsevier Inc. All rights reserved.

Name ______________________________ Date ______________

PRETEST

True or False

_____ 1. A complete patient examination consists of a physical examination and laboratory tests.

_____ 2. Arthritis is an example of a chronic illness.

_____ 3. An otoscope is used to examine the eyes.

_____ 4. A patient should be identified by name and date of birth.

_____ 5. The reason for weighing a prenatal patient is to determine the baby's due date.

_____ 6. The height of an adult is measured during every office visit.

_____ 7. The lithotomy position is used to examine the vagina.

_____ 8. Inspection involves the observation of the patient for any signs of disease.

_____ 9. Measuring blood pressure is an example of auscultation.

_____ 10. The supine position is used to examine the back.

POSTTEST

True or False

_____ 1. The prognosis is what is wrong with the patient.

_____ 2. A risk factor means that a patient will develop a certain disease.

_____ 3. A CT scan is an example of a therapeutic procedure.

_____ 4. The function of a speculum is to open a body orifice for viewing.

_____ 5. The process of measuring the patient is called mensuration.

_____ 6. A reason for weighing a child is to determine drug dosage.

_____ 7. The purpose of draping a patient is to make it easier for the physician to examine the patient.

_____ 8. Sims position is used for flexible sigmoidoscopy.

_____ 9. Measuring pulse is an example of percussion.

_____ 10. BMI is the abbreviation for body mass index.

Copyright © 2008, 2004, 2000, 1995, 1990 by Saunders, an imprint of Elsevier Inc. All rights reserved.

KEY TERM ASSESSMENT

Directions: Match each medical term with its definition.

_______ 1. Audiometer
_______ 2. Auscultation
_______ 3. Bariatrics
_______ 4. Clinical diagnosis
_______ 5. Diagnosis
_______ 6. Differential diagnosis
_______ 7. Inspection
_______ 8. Mensuration
_______ 9. Ophthalmoscope
_______ 10. Otoscope
_______ 11. Palpation
_______ 12. Percussion
_______ 13. Percussion hammer
_______ 14. Prognosis
_______ 15. Speculum
_______ 16. Symptom

A. An instrument for examining the interior of the eye
B. A tentative diagnosis obtained through the evaluation of the health history and the physical examination, without the benefit of laboratory or diagnostic tests
C. An instrument for opening a body orifice or cavity for viewing
D. An instrument used to measure hearing
E. The process of measuring the patient
F. The scientific method for determining and identifying a patient's condition
G. The process of tapping the body to detect disease
H. The process of observing a patient to detect any signs of disease
I. Any change in the body or its functioning that indicates that a disease might be present
J. The process of listening to the sounds produced within the body to detect signs of disease
K. A determination of which of two or more diseases with similar symptoms is producing the patient's symptoms
L. An instrument for examining the external ear canal and tympanic membrane
M. The process of feeling with the hands to detect signs of disease
N. An instrument with a rubber head, used for testing reflexes
O. The probable course and outcome of a patient's condition and the patient's prospects for recovery
P. The branch of medicine that deals with the treatment and control of obesity

Copyright © 2008, 2004, 2000, 1995, 1990 by Saunders, an imprint of Elsevier Inc. All rights reserved.

EVALUATION OF LEARNING

Directions: Fill in each blank with the correct answer.

1. What are the three parts of a complete patient examination?

2. List two functions of the patient examination.

3. What is the purpose of establishing a final diagnosis?

4. Why is there a space for indicating the clinical diagnosis on the laboratory request form?

5. What is a risk factor?

6. What is an acute illness? List two examples of acute illnesses.

7. What is a chronic illness? List two examples of chronic illnesses.

8. What is the difference between a therapeutic procedure and a diagnostic procedure?

9. How can patient apprehension be reduced during a physical examination?

10. Why should the patient be asked if he or she needs to empty the bladder before a physical examination?

Copyright © 2008, 2004, 2000, 1995, 1990 by Saunders, an imprint of Elsevier Inc. All rights reserved.

11. What is the purpose for measuring weight?

12. What is the purpose of positioning and draping?

13. Indicate three types of examinations for which the supine position is used.

14. Indicate two types of examinations for which the lithotomy position is used.

15. Indicate one type of examination for which the knee-chest position is used.

16. List four types of assessments that can be made through inspection.

17. List four types of assessments that can be made through palpation.

18. Explain what can be assessed through the use of percussion.

19. What type of assessment can be made using auscultation?

20. What type of stethoscope chestpiece should be used to assess the heart?

Copyright © 2008, 2004, 2000, 1995, 1990 by Saunders, an imprint of Elsevier Inc. All rights reserved.

CRITICAL THINKING ACTIVITIES

A. READING WEIGHT MEASUREMENTS

The diagram below is an illustration of a portion of the calibration bar of an upright balance beam scale. In the spaces provided, record the weight measurements indicated on the calibration bar. In all cases, assume that the lower weight is resting in the 100-lb notched groove.

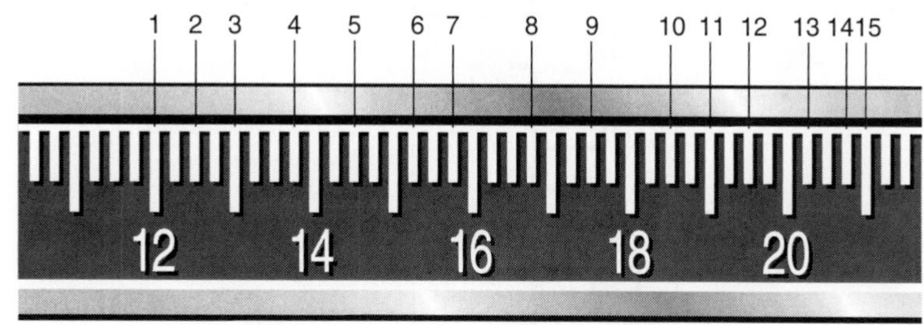

1. _______
2. _______
3. _______
4. _______
5. _______
6. _______
7. _______
8. _______
9. _______
10. _______
11. _______
12. _______
13. _______
14. _______
15. _______

Copyright © 2008, 2004, 2000, 1995, 1990 by Saunders, an imprint of Elsevier Inc. All rights reserved.

B. READING HEIGHT MEASUREMENTS

The diagram below is an illustration of a portion of the calibration rod of an upright balance beam scale. In the spaces provided, indicate the height measurement in feet and inches indicated on the calibration rod.

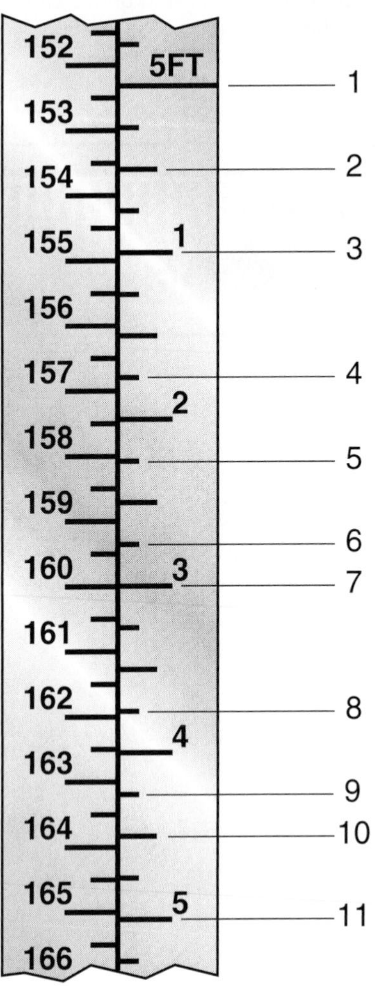

1. _______
2. _______
3. _______
4. _______
5. _______
6. _______
7. _______
8. _______
9. _______
10. _______
11. _______

Copyright © 2008, 2004, 2000, 1995, 1990 by Saunders, an imprint of Elsevier Inc. All rights reserved.

C. CALCULATING BMI

1. Using the Highlight on Interpreting Body Weight box on page 179 of your textbook, calculate and interpret your BMI and record the results below.

___

2. List the diseases that an individual with an above-normal BMI has an increased chance of developing.

___

___

___

___

D. DEAR GABBY

Gabby is attending a writer's convention and wants you to fill in for her. In the space provided, respond to the following letter using the knowledge you have acquired in this chapter.

Dear Gabby:

I have been reading your column in the local newspaper for many years. I had a problem with this young doctor that I saw recently and it has me very concerned. I am 67 years "young" and am very active. I drink herbal teas, eat lots of fruits and vegetables, and do housework and gardening. I rarely have a cold or get sick, so it has been many years since I have been to see a doctor.

This young doctor did something called a BMI. I know it is probably one of those new-fangled tests they do, and I hope it was covered by my health insurance policy. Anyway, the doctor told me that I have a BMI of 27 and that I should exercise more and eat a little less. His medical assistant came in afterward and gave me some information on a healthy diet and exercise, but I was so upset at that point, I think I threw the information away when I got home!

There used to be an insurance company table that showed whether or not you were within your ideal weight. It seems to me that the last time I checked it, I was not a bit overweight. But now this young doctor and his assistant are trying to tell me that I need to lose weight. Gabby, what should I do?

Confused and Concerned in Connecticut

___

___

___

___

___

___

___

___

___

___

___

___

E. PATIENT POSITIONS

In which position would you place the patient for the following examinations or procedures?

1. Measurement of rectal temperature of an adult ___
2. Examination of the back ___
3. Measurement of vital signs ___
4. Pelvic examination ___

Copyright © 2008, 2004, 2000, 1995, 1990 by Saunders, an imprint of Elsevier Inc. All rights reserved.

5. Examination of the upper extremities ______________________________

6. Examination of the eyes, ears, nose, and throat ______________________________

7. Examination of the breasts ______________________________

8. Flexible sigmoidoscopy ______________________________

9. Administration of an enema ______________________________

10. Examination of the upper body of a patient with emphysema ______________________________

F. EXAMINATION TECHNIQUES

List the examination technique (inspection, palpation, percussion, auscultation) that is used in each of the following situations.

1. A patient with a stutter ______________________________

2. Taking the radial pulse ______________________________

3. Finding the location of the apical pulse ______________________________

4. Taking the apical pulse ______________________________

5. Taking respiration (may be two answers, depending on method) ______________________________

6. A patient with cracked lips ______________________________

7. Checking for lumps in the breast ______________________________

8. Checking reflexes ______________________________

9. Obtaining the fetal heart rate ______________________________

10. A patient with a fever (may be several methods) ______________________________

G. OTOSCOPE

Obtain an otoscope and an ophthalmoscope. Following the manufacturer's instructions, perform the following. Place a check mark next to each task upon completion.

_______ 1. Turn the otoscope on and off.

_______ 2. Change the bulb in the otoscope.

_______ 3. Change the batteries or recharge the otoscope.

_______ 4. Change the speculum of the otoscope.

Copyright © 2008, 2004, 2000, 1995, 1990 by Saunders, an imprint of Elsevier Inc. All rights reserved.

H. CROSSWORD PUZZLE
The Physical Examination

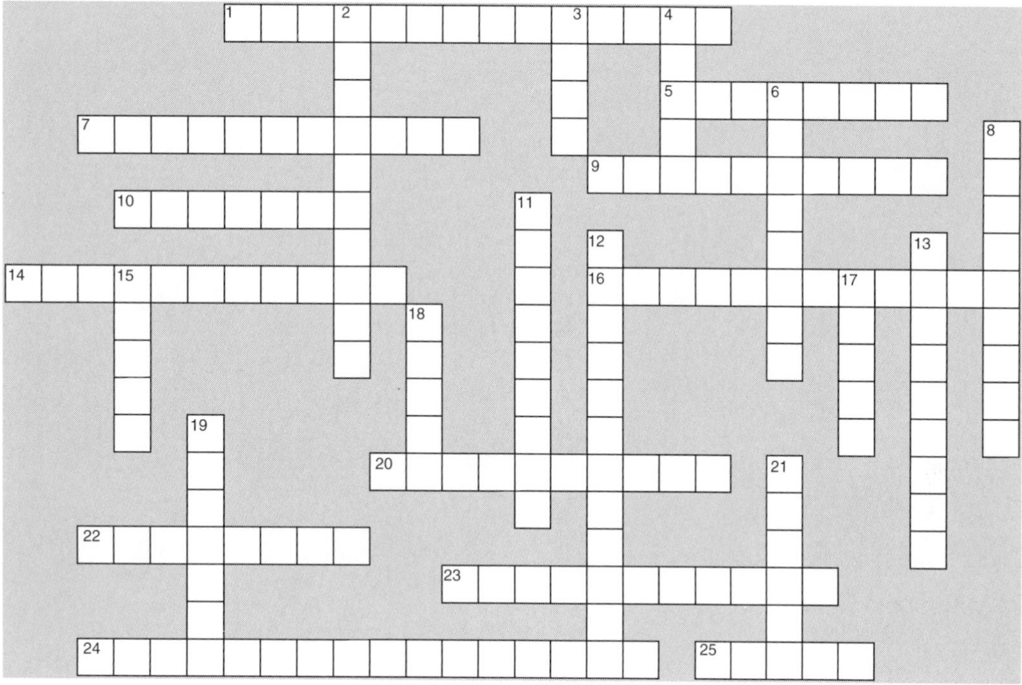

Directions: Complete the crossword puzzle using the clues presented below.

ACROSS
1 Eye examiner
5 Ear examiner
7 BMI: below 18.5
9 BMI: 25 to 29.9
10 "Listen to heart" position
14 Measuring the patient
16 I am listening
20 Metric unit of height
22 Metric unit of weight
23 Curative procedure
24 Reflex tester
25 BMI: 30 or more

DOWN
2 Hearing tester
3 Flex sigmoid position
4 Face-down
6 Orifice opener
8 What is the probable outcome?
11 What is wrong with you?
12 Before you measure weight
13 GYN position
15 Five feet in inches
17 Severe and intense condition
18 Provides warmth and modesty
19 Long-time illness
21 Face-up

Copyright © 2008, 2004, 2000, 1995, 1990 by Saunders, an imprint of Elsevier Inc. All rights reserved.

Notes

Copyright © 2008, 2004, 2000, 1995, 1990 by Saunders, an imprint of Elsevier Inc. All rights reserved.

PRACTICE FOR COMPETENCY

Procedure 5-1: Weight and Height. Take weight and height measurements. Record results in the chart provided.

Procedures 5-2 to 5-9: Positioning and Draping. Position and drape an individual in each of the following positions: Sitting, Supine, Prone, Dorsal Recumbent, Lithotomy, Sims, Knee-Chest, and Fowler's.

Procedure 5-10: Assisting with the Physical Examination. Prepare the patient and assist with a physical examination. In the chart provided, record the results of the procedures you performed while assisting with the examination (e.g., vital signs, height, and weight).

CHART	
Date	

Copyright © 2008, 2004, 2000, 1995, 1990 by Saunders, an imprint of Elsevier Inc. All rights reserved.

Chart	
Date	

Copyright © 2008, 2004, 2000, 1995, 1990 by Saunders, an imprint of Elsevier Inc. All rights reserved.

EVALUATION OF COMPETENCY

Procedure 5-1: Measuring Weight and Height

Name: ______________________________ Date: ______________

Evaluated By: ______________________________ Score: ______________

Performance Objective

Outcome:	Measure weight and height.
Conditions:	Given a paper towel.
	Using an upright balance scale.
Standards:	Time: 5 minutes. Student completed procedure in ____ minutes.
	Accuracy: Satisfactory score on the Performance Evaluation Checklist.

Performance Evaluation Checklist

Trial 1	*Trial 2*	*Point Value*	*Performance Standards*
			WEIGHT
		•	Sanitized hands.
			Checked the balance scale for accuracy
		•	Verified that the upper and lower weights were on zero.
		•	Looked at the indicator point to make sure the scale is balanced.
		▷	Stated what will be observed if the scale is balanced.
		▷	Explained what to do if the indicator point rests below the center.
		▷	Explained what to do if the indicator point rests above the center.
		▷	Stated what occurs if the scale is not balanced.
		•	Greeted the patient and introduced yourself.
		•	Identified the patient and explained the procedure.
		•	Instructed patient to remove shoes and heavy outer clothing.
		•	Placed paper towel on the scale.
		•	Assisted patient onto the scale.
		•	Instructed patient not to move.
			Balanced the scale
		•	Moved the lower weight to the groove that did not cause the indicator point to drop to the bottom of the balance area.
		▷	Stated why the lower weight should be seated firmly in its groove.

Copyright © 2008, 2004, 2000, 1995, 1990 by Saunders, an imprint of Elsevier Inc. All rights reserved.

Trial 1	Trial 2	Point Value	Performance Standards
		•	Slid the upper weight slowly until the indicator point came to a rest at the center of the balance area.
		•	Read the results to the nearest quarter pound. Jotted down this value or made a mental note of it.
		*	The reading was identical to the evaluator's reading.
		•	Asked the patient to step off the scale.
			HEIGHT
		•	Slid the calibration rod until it was above the patient's height.
		•	Opened the measuring bar to its horizontal position.
		•	Instructed the patient to step onto the scale platform with his/her back to the scale.
		•	Instructed patient to stand erect and to look straight ahead.
		•	Carefully lowered the measuring bar until it rested gently on top of the patient's head.
		•	Verified that the bar was in a horizontal position.
		•	Instructed the patient to step down and put on his/her shoes.
		•	Read the marking to the nearest quarter inch. Jotted down this value or made a mental note of it.
		*	The reading was identical to the evaluator's reading.
		•	Returned the measuring bar to its vertical position.
		•	Slid the calibration rod to its lowest position.
		•	Returned the weights to zero.
		•	Sanitized hands.
		•	Charted the results correctly.
		*	Completed the procedure within 5 minutes.
			TOTALS

CHART	
Date	

Copyright © 2008, 2004, 2000, 1995, 1990 by Saunders, an imprint of Elsevier Inc. All rights reserved.

Evaluation of Student Performance

EVALUATION CRITERIA			COMMENTS
Symbol	Category	Point Value	
✶	Critical Step	16 points	
●	Essential Step	6 points	
▷	Theory Question	2 points	
Score calculation: 100 points – ______ points missed ____ Score Satisfactory score: 85 or above			

AAMA/CAAHEP Competency Achieved:

☑ III. C. 3. b. (4) (e): Prepare patient for and assist with routine and specialty examinations.

Copyright © 2008, 2004, 2000, 1995, 1990 by Saunders, an imprint of Elsevier Inc. All rights reserved.

Notes

Copyright © 2008, 2004, 2000, 1995, 1990 by Saunders, an imprint of Elsevier Inc. All rights reserved.

EVALUATION OF COMPETENCY

Procedure 5-2: Sitting Position

Name: ______________________________ Date: ______________

Evaluated By: ______________________________ Score: ______________

Performance Objective

Outcome: Position and drape an individual in the sitting position.

Conditions: Using an examining table.

Given the following: a patient gown and a drape.

Standards: Time: 5 minutes. Student completed procedure in ____ minutes.

Accuracy: Satisfactory score on the Performance Evaluation Checklist.

Performance Evaluation Checklist

Trial 1	*Trial 2*	*Point Value*	*Performance Standards*
		•	Sanitized hands.
		•	Greeted the patient and introduced yourself.
		•	Identified the patient.
		•	Explained what type of examination or procedure will be performed.
		•	Provided patient with a patient gown.
		•	Instructed patient to remove clothing and to put on a patient gown with the opening in front.
		▷	Stated what qualities the disrobing facility should have.
		•	Pulled out the footrest and assisted the patient into a sitting position.
		•	The patient's buttocks and thighs were firmly supported on the edge of the table.
		•	Placed a drape over the patient's thighs and legs.
		•	Assisted the patient off the table after the exam.
		•	Returned the footrest to its normal position.
		•	Instructed the patient to get dressed.
		•	Discarded the gown and drape in a waste container.
		▷	Stated one use of the sitting position.
		*	Completed the procedure within 5 minutes.
			TOTALS

Copyright © 2008, 2004, 2000, 1995, 1990 by Saunders, an imprint of Elsevier Inc. All rights reserved.

Evaluation of Student Performance

EVALUATION CRITERIA			COMMENTS
Symbol	**Category**	**Point Value**	
✶	Critical Step	16 points	
●	Essential Step	6 points	
▷	Theory Question	2 points	
Score calculation: 100 points – ______ points missed ____ Score Satisfactory score: 85 or above			

AAMA/CAAHEP Competency Achieved:

☑ III. C. 3. b. (4) (e): Prepare patient for and assist with routine and specialty examinations.

Copyright © 2008, 2004, 2000, 1995, 1990 by Saunders, an imprint of Elsevier Inc. All rights reserved.

EVALUATION OF COMPETENCY

Procedure 5-3: Supine Position

Name: ______________________________ Date: ______________

Evaluated By: ______________________________ Score: ______________

Performance Objective

Outcome:	Position and drape and individual in the supine position.
Conditions:	Using an examining table.
	Given the following: a patient gown and a drape.
Standards:	Time: 5 minutes. Student completed procedure in ____ minutes.
	Accuracy: Satisfactory score on the Performance Evaluation Checklist.

Performance Evaluation Checklist

Trial 1	*Trial 2*	*Point Value*	*Performance Standards*
		•	Sanitized hands.
		•	Greeted the patient and introduced yourself.
		•	Identified the patient.
		•	Explained what type of examination or procedure will be performed.
		•	Provided patient with a patient gown.
		•	Instructed patient to remove clothing and to put on a patient gown with the opening in front.
		•	Pulled out the footrest and assisted the patient into a sitting position.
		•	Placed a drape over the patient's thighs and legs.
		•	Asked the patient to move back on the table.
		•	Pulled out the table extension while supporting the patient's lower legs.
		•	Asked the patient to lie down on his/her back with the legs together.
		•	Placed the patient's arms above the head or alongside their body.
		•	Positioned the drape lengthwise over the patient.
		▷	Stated the purpose of the drape.
		•	Moved the drape according to the body parts being examined.
		•	Assisted the patient back into a sitting position after the exam.
		•	Slid the table extension back into place while supporting the patient's lower legs.
		•	Assisted the patient from the examining table.
		•	Returned the footrest to its normal position.

Copyright © 2008, 2004, 2000, 1995, 1990 by Saunders, an imprint of Elsevier Inc. All rights reserved.

Trial 1	Trial 2	Point Value	*Performance Standards*
		•	Instructed the patient to get dressed.
		•	Discarded the gown and drape in a waste container.
		▷	Stated one use of the supine position.
		✶	Completed the procedure within 5 minutes.
			TOTALS

Evaluation of Student Performance

EVALUATION CRITERIA			COMMENTS
Symbol	Category	Point Value	
✶	Critical Step	16 points	
•	Essential Step	6 points	
▷	Theory Question	2 points	
Score calculation: 100 points – ____ points missed ____ Score Satisfactory score: 85 or above			

AAMA/CAAHEP Competency Achieved:

☑ III. C. 3. b. (4) (e): Prepare patient for and assist with routine and specialty examinations.

Copyright © 2008, 2004, 2000, 1995, 1990 by Saunders, an imprint of Elsevier Inc. All rights reserved.

EVALUATION OF COMPETENCY

Procedure 5-4: Prone Position

Name: ______________________________ Date: ______________

Evaluated By: ______________________________ Score: ______________

Performance Objective

Outcome:	Position and drape an individual in the prone position.
Conditions:	Using an examining table.
	Given the following: a patient gown and a drape.
Standards:	Time: 5 minutes. Student completed procedure in ____ minutes.
	Accuracy: Satisfactory score on the Performance Evaluation Checklist.

Performance Evaluation Checklist

Trial 1	*Trial 2*	*Point Value*	*Performance Standards*
		•	Sanitized hands.
		•	Greeted the patient and introduced yourself.
		•	Identified the patient.
		•	Explained what type of examination or procedure will be performed.
		•	Provided patient with a patient gown.
		•	Instructed patient to remove clothing and to put on a patient gown with the opening in back.
		•	Pulled out the footrest and assisted the patient into a sitting position.
		•	Placed a drape over the patient's thighs and legs.
		•	Asked the patient to move back on the table.
		•	Pulled out the table extension while supporting the patient's lower legs.
		•	Asked the patient to lie down on his/her back.
		•	Positioned the drape lengthwise over the patient.
		•	Asked the patient to turn onto his or her stomach by rolling toward you.
		•	Provided assistance.
		▷	Stated the reason for providing assistance.
		•	Positioned the patient with his/her legs together and the head turned to one side.
		•	Placed the patient's arms above their head or alongside their body.
		•	Adjusted the drape as needed.
		•	Moved the drape according to the body parts being examined.

Copyright © 2008, 2004, 2000, 1995, 1990 by Saunders, an imprint of Elsevier Inc. All rights reserved.

Trial 1	Trial 2	Point Value	*Performance Standards*
		•	Assisted the patient into the supine position after the exam.
		•	Assisted the patient into a sitting position.
		•	Slid the table extension back into place while supporting the patient's lower legs.
		•	Assisted the patient from the examining table.
		•	Returned the footrest to its normal position.
		•	Instructed the patient to get dressed.
		•	Discarded the gown and drape in a waste container.
		▷	Stated one use of the prone position.
		✶	Completed the procedure within 5 minutes.
			TOTALS

Evaluation of Student Performance

EVALUATION CRITERIA			COMMENTS
Symbol	Category	Point Value	
✶	Critical Step	16 points	
•	Essential Step	6 points	
▷	Theory Question	2 points	
Score calculation: 100 points – ______ points missed ____ Score Satisfactory score: 85 or above			

AAMA/CAAHEP Competency Achieved:

☑ III. C. 3. b. (4) (e): Prepare patient for and assist with routine and specialty examinations.

Copyright © 2008, 2004, 2000, 1995, 1990 by Saunders, an imprint of Elsevier Inc. All rights reserved.

EVALUATION OF COMPETENCY

Procedure 5-5: Dorsal Recumbent Position

Name: ______________________________ Date: ____________

Evaluated By: ______________________________ Score: ____________

Performance Objective

Outcome:	Position and drape an individual in the dorsal recumbent position.
Conditions:	Using an examining table.
	Given the following: a patient gown and a drape.
Standards:	Time: 5 minutes. Student completed procedure in ____ minutes.
	Accuracy: Satisfactory score on the Performance Evaluation Checklist.

Performance Evaluation Checklist

Trial 1	*Trial 2*	*Point Value*	*Performance Standards*
		•	Sanitized hands.
		•	Greeted the patient and introduced yourself.
		•	Identified the patient.
		•	Explained what type of examination or procedure will be performed.
		•	Provided patient with a patient gown.
		•	Instructed patient to remove clothing and to put on a patient gown with the opening in front.
		•	Pulled out the footrest and assisted the patient into a sitting position.
		•	Placed a drape over the patient's thighs and legs.
		•	Asked the patient to move back on the table.
		•	Pulled out the table extension while supporting the patient's lower legs.
		•	Asked the patient to lie down on their back.
		•	Placed the patient's arms above their head or alongside their body.
		•	Positioned the drape diagonally over the patient.
		•	Asked the patient to bend their knees and place each foot at the edge of the table with the soles of their feet flat on the table.
		•	Provided assistance.
		•	Pushed in the table extension and the footrest.
		•	Adjusted the drape as needed.
		•	Folded back the center corner of the drape when the physician was ready to examine the patient.
		•	Pulled out the footrest and the table extension after the exam.

Copyright © 2008, 2004, 2000, 1995, 1990 by Saunders, an imprint of Elsevier Inc. All rights reserved.

Trial 1	Trial 2	Point Value	Performance Standards
		•	Assisted the patient back into a supine position and then into a sitting position.
		•	Slid the table extension back into place while supporting the patient's lower legs.
		•	Assisted the patient from the examining table.
		•	Returned the footrest to its normal position.
		•	Instructed the patient to get dressed.
		•	Discarded the gown and drape in a waste container.
		▷	Stated one use of the dorsal recumbent position.
		✶	Completed the procedure within 5 minutes.
			TOTALS

Evaluation of Student Performance

EVALUATION CRITERIA			COMMENTS
Symbol	Category	Point Value	
✶	Critical Step	16 points	
•	Essential Step	6 points	
▷	Theory Question	2 points	
Score calculation: 100 points – ______ points missed ____ Score Satisfactory score: 85 or above			

AAMA/CAAHEP Competency Achieved:

☑ III. C. 3. b. (4) (e): Prepare patient for and assist with routine and specialty examinations.

Copyright © 2008, 2004, 2000, 1995, 1990 by Saunders, an imprint of Elsevier Inc. All rights reserved.

EVALUATION OF COMPETENCY

Procedure 5-6: Lithotomy Position

Name: ______________________________ Date: ______________

Evaluated By: ______________________________ Score: ______________

Performance Objective

Outcome:	Position and drape an individual in the lithotomy position.
Conditions:	Using an examining table.
	Given the following: a patient gown and a drape.
Standards:	Time: 5 minutes. Student completed procedure in ____ minutes.
	Accuracy: Satisfactory score on the Performance Evaluation Checklist.

Performance Evaluation Checklist

Trial 1	*Trial 2*	*Point Value*	*Performance Standards*
		•	Sanitized hands.
		•	Greeted the patient and introduced yourself.
		•	Identified the patient.
		•	Explained what type of examination or procedure will be performed.
		•	Provided patient with a patient gown.
		•	Instructed patient to remove clothing and to put on a patient gown with the opening in front.
		•	Pulled out the footrest and assisted the patient into a sitting position.
		•	Placed a drape over the patient's thighs and legs.
		•	Asked the patient to move back on the table.
		•	Pulled out the table extension while supporting the patient's lower legs.
		•	Asked the patient to lie down on their back.
		•	Placed the patient's arms above head or alongside body.
		•	Positioned the drape diagonally over the patient.
		•	Pulled out the stirrups and position them at an angle.
		•	Positioned the stirrups so that they were level with the examining table and pulled out approximately 1 foot from the edge of the table.
		•	Asked the patient to bend the knees and place each foot into a stirrup.
		•	Provided assistance.
		•	Pushed in the table extension and the footrest.

Copyright © 2008, 2004, 2000, 1995, 1990 by Saunders, an imprint of Elsevier Inc. All rights reserved.

Trial 1	Trial 2	Point Value	*Performance Standards*
			Instructed the patient to slide buttocks to the edge of the table and to rotate thighs outward as far as is comfortable.
		•	Repositioned the drape as needed.
		•	Folded back the center corner of the drape when the physician was ready to examine the genital area.
		•	After completion of the exam, pulled out the footrest and the table extension.
		•	Asked the patient to slide their buttocks back from the end of the table.
		•	Lifted the patient's legs out of the stirrups at the same time and placed them on the table extension.
		▷	Stated why both legs should be lifted at the same time.
		•	Returned stirrups to the normal position.
		•	Assisted the patient back into a sitting position.
		•	Slid the table extension back into place while supporting the patient's lower legs.
		•	Assisted the patient from the examining table.
		•	Returned the footrest to its normal position.
		•	Instructed the patient to get dressed.
		•	Discarded the gown and drape in a waste container.
		▷	Stated one use of the lithotomy position.
		*	Completed the procedure within 5 minutes.
			TOTALS

Evaluation of Student Performance

EVALUATION CRITERIA			COMMENTS
Symbol	Category	Point Value	
*	Critical Step	16 points	
•	Essential Step	6 points	
▷	Theory Question	2 points	
Score calculation: 100 points – _____ points missed _____ Score Satisfactory score: 85 or above			

AAMA/CAAHEP Competency Achieved:

☑ III. C. 3. b. (4) (e): Prepare patient for and assist with routine and specialty examinations.

Copyright © 2008, 2004, 2000, 1995, 1990 by Saunders, an imprint of Elsevier Inc. All rights reserved.

EVALUATION OF COMPETENCY

Procedure 5-7: Sims Position

Name: ______________________________ Date: ____________

Evaluated By: ______________________________ Score: ____________

Performance Objective

Outcome:	Position and drape an individual in the Sims position.
Conditions:	Using an examining table.
	Given the following: a patient gown and a drape.
Standards:	Time: 5 minutes. Student completed procedure in ____ minutes.
	Accuracy: Satisfactory score on the Performance Evaluation Checklist.

Performance Evaluation Checklist

Trial 1	*Trial 2*	*Point Value*	*Performance Standards*
		•	Sanitized hands.
		•	Greeted the patient and introduced yourself.
		•	Identified the patient.
		•	Explained what type of examination or procedure will be performed.
		•	Provided patient with a patient gown.
		•	Instructed patient to remove clothing and to put on a patient gown with the opening in back.
		•	Pulled out the footrest and assisted the patient into a sitting position.
		•	Placed a drape over the patient's thighs and legs.
		•	Asked the patient to move back on the table.
		•	Pulled out the table extension while supporting the patient's lower legs.
		•	Asked the patient to lie down on their back.
		•	Positioned the drape lengthwise over the patient.
		•	Asked the patient to turn onto their left side.
		•	Provided assistance.
		•	Positioned the left arm behind the body and the right arm forward with the elbow bent.
		•	Assisted the patient in flexing the legs with the right leg flexed sharply and the left leg flexed slightly.
		•	Adjusted the drape by folding back the drape to expose the anal area when the physician was ready to examine the patient.

Copyright © 2008, 2004, 2000, 1995, 1990 by Saunders, an imprint of Elsevier Inc. All rights reserved.

Trial 1	Trial 2	Point Value	*Performance Standards*
		•	Assisted the patient into a supine position and then into a sitting position following the exam.
		•	Slid the table extension back into place while supporting the patient's lower legs.
		•	Assisted the patient from the examining table.
		•	Returned the footrest to its normal position.
		•	Instructed the patient to get dressed.
		•	Discarded the gown and drape in a waste container.
		▷	Stated one use of the Sims position.
		*	Completed the procedure within 5 minutes.
			TOTALS

Evaluation of Student Performance

EVALUATION CRITERIA			COMMENTS
Symbol	Category	Point Value	
*	Critical Step	16 points	
•	Essential Step	6 points	
▷	Theory Question	2 points	
Score calculation: 100 points – ______ points missed ____ Score Satisfactory score: 85 or above			

AAMA/CAAHEP Competency Achieved:

☑ III. C. 3. b. (4) (e): Prepare patient for and assist with routine and specialty examinations.

Copyright © 2008, 2004, 2000, 1995, 1990 by Saunders, an imprint of Elsevier Inc. All rights reserved.

EVALUATION OF COMPETENCY

Procedure 5-8: Knee-Chest Position

Name: ______________________ Date: __________

Evaluated By: ______________________ Score: __________

Performance Objective

Outcome:	Position and drape an individual in the knee-chest position.	
Conditions:	Using an examining table.	
	Given the following: a patient gown and a drape.	
Standards:	Time: 5 minutes.	Student completed procedure in ____ minutes.
	Accuracy: Satisfactory score on the Performance Evaluation Checklist.	

Performance Evaluation Checklist

Trial 1	*Trial 2*	*Point Value*	*Performance Standards*
		•	Sanitized hands.
		•	Greeted the patient and introduced yourself.
		•	Identified the patient.
		•	Explained what type of examination or procedure will be performed.
		•	Provided patient with a patient gown.
		•	Instructed patient to remove clothing and to put on a patient gown with the opening in back.
		•	Pulled out the footrest and assisted the patient into a sitting position.
		•	Placed a drape over the patient's thighs and legs.
		•	Asked the patient to move back on the table.
		•	Pulled out the table extension while supporting the patient's lower legs.
		•	Assisted the patient into the supine position and then into the prone position.
		•	Positioned the drape diagonally over the patient.
		•	Asked the patient to bend their arms at the elbows and rest them alongside their head.
		•	Asked the patient to elevate the buttocks while keeping their back straight.
		•	Turned the patient's head to one side, with the weight of their body supported by their chest.
		•	Used a pillow for additional support, if needed.
		•	Separated the knees and lower legs approximately 12 inches.
		•	Adjusted the drape diagonally as needed.

Copyright © 2008, 2004, 2000, 1995, 1990 by Saunders, an imprint of Elsevier Inc. All rights reserved.

Trial 1	Trial 2	Point Value	*Performance Standards*
		•	Folded back a small portion of the drape to expose the anal area when the physician was ready to examine the patient.
		•	Assisted the patient into a prone position and then into a supine position after the exam.
		•	Allowed the patient to rest in a supine position before sitting up.
		▷	Stated why the patient should be allowed to rest.
		•	Assisted the patient into a sitting position.
		•	Slid the table extension back into place while supporting the patient's lower legs.
		•	Assisted the patient from the examining table.
		•	Returned the footrest to its normal position.
		•	Instructed the patient to get dressed.
		•	Discarded the gown and drape in a waste container.
		▷	Stated one use of the knee-chest position.
		*	Completed the procedure within 5 minutes.
			TOTALS

Evaluation of Student Performance

EVALUATION CRITERIA			COMMENTS
Symbol	Category	Point Value	
*	Critical Step	16 points	
•	Essential Step	6 points	
▷	Theory Question	2 points	
Score calculation: 100 points – ______ points missed ______ Score Satisfactory score: 85 or above			

AAMA/CAAHEP Competency Achieved:

☑ III. C. 3. b. (4) (e): Prepare patient for and assist with routine and specialty examinations.

Copyright © 2008, 2004, 2000, 1995, 1990 by Saunders, an imprint of Elsevier Inc. All rights reserved.

EVALUATION OF COMPETENCY

Procedure 5-9: Fowler's Position

Name: ______________________________ Date: ______________

Evaluated By: ______________________________ Score: ______________

Performance Objective

Outcome:	Position and drape an individual in the Fowler's position.
Conditions:	Using an examining table.
	Given the following: a patient gown and a drape.
Standards:	Time: 5 minutes. Student completed procedure in ____ minutes.
	Accuracy: Satisfactory score on the Performance Evaluation Checklist.

Performance Evaluation Checklist

Trial 1	*Trial 2*	*Point Value*	*Performance Standards*
		•	Sanitized hands.
		•	Greeted the patient and introduced yourself.
		•	Identified the patient.
		•	Explained what type of examination or procedure will be performed.
		•	Provided patient with a patient gown.
		•	Instructed patient to remove clothing and to put on a patient gown with the opening in front.
		•	Positioned the head of the table at a 45-degree angle for a semi-Fowler's position or at a 90-degree angle for a full Fowler's position.
		•	Pulled out the footrest and assisted the patient into a sitting position.
		•	Placed a drape over the patient's thighs and legs.
		•	Pulled out the table extension while supporting the patient's lower legs.
		•	Asked the patient to lean back against the table head.
		•	Provided assistance.
		•	Positioned the drape over the patient.
		•	Moved the drape according to the body parts being examined.
		•	Assisted the patient into a sitting position after the exam.
		•	Slid the table extension back into place while supporting the patient's lower legs.
		•	Assisted the patient from the examining table.
		•	Instructed the patient to get dressed.

Copyright © 2008, 2004, 2000, 1995, 1990 by Saunders, an imprint of Elsevier Inc. All rights reserved.

Trial 1	Trial 2	Point Value	*Performance Standards*
		•	Returned the head of the table and the footrest to their normal positions.
		•	Discarded the gown and drape in a waste container.
		▷	Stated one use of the Fowler's position.
		✶	Completed the procedure within 5 minutes.
			TOTALS

Evaluation of Student Performance

EVALUATION CRITERIA			COMMENTS
Symbol	Category	Point Value	
✶	Critical Step	16 points	
•	Essential Step	6 points	
▷	Theory Question	2 points	
Score calculation: 100 points – ______ points missed ____ Score Satisfactory score: 85 or above			

AAMA/CAAHEP Competency Achieved:

☑ III. C. 3. b. (4) (e): Prepare patient for and assist with routine and specialty examinations.

Copyright © 2008, 2004, 2000, 1995, 1990 by Saunders, an imprint of Elsevier Inc. All rights reserved.

EVALUATION OF COMPETENCY

Procedure 5-10: Assisting with the Physical Examination

Name: ______________________________ Date: ______________

Evaluated By: ______________________________ Score: ______________

Performance Objective

Outcome:	Prepare the patient and assist with a physical examination.
Conditions:	Using an examining table.
	Given the following: equipment for the type of examination to be performed, patient examination gown, and drapes.
Standards:	Time: 20 minutes. Student completed procedure in ____ minutes.
	Accuracy: Satisfactory score on the Performance Evaluation Checklist.

Performance Evaluation Checklist

Trial 1	*Trial 2*	*Point Value*	*Performance Standards*
		•	Prepared examining room.
		•	Sanitized hands.
		•	Assembled all necessary equipment.
		•	Arranged instruments in a neat and orderly manner.
		•	Obtained the patient's medical record.
		•	Went to the waiting room and asked the patient to come back.
		•	Escorted the patient to the examining room.
		•	Asked the patient to be seated.
		•	Greeted the patient and introduced yourself.
		•	Identified the patient by full name and date of birth.
		▷	Stated why a calm and friendly manner should be used.
		•	Seated yourself facing the patient at a distance of 3 to 4 feet.
		•	Obtained and recorded patient symptoms.
		•	Measured vital signs and charted results.
		▷	State the adult normal range for temperature (97° to 99° F), pulse (60 to 100 b/m), respiration (12 to 20/min), and blood pressure (<120/80).
		•	Measured weight and height, and charted results.
		•	Asked patient if he or she needs to void.
		▷	Stated why the patient should be asked to void.
		•	Instructed patient to remove all clothing and put on an examining gown.

Copyright © 2008, 2004, 2000, 1995, 1990 by Saunders, an imprint of Elsevier Inc. All rights reserved.

Trial 1	Trial 2	Point Value	*Performance Standards*
		•	Informed the patient that the physician will be in soon.
		•	Left the room to provide patient with privacy.
		•	Made patient's medical record available to the physician.
		•	Checked to make sure patient is ready to be seen.
		•	Informed physician that the patient is ready.
		•	***Assisted the physician***
			Ensured the patient was in a sitting position on exam table.
		•	Handed the ophthalmoscope to the physician when requested.
		•	Dimmed the lights when the physician was ready to use the ophthalmoscope.
		▷	Stated why the lights are dimmed.
		▷	Stated the proper use of the ophthalmoscope.
		•	Handed the otoscope to the examiner when requested.
		▷	Stated the proper use of the otoscope.
		•	Is able to change the speculum and bulb in the otoscope.
		•	Handed the tongue depressor to the examiner when requested.
		•	Offered reassurance to patient as needed.
		•	Positioned patient as required for examination of the remaining body systems.
			Assisted and instructed patient
		•	Allowed patient to rest in a sitting position before getting off the examining table.
		▷	Stated why the patient should be allowed to rest before getting off the table.
		•	Assisted patient off the examining table.
		•	Instructed patient to get dressed.
		•	Provided patient with any necessary instructions.
		▷	Stated what type of instructions may need to be relayed to the patient.
		•	Sanitized hands and charted any instructions given to the patient.
		•	Escorted the patient to the reception area.
			Cleaned the examining room
		•	Discarded paper on the examining table and unrolled a fresh length.
		•	Discarded all disposable supplies into an appropriate waste container.
		•	Checked to make sure ample supplies are available.
		•	Removed reusable equipment for sanitization, sterilization, or disinfection.
		*	Completed the procedure within 20 minutes.
			TOTALS

CHART	
Date	

Copyright © 2008, 2004, 2000, 1995, 1990 by Saunders, an imprint of Elsevier Inc. All rights reserved.

Evaluation of Student Performance

EVALUATION CRITERIA			COMMENTS
Symbol	Category	Point Value	
✶	Critical Step	16 points	
●	Essential Step	6 points	
▷	Theory Question	2 points	
Score calculation: 100 points – _____ points missed ____ Score Satisfactory score: 85 or above			

AAMA/CAAHEP Competency Achieved:

☑ III. C. 3. b. (4) (d): Prepare and maintain examination and treatment areas.
☑ III. C. 3. b. (4) (e): Prepare patient for and assist with routine and specialty examinations.
☑ III. C. 3. c. (3) (b): Instruct individuals according to their needs.
☑ III. C. 3. c. (3) (c): Provide instruction for health maintenance and disease prevention.
☑ III. C. 3. c. (3) (d): Identify community resources.
☑ III. C. 3. c. (4) (a): Perform an inventory of supplies and equipment.
☑ III. C. 3. c. (4) (b): Perform routine maintenance of administrative and clinical equipment.

Copyright © 2008, 2004, 2000, 1995, 1990 by Saunders, an imprint of Elsevier Inc. All rights reserved.

Notes

Copyright © 2008, 2004, 2000, 1995, 1990 by Saunders, an imprint of Elsevier Inc. All rights reserved.

6

Eye and Ear Assessment and Procedures

CHAPTER ASSIGNMENTS

√ After Completing	Date Due	Textbook Page(s)	TEXTBOOK ASSIGNMENTS	Possible Points	Points You Earned
		204-232	Read Chapter 6: Eye and Ear Assessment and Procedures		
		210 228	Read Case Study 1 Case Study 1 questions	 5	
		214 228	Read Case Study 2 Case Study 2 questions	 5	
		219 228-229	Read Case Study 3 Case Study 3 questions	 5	
		229-230	Apply Your Knowledge questions	10	
			TOTAL POINTS		

√ After Completing	Date Due	Study Guide Page(s)	STUDY GUIDE ASSIGNMENTS (CTA: Critical Thinking Activity)	Possible Points	Points You Earned
		225	Pretest	10	
		225	Key Term Assessment	11	
		226-228	Evaluation of Learning questions	31	
			CD Activity: Chapter 6 Eye-Dentify! (Record points earned)		
		229	CTA A: Measuring Distance Visual Acuity	6	
		229	CTA B: Interpreting Visual Acuity Results	4	
		229	CTA C: Charting Visual Acuity Results	4	

Copyright © 2008, 2004, 2000, 1995, 1990 by Saunders, an imprint of Elsevier Inc. All rights reserved.

√ After Completing	Date Due	Study Guide Page(s)	STUDY GUIDE ASSIGNMENTS (CTA: Critical Thinking Activity)	Possible Points	Points You Earned
			CD Activity: Chapter 6 Can you Hear Me Now? (Record points earned)		
		230	CTA D: Ear Procedures	8	
		231	CTA E: Dear Gabby	10	
		232	CTA F: Crossword Puzzle	23	
		234	CTA G: Eye and Ear Conditions	40	
			CD Activity: Chapter 6 Animations	20	
		225	Posttest	10	
			ADDITIONAL ASSIGNMENTS		
			TOTAL POINTS		

Copyright © 2008, 2004, 2000, 1995, 1990 by Saunders, an imprint of Elsevier Inc. All rights reserved.

√ When Assigned By Your Instructor	Study Guide Page(s)	Practices Required	LABORATORY ASSIGNMENTS (Procedure Number and Name)	*Score
	237	5	**Practice for Competency** 6-1: Assessing Distance Visual Acuity—Snellen Chart Textbook reference: pp. 212-213	
	239-240		**Evaluation of Competency** 6-1: Assessing Distance Visual Acuity—Snellen Chart	*
	237	3	**Practice for Competency** 6-2: Assessing Color Vision—Ishihara Test Textbook reference: pp. 213-214	
	241-242		**Evaluation of Competency** 6-2: Assessing Color Vision—Ishihara Test	*
	237	3	**Practice for Competency** 6-3: Performing an Eye Irrigation Textbook reference: pp. 215-217	
	243-244		**Evaluation of Competency** 6-3: Performing an Eye Irrigation	*
	237	3	**Practice for Competency** 6-4: Performing an Eye Instillation Textbook reference: pp. 217-218	
	245-246		**Evaluation of Competency** 6-4: Performing an Eye Instillation	*
	237	3	**Practice for Competency** 6-5: Performing an Ear Irrigation Textbook reference: pp. 224-226	
	247-249		**Evaluation of Competency** 6-5: Performing an Ear Irrigation	*
	237	3	**Practice for Competency** 6-6: Performing an Ear Instillation Textbook reference: pp. 226-227	
	251-252		**Evaluation of Competency** 6-6: Performing an Ear Instillation	*
			ADDITIONAL ASSIGNMENTS	

Copyright © 2008, 2004, 2000, 1995, 1990 by Saunders, an imprint of Elsevier Inc. All rights reserved.

Notes

Copyright © 2008, 2004, 2000, 1995, 1990 by Saunders, an imprint of Elsevier Inc. All rights reserved.

Name ______________________________ Date ______________

PRETEST

True or False

_____ 1. The outer layer of the eye composed of white connective tissue is known as the sclera.

_____ 2. A person who is farsighted has a condition known as myopia.

_____ 3. An optometrist can perform eye surgery.

_____ 4. The Snellen eye test is conducted at a distance of 20 feet.

_____ 5. The eustachian tube connects the nasopharynx to the inner ear.

_____ 6. An eye instillation may be performed to treat an eye infection.

_____ 7. The function of cerumen is to inhibit the growth of pathogens.

_____ 8. The most specific type of hearing test is the tuning fork test.

_____ 9. Serous otitis media can result in a conductive hearing loss.

_____10. An ear instillation may be performed to treat an ear infection.

POST TEST

True or False

_____ 1. The function of the lens is to permit the entrance of light rays into the eye.

_____ 2. Visual acuity refers to sharpness of vision.

_____ 3. Presbyopia is a decrease in the elasticity of the lens due to the aging process.

_____ 4. An optician fills prescriptions for eyeglasses.

_____ 5. The Snellen Big E chart is used with school-aged children.

_____ 6. The most common color vision defects are congenital in nature.

_____ 7. The cochlea functions in maintaining equilibrium.

_____ 8. The range of frequencies for normal speech is 300 to 4000 Hz.

_____ 9. Intense noise can result in a sensorineural hearing loss.

_____10. Tympanometry is used to diagnose patients with auditory nerve damage.

KEY TERM ASSESSMENT

Directions: Match each medical term with its definition.

_______ 1. Audiometer

_______ 2. Canthus

_______ 3. Cerumen

_______ 4. Hyperopia

_______ 5. Instillation

_______ 6. Irrigation

_______ 7. Myopia

_______ 8. Otoscope

_______ 9. Presbyopia

_______10. Refraction

_______11. Tympanic membrane

A. The washing of a body canal with a flowing solution

B. A decrease in the elasticity of the lens that occurs with aging, resulting in a decreased ability to focus on close objects

C. Farsightedness

D. The deflection or bending of light rays by a lens

E. The junction of the eyelids at either corner of the eye

F. Nearsightedness

G. The dropping of a liquid into a body cavity

H. An instrument for examining the external ear canal and tympanic membrane

I. Earwax

J. An instrument used to quantitatively measure hearing acuity for the various frequencies of sound waves

K. A thin, semitransparent membrane located between the external ear canal and the middle ear that receives and transmits sound waves

Copyright © 2008, 2004, 2000, 1995, 1990 by Saunders, an imprint of Elsevier Inc. All rights reserved.

EVALUATION OF LEARNING

Directions: Fill in each blank with the correct answer.

1. What is the name of the tough white outer covering of the eye?

 ____

2. What is the function of the lens?

 ____

3. What is the function of the retina?

 ____

4. What parts of the eye are covered with conjunctiva?

 ____

 ____

5. What are each of the following eye professionals qualified to perform?

 a. Ophthalmologist

 ____

 ____

 b. Optometrist

 ____

 ____

 c. Optician

 ____

 ____

6. What is visual acuity?

 ____

 ____

7. What condition can be detected by measuring distance visual acuity?

 ____

8. What type of patient would warrant use of the Snellen Big E eye chart? (Give two examples.)

 ____

 ____

9. Explain the significance of the top number and bottom number next to each line of letters of the Snellen eye chart.

 ____

 ____

10. List two conditions that can be detected by measuring near visual acuity.

 ____

 ____

Copyright © 2008, 2004, 2000, 1995, 1990 by Saunders, an imprint of Elsevier Inc. All rights reserved.

11. Explain the difference between congenital and acquired color vision defects.

12. What is a polychromatic plate?

13. List three reasons for performing eye irrigation.

14. List three reasons for performing eye instillation.

15. What is the function of the ear auricle?

16. What is the function of cerumen?

17. Explain why the external auditory canal must be straightened when viewing it with an otoscope.

18. What is the normal appearance of the tympanic membrane?

19. What is the purpose of the eustachian tube?

20. What is the function of the semicircular canals?

21. What is the range of frequencies for normal speech?

Copyright © 2008, 2004, 2000, 1995, 1990 by Saunders, an imprint of Elsevier Inc. All rights reserved.

22. List five conditions that may cause conductive hearing loss.

23. List four conditions that may result in sensorineural hearing loss.

24. How is hearing acuity tested with the gross screening test?

25. What are the names of the hearing acuity tests that require the use of a tuning fork?

26. What information is obtained through audiometry?

27. What information is obtained through tympanometry?

28. List three reasons for performing ear irrigation.

29. List three reasons for performing ear instillation.

30. Explain how impacted cerumen is removed from the ear.

31. Explain how to straighten the external auditory canal in an adult and in children 3 years of age and younger.

Copyright © 2008, 2004, 2000, 1995, 1990 by Saunders, an imprint of Elsevier Inc. All rights reserved.

CRITICAL THINKING ACTIVITIES

A. MEASURING DISTANCE VISUAL ACUITY

For each of the following situations, write C if the technique is correct and I if the technique is incorrect.

_______ 1. The patient is not given an opportunity to study the Snellen chart before beginning the test.

_______ 2. The Snellen chart is positioned at the medical assistant's eye level.

_______ 3. The patient is instructed to use his hand to cover the eye that is not being tested.

_______ 4. The medical assistant instructs the patient to close the eye that is not being tested.

_______ 5. The first line that the medical assistant asks the patient to identify is the 20/20 line.

_______ 6. The medical assistant observes the patient for signs of squinting or leaning forward during the test.

B. INTERPRETING VISUAL ACUITY RESULTS

1. A patient has a distance visual acuity reading of 20/30 in the right eye. Using this information, answer the following questions:

   a. How far was the patient from the eye chart?

   ____

   b. At what distance would a person with normal acuity be able to read this line?

   ____

2. A patient has a distance visual acuity reading of 20/10 in the left eye. Using this information, answer the following questions:

   a. How far was the patient from the eye chart?

   ____

   b. At what distance would a person with normal acuity be able to read this line?

   ____

C. CHARTING VISUAL ACUITY RESULTS

Properly chart the distance visual acuity results in the spaces provided. In all cases, the line indicated is the smallest line the patient could read at a distance of 20 feet.

1. The patient read the line marked 20/30 with the right eye with two errors, and with the left eye read the line marked 20/30 with one error. The patient was wearing corrective lenses.

   ____

   ____

2. The patient read the line marked 20/20 with the right eye with one error, and with the left eye read the line marked 20/20 with no errors. The patient was wearing corrective lenses.

   ____

   ____

3. The patient read the line marked 20/40 with the right eye with two errors, and with the left eye read the line marked 20/30 with one error. The patient exhibited squinting and frowning during the test. The patient was not wearing corrective lenses.

   ____

   ____

4. The patient read the line marked 20/15 with the right eye with no errors, and with the left eye read the line marked 20/20 with one error. The patient was not wearing corrective lenses.

   ____

   ____

Copyright © 2008, 2004, 2000, 1995, 1990 by Saunders, an imprint of Elsevier Inc. All rights reserved.

D. EAR PROCEDURES

Explain the principle for each of the following:

Ear Irrigation

1. Positioning the patient's head so that it is tilted toward the affected ear

____

____

2. Cleansing the outer ear before irrigating

____

____

3. Straightening the external auditory canal

____

____

4. Injecting the irrigating solution toward the roof of the ear canal

____

____

5. Making sure not to obstruct the canal opening

____

____

Ear Instillation

6. Positioning the patient's head so that it is tilted toward the unaffected ear

____

____

7. Instructing the patient to lie on the unaffected side after the instillation

____

____

8. Placing a cotton wick in the patient's ear

____

____

Copyright © 2008, 2004, 2000, 1995, 1990 by Saunders, an imprint of Elsevier Inc. All rights reserved.

E. DEAR GABBY

Gabby has a middle ear infection and is not feeling well. She wants you to fill in for her. In the space provided, respond to the following letter.

Dear Gabby:

I am dating the sweetest and dearest man. "Mike" has only one flaw. He likes loud music. He had those big boom boxes installed in his car. When we drive somewhere in his car, he blasts the music. Sometimes when we are driving down a street, people even turn around to see where the loud music is coming from. The music hurts my ears and I cannot think straight. My ears even start ringing when we go on a trip. When I am talking to Mike, he says I mumble, and so I have to speak extra loud around him. I keep telling Mike that the loud music is going to damage our hearing, but he says that we are way too young for that and that only old people have trouble hearing. Please help me Gabby, because I love going on trips with Mike, but not if my ears hurt afterward.

Signed, Ears are Ringing

____

____

____

____

____

____

____

____

____

____

____

Copyright © 2008, 2004, 2000, 1995, 1990 by Saunders, an imprint of Elsevier Inc. All rights reserved.

F. CROSSWORD PUZZLE

Eye and Ear

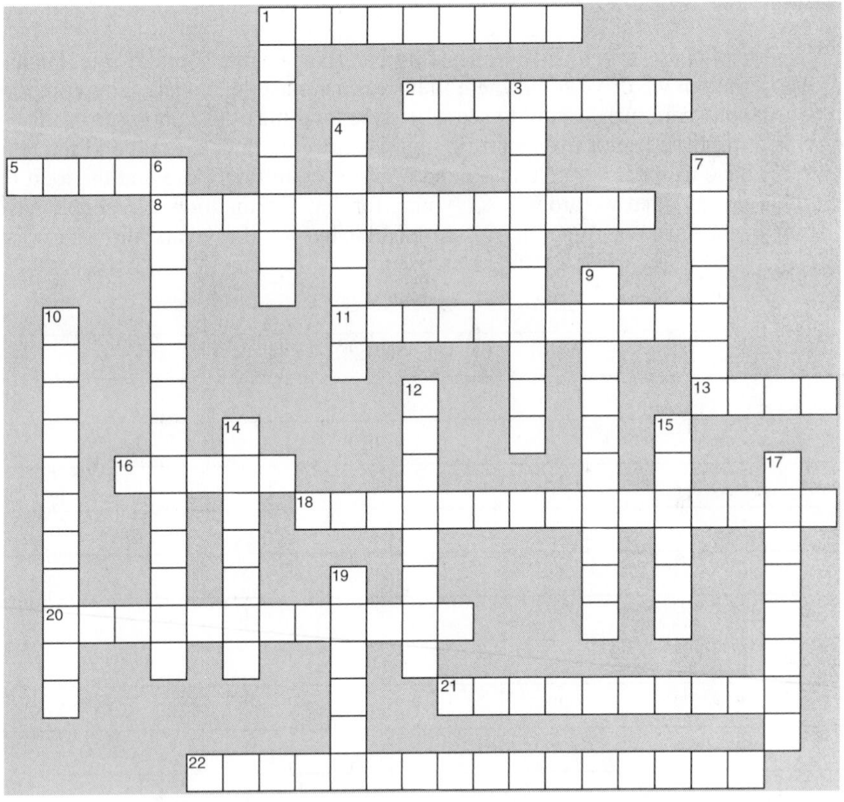

Directions: Complete the crossword puzzle using the clues provided below.

ACROSS

1 Symptom of pink eye
2 Has an S-shape
5 Eye opening
8 Middle ear to the nasopharynx
11 Function of semicircular canals
13 Music that is too loud may cause this
16 An ossicle
18 Dr. that dx and tx eye disorders
20 Fixed stapes
21 Instrument that measures hearing
22 Drum in your ear

DOWN

1 Risk factor for eye disorders
3 Caught it!
4 Measurement unit for sound
6 20/200 OU $\bar{c}$c
7 Earwax
9 Decreased lens elasticity
10 Controls shape of the lens
12 A cause of pink eye
14 Sound wave collector
15 Cannot see far away
17 Color-blind test
19 Transparent cover of the iris

Copyright © 2008, 2004, 2000, 1995, 1990 by Saunders, an imprint of Elsevier Inc. All rights reserved.

Notes

Copyright © 2008, 2004, 2000, 1995, 1990 by Saunders, an imprint of Elsevier Inc. All rights reserved.

G. EYE AND EAR CONDITIONS

1. You and your classmates work at a large clinic. It is National Eye and Ear Week. The physicians at your clinic ask you to develop for their patients informative, creative, and colorful brochures relating to eye and ear conditions. Choose a condition below and design a brochure using the blank FAQ (Frequently Asked Questions) brochure provided on the following page. Each student in the class should select a different topic. On a separate sheet of paper, write three true/false questions relating to the information in your brochure.
2. Present your brochure to the class. After all the brochures have been presented, each student should ask their three questions to the entire class to see how well the class understands eye and ear conditions. (Note: You can take notes during the presentations and refer to them when answering the questions.)

Eye

1. Amblyopia (lazy eye)
2. Age-related macular degeneration
3. Astigmatism
4. Blepharitis
5. Cataracts
6. CMV retinitis
7. Corneal ulcer
8. Corneal abrasion
9. Strabismus (crossed-eyed)
10. Diabetic retinopathy
11. Drooping eyelids (ptosis)
12. Dry eyes
13. Floaters and spots
14. Glaucoma
15. Keratoconus
16. Ocular hypertension
17. Retinal detachment
18. Retinitis pigmentosa
19. Stye

Ear

1. Acute mastoiditis
2. External otitis
3. Meniere's disease
4. Noise-induced hearing loss
5. Serous otitis media

Copyright © 2008, 2004, 2000, 1995, 1990 by Saunders, an imprint of Elsevier Inc. All rights reserved.

FAQ on:

Q: A:

Q: A:

Q: A:

Q: A:

Copyright © 2008, 2004, 2000, 1995, 1990 by Saunders, an imprint of Elsevier Inc. All rights reserved.

Q:

A:

Q:

A:

Illustration

Q:

A:

Q:

A:

Copyright © 2008, 2004, 2000, 1995, 1990 by Saunders, an imprint of Elsevier Inc. All rights reserved.

PRACTICE FOR COMPETENCY

Eye Assessment and Procedures

Procedure 6-1: Distance Visual Acuity. Assess distance visual acuity using a Snellen eye chart and record results in the chart provided. Circle any readings that indicate distance visual acuity above or below average.

Procedure 6-2: Color Vision. Assess color vision and record results in the chart provided. Circle any abnormal results.

Procedure 6-3: Eye Irrigation. Perform an eye irrigation and record the procedure in the chart provided.

Procedure 6-4: Eye Instillation. Perform an eye instillation and record the procedure in the chart provided.

Ear Procedures

Procedure 6-5: Ear Irrigation. Perform an ear irrigation and record the procedure in the chart provided.

Procedure 6-6: Ear Instillation. Perform an ear instillation and record the procedure in the chart provided.

CHART	
Date	

Copyright © 2008, 2004, 2000, 1995, 1990 by Saunders, an imprint of Elsevier Inc. All rights reserved.

Chart	
Date	

Copyright © 2008, 2004, 2000, 1995, 1990 by Saunders, an imprint of Elsevier Inc. All rights reserved.

EVALUATION OF COMPETENCY

Procedure 6-1: Assessing Distance Visual Acuity—Snellen Chart

Name: ______________________________ Date: ______________

Evaluated By: ______________________________ Score: ______________

Performance Objective

Outcome:	Assess distance visual acuity.
Conditions:	Given the following: Snellen eye chart, eye occluder, and an antiseptic wipe.
Standards:	Time: 5 minutes. Student completed procedure in ____ minutes.
	Accuracy: Satisfactory score on the Performance Evaluation Checklist.

Performance Evaluation Checklist

Trial 1	*Trial 2*	*Point Value*	*Performance Standards*
		•	Sanitized hands.
		•	Assembled equipment.
		•	Disinfected the eye occluder with an antiseptic wipe.
		•	Greeted the patient and introduced yourself.
		•	Identified the patient and explained the procedure.
		•	Determined if patient wears corrective lenses and instructed patient to leave them on during the test.
		•	Positioned patient 20 feet from the eye chart.
		•	Positioned the center of the eye chart at patient's eye level.
		•	Instructed patient to cover the left eye with the occluder and to keep the left eye open.
		▷	Stated how the occluder should be positioned if the patient wears glasses.
		▷	Explained why the patient's left eye should remain open.
		•	Instructed patient not to squint during the test.
		▷	Explained why patient should not squint during the test.
		•	Asked patient to identify the 20/70 line, using the right eye.
		▷	Stated why the test should begin with a line that is above the 20/20 line.
		•	Proceeded down the chart if the patient identified the 20/70 line or proceeded up the chart if the patient was unable to identify the 20/70 line.
		•	Continued until the smallest line of letters that the patient could read was reached.

Copyright © 2008, 2004, 2000, 1995, 1990 by Saunders, an imprint of Elsevier Inc. All rights reserved.

Trial 1	Trial 2	Point Value	*Performance Standards*
		•	Observed patient for any unusual symptoms.
		•	Jotted down the numbers next to the smallest line read by the patient.
		•	Asked patient to cover the right eye and to keep the right eye open.
		•	Measured visual acuity in the left eye.
		•	Jotted down the numbers next to the smallest line read by the patient.
		*	The visual acuity measurements were identical to the evaluator's measurements.
		•	Charted the results correctly.
		•	Disinfected the occluder with an antiseptic wipe.
		•	Sanitized hands.
		*	Completed the procedure within 5 minutes.
			TOTALS

CHART	
Date	

Evaluation of Student Performance

EVALUATION CRITERIA			COMMENTS
Symbol	Category	Point Value	
*	Critical Step	16 points	
•	Essential Step	6 points	
▷	Theory Question	2 points	
Score calculation: 100 points - ______ points missed ____ Score Satisfactory score: 85 or above			

AAMA/CAAHEP Competency Achieved:

☑ III. C. 3. b. (4) (e): Prepare patient for and assist with routine and specialty examinations.

Copyright © 2008, 2004, 2000, 1995, 1990 by Saunders, an imprint of Elsevier Inc. All rights reserved.

EVALUATION OF COMPETENCY

Procedure 6-2: Assessing Color Vision—Ishihara Test

Name: ______________________________ Date: ____________

Evaluated By: ______________________________ Score: ____________

Performance Objective

Outcome:	Assess color vision.
Conditions:	Given an Ishihara book of color plates and a cotton swab.
Standards:	Time: 10 minutes. Student completed procedure in ____ minutes.
	Accuracy: Satisfactory score on the Performance Evaluation Checklist.

Performance Evaluation Checklist

Trial 1	Trial 2	Point Value	*Performance Standards*
		•	Sanitized hands.
		•	Assembled equipment.
		•	Conducted the test in a quiet room illuminated by natural daylight.
		▷	Stated why natural daylight should be used.
		•	Greeted the patient and introduced yourself.
		•	Identified the patient.
		•	Explained the procedure using the practice plate.
		▷	Stated the purpose of the practice plate.
		•	Held the first plate 30 inches from the patient at a right angle to the patient's line of vision.
		•	Instructed patient to keep both eyes open.
		•	Told patient that he/she would have 3 seconds to identify each plate.
		•	Asked the patient to identify the number on the plate.
		•	Asked the patient to trace plates with winding lines with a cotton swab.
		▷	Stated why a cotton swab should be used to make the tracing.
		•	Recorded the results after identification of each plate.
		•	Continued until the patient viewed all plates.
		•	Charted the results correctly.
		*	The results were identical to the evaluator's results.
		•	Returned the Ishihara book to its proper place, storing it in a closed position.
		▷	Explained why the book should be stored in a closed position.
		*	Completed the procedure within 10 minutes.
			TOTALS

Copyright © 2008, 2004, 2000, 1995, 1990 by Saunders, an imprint of Elsevier Inc. All rights reserved.

CHART	
Date	

CHART		
Plate No.	Normal Person	Results
1	12	
2	8	
3	5	
4	29	
5	74	
6	7	
7	45	
8	2	
9	X	
10	16	
11	Traceable	
Date :		
Evaluated by :		

Evaluation of Student Performance

EVALUATION CRITERIA			COMMENTS
Symbol	Category	Point Value	
✶	Critical Step	16 points	
●	Essential Step	6 points	
▷	Theory Question	2 points	
Score calculation: 100 points – ______ points missed ______ Score Satisfactory score: 85 or above			

AAMA/CAAHEP Competency Achieved:

☑ III. C. 3. b. (4) (e): Prepare patient for and assist with routine and specialty examinations.

Copyright © 2008, 2004, 2000, 1995, 1990 by Saunders, an imprint of Elsevier Inc. All rights reserved.

EVALUATION OF COMPETENCY

Procedure 6-3: Performing an Eye Irrigation

Name: ______________________________ Date: ______________

Evaluated By: ______________________________ Score: ______________

Performance Objective

Outcome:	Perform an eye irrigation.
Conditions:	Given the following: disposable (nonpowdered) gloves, irrigating solution, solution container, disposable rubber bulb syringe, basin, moisture-resistant towel, and sterile gauze pads.
Standards:	Time: 5 minutes. Student completed procedure in ____ minutes.
	Accuracy: Satisfactory score on the Performance Evaluation Checklist.

Performance Evaluation Checklist

Trial 1	*Trial 2*	*Point Value*	*Performance Standards*
		•	Sanitized hands.
		•	Assembled equipment.
		•	Checked the solution label with the physician's instructions.
		•	Checked expiration date of the solution.
		▷	Stated the reason for checking the expiration date.
		•	Warmed the irrigating solution to body temperature.
		▷	Explained why the solution should be at body temperature.
		•	Checked the label a second time and poured the solution into a basin.
		•	Checked the label a third time before returning the container to storage.
		•	Greeted the patient and introduced yourself.
		•	Identified the patient and explained the procedure.
		•	Asked patient to remove glasses or contact lenses.
		•	Positioned patient in a lying or sitting position.
		•	Placed a moisture-resistant towel on the patient's shoulder.
		•	Positioned a basin tightly against the patient's cheek.
		•	Asked patient to tilt head in the direction of the affected eye and hold the basin in place.
		▷	Explained why patient's head is turned in the direction of the affected eye.
		•	Applied nonpowdered gloves.
		▷	Stated why nonpowdered gloves should be used.
		•	Cleansed the eyelids from inner to outer canthus.

Copyright © 2008, 2004, 2000, 1995, 1990 by Saunders, an imprint of Elsevier Inc. All rights reserved.

Trial 1	Trial 2	Point Value	*Performance Standards*
		▷	Stated why eyelids are cleansed.
		•	Filled irrigating syringe.
		•	Instructed patient to keep both eyes open and to look at a focal point.
		▷	Stated the reason for looking at a focal point.
		•	Separated eyelids.
		•	Held tip of syringe 1 inch above the eye at the inner canthus.
		•	Allowed solution to flow over the eye at a moderate rate from the inner canthus to the outer canthus and directed solution to the lower conjunctiva.
		▷	Explained why the syringe should be directed toward the lower conjunctiva.
		•	Did not allow syringe to touch the eye.
		•	Refilled the syringe and continued irrigating until the desired results were obtained or all the solution was used.
		•	Dried eyelids with gauze pad from inner to outer canthus.
		•	Removed gloves and sanitized hands.
		•	Charted the procedure correctly.
		▷	Stated the abbreviation for both eyes (OU), the right eye (OD), and the left eye (OS).
		•	Returned equipment.
		*	Completed the procedure within 5 minutes.
			TOTALS

CHART	
Date	

Evaluation of Student Performance

EVALUATION CRITERIA			COMMENTS
Symbol	Category	Point Value	
*	Critical Step	16 points	
•	Essential Step	6 points	
▷	Theory Question	2 points	
Score calculation: 100 points – ____ points missed ____ Score Satisfactory score: 85 or above			

AAMA/CAAHEP Competency Achieved:

☑ III. C. 3. b. (4) (f): Prepare patient for and assist with procedures, treatments, and minor office surgeries.

Copyright © 2008, 2004, 2000, 1995, 1990 by Saunders, an imprint of Elsevier Inc. All rights reserved.

EVALUATION OF COMPETENCY

Procedure 6-4: Performing an Eye Instillation

Name: ______________________________ Date: ______________

Evaluated By: ______________________________ Score: ______________

Performance Objective

Outcome:	Perform an eye instillation.
Conditions:	Given the following: disposable (nonpowdered) gloves, ophthalmic medication, tissues, and gauze pads.
Standards:	Time: 5 minutes. Student completed procedure in ____ minutes.
	Accuracy: Satisfactory score on the Performance Evaluation Checklist.

Performance Evaluation Checklist

Trial 1	*Trial 2*	*Point Value*	*Performance Standards*
		•	Sanitized hands.
		•	Assembled equipment.
		•	Checked the drug label when removing it from storage.
		▷	Stated what word must appear on the medication label.
		•	Checked drug label and dosage against the physician's instructions.
		•	Checked the expiration date of the medication.
		•	Greeted the patient and introduced yourself.
		•	Identified the patient and explained the procedure.
		•	Positioned patient in a sitting or supine position.
		•	Applied nonpowdered gloves.
		•	Prepared the medication.
		•	Checked the drug label and removed the cap.
		•	Asked patient to look up and exposed the lower conjunctival sac.
		▷	Explained the reason for asking patient to look up.
		•	Drew the skin of the cheek downward and exposed the conjunctival sac.
		•	Inserted the medication correctly.
		▷	Explained how to instill eyedrops and ointment.
		•	Instructed patient to close eyes gently and move eyeballs.
		▷	Stated the reason for closing the eyes and moving the eyeballs.
		•	Told patient that the instillation may temporarily blur vision.

Copyright © 2008, 2004, 2000, 1995, 1990 by Saunders, an imprint of Elsevier Inc. All rights reserved.

Trial 1	Trial 2	Point Value	*Performance Standards*
		•	Dried eyelids with a gauze pad from inner to outer canthus.
		•	Removed gloves and sanitized hands.
		•	Charted the procedure correctly.
		•	Returned equipment.
		*	Completed the procedure within 5 minutes.
			TOTALS

CHART	
Date	

Evaluation of Student Performance

EVALUATION CRITERIA			COMMENTS
Symbol	Category	Point Value	
*	Critical Step	16 points	
•	Essential Step	6 points	
▷	Theory Question	2 points	
Score calculation: 100 points – ______ points missed ____ Score Satisfactory score: 85 or above			

AAMA/CAAHEP Competency Achieved:

☑ III. C. 3. b. (4) (f): Prepare patient for and assist with procedures, treatments, and minor office surgeries.

Copyright © 2008, 2004, 2000, 1995, 1990 by Saunders, an imprint of Elsevier Inc. All rights reserved.

EVALUATION OF COMPETENCY

Procedure 6-5: Performing an Ear Irrigation

Name: ______________________________ Date: ______________

Evaluated By: ______________________________ Score: ______________

Performance Objective

Outcome: Perform an ear irrigation.

Conditions: Given the following: disposable gloves, irrigating solution, solution container, irrigating syringe, ear basin, moisture-resistant towel, gauze pads, and ear wick.

Standards: Time: 10 minutes. Student completed procedure in ____ minutes.

Accuracy: Satisfactory score on the Performance Evaluation Checklist.

Performance Evaluation Checklist

Trial 1	*Trial 2*	*Point Value*	*Performance Standards*
		•	Sanitized hands.
		•	Assembled equipment.
		•	Checked the label of the irrigating solution with the physician's instructions.
		•	Checked expiration date of the solution.
		•	Warmed the irrigating solution to body temperature.
		▷	Stated the reason for warming the irrigating solution.
		•	Check the label a second time and poured the solution into a basin.
		•	Check the label a third time before returning the container to storage.
		•	Greeted the patient and introduced yourself.
		•	Identified the patient and explained the procedure.
		•	Positioned patient, with the head tilted toward the affected ear.
		▷	Explained why the head should be tilted toward the affected ear.
		•	Placed a towel on patient's shoulder and instructed patient to hold the ear basin under the affected ear.
		•	Applied gloves.
		•	Cleansed the outer ear.
		▷	Explained why the outer ear should be cleansed.
		•	Filled the irrigating syringe.
		•	Expelled air from syringe.
		▷	Explained why air should be expelled from syringe.
		•	Properly straightened the ear canal.
		▷	Stated why the canal must be straightened.

Copyright © 2008, 2004, 2000, 1995, 1990 by Saunders, an imprint of Elsevier Inc. All rights reserved.

Trial 1	Trial 2	Point Value	*Performance Standards*
		•	Inserted syringe tip into the ear.
		•	Did not insert the syringe too deeply.
		•	Made sure that tip of syringe did not obstruct the canal opening.
		▷	Stated why the canal should not be obstructed.
		•	Injected the irrigating solution toward the roof of the ear canal.
		▷	Stated why solution should be injected toward roof of the canal.
		•	Refilled the syringe and continued irrigating until the desired results were obtained or all the solution was used.
		•	Observed the returning solution to note the material present and the amount.
		•	Dried outside of the ear with a gauze pad.
		•	Informed patient that the ear will feel sensitive.
		•	Instructed patient to lie on the affected side on treatment table.
		▷	Explained why patient should lie on the affected side.
		•	Inserted a cotton wick loosely in the ear canal for 15 minutes.
		▷	Stated the purpose of the cotton wick.
		•	Removed gloves and sanitized hands.
		•	Charted the procedure correctly.
		▷	Stated the abbreviation for both ears (AU), the right ear (AD), and the left ear (AS).
		•	Returned equipment.
		*	Completed the procedure within 10 minutes.
			TOTALS

CHART	
Date	

Copyright © 2008, 2004, 2000, 1995, 1990 by Saunders, an imprint of Elsevier Inc. All rights reserved.

Evaluation of Student Performance

EVALUATION CRITERIA			COMMENTS
Symbol	Category	Point Value	
*	Critical Step	16 points	
•	Essential Step	6 points	
▷	Theory Question	2 points	
Score calculation: 100 points – ______ points missed ____ Score Satisfactory score: 85 or above			

AAMA/CAAHEP Competency Achieved:

☑ III. C. 3. b. (4) (f): Prepare patient for and assist with procedures, treatments, and minor office surgeries.

Copyright © 2008, 2004, 2000, 1995, 1990 by Saunders, an imprint of Elsevier Inc. All rights reserved.

Notes

Copyright © 2008, 2004, 2000, 1995, 1990 by Saunders, an imprint of Elsevier Inc. All rights reserved.

EVALUATION OF COMPETENCY

Procedure 6-6: Performing an Ear Instillation

Name: ______________________________ Date: ______________

Evaluated By: ______________________________ Score: ______________

Performance Objective

Outcome:	Perform an ear instillation.
Conditions:	Given the following: disposable gloves, otic medication, and gauze pad.
Standards:	Time: 5 minutes. Student completed procedure in ____ minutes.
	Accuracy: Satisfactory score on the Performance Evaluation Checklist.

Performance Evaluation Checklist

Trial 1	*Trial 2*	*Point Value*	*Performance Standards*
		•	Sanitized hands.
		•	Assembled equipment.
		•	Checked the drug label when removing the medication from storage.
		▷	Stated what word must appear on the medication label.
		•	Checked the drug label and dosage against the physician's instructions.
		•	Checked the expiration date of the medication.
		▷	Explained what might occur if the medication is outdated.
		•	Greeted the patient and introduced yourself.
		•	Identified the patient and explained the procedure.
		•	Positioned patient in a sitting position.
		•	Warmed the ear drops with your hands.
		•	Applied gloves.
		•	Mixed medication if required.
		•	Checked the drug label and removed the cap.
		•	Asked the patient to tilt the head tilted in the direction of the unaffected ear.
		•	Properly straightened the ear canal.
		▷	Stated the reason for straightening the canal.
		•	Placed tip of dropper at the opening of the ear canal and inserted the proper amount of medication.
		•	Instructed patient to lie on the unaffected side for 2 to 3 minutes.
		▷	Explained why patient should lie on the unaffected side.
		•	Placed a moistened cotton wick loosely in the ear canal for 15 minutes.

Copyright © 2008, 2004, 2000, 1995, 1990 by Saunders, an imprint of Elsevier Inc. All rights reserved.

Trial 1	Trial 2	Point Value	Performance Standards
		▷	Stated the reason for moistening the wick.
		•	Removed gloves and sanitized hands.
		•	Charted the procedure correctly.
		•	Returned equipment.
		✶	Completed the procedure within 5 minutes.
			TOTALS

CHART	
Date	

Evaluation of Student Performance

EVALUATION CRITERIA			COMMENTS
Symbol	Category	Point Value	
✶	Critical Step	16 points	
•	Essential Step	6 points	
▷	Theory Question	2 points	
Score calculation: 100 points – ______ points missed ______ Score Satisfactory score: 85 or above			

AAMA/CAAHEP Competency Achieved:

☑ III. C. 3. b. (4) (f): Prepare patient for and assist with procedures, treatments, and minor office surgeries.

Copyright © 2008, 2004, 2000, 1995, 1990 by Saunders, an imprint of Elsevier Inc. All rights reserved.

7

Physical Agents to Promote Tissue Healing

CHAPTER ASSIGNMENTS

√ After Completing	Date Due	Textbook Page(s)	TEXTBOOK ASSIGNMENTS	Possible Points	Points You Earned
		233-264	Read Chapter 7: Physical Agents to Promote Tissue Healing		
		237 261	Read Case Study 1 Case Study 1 questions	5	
		251 261	Read Case Study 2 Case Study 2 questions	5	
		255 261	Read Case Study 3 Case Study 3 questions	5	
		262	Apply Your Knowledge questions	10	
			TOTAL POINTS		
√ After Completing	**Date Due**	**Study Guide Page(s)**	**STUDY GUIDE ASSIGNMENTS (CTA: Critical Thinking Activity)**	**Possible Points**	**Points You Earned**
		257	Pretest	10	
		258	Key Term Assessment	15	
		260-263	Evaluation of Learning questions	35	
		263	CTA A: Dear Gabby	10	
		264-265	CTA B: Fractures and Sprains	12	
		265-267	CTA C: Cast Care	20	
		269	CTA D: Crutch Guidelines	8	
		270	CTA E: Accessibility for Physical Disabilities	7	
		271	CTA F: Crossword Puzzle	26	
		272	CTA G: Bone and Joint Conditions	40	

Copyright © 2008, 2004, 2000, 1995, 1990 by Saunders, an imprint of Elsevier Inc. All rights reserved.

√ After Completing	Date Due	Study Guide Page(s)	STUDY GUIDE ASSIGNMENTS (CTA: Critical Thinking Activity)	Possible Points	Points You Earned
			CD Activity: Chapter 7 Animations	20	
			CD Activity: Chapter 7 Quiz Show (Record points earned)		
		257	Posttest	10	
			ADDITIONAL ASSIGNMENTS		
			TOTAL POINTS		

Copyright © 2008, 2004, 2000, 1995, 1990 by Saunders, an imprint of Elsevier Inc. All rights reserved.

√ When Assigned By Your Instructor	Study Guide Page(s)	Practices Required	LABORATORY ASSIGNMENTS (Procedure Number and Name)	*Score
	275	3	DVD **Practice for Competency** 7-1: Applying a Heating Pad Textbook reference: p. 238	
	277-278		**Evaluation of Competency** 7-1: Applying a Heating Pad	*
	275	3	DVD **Practice for Competency** 7-2: Applying a Hot Soak Textbook reference: pp. 238-239	
	279-280		**Evaluation of Competency** 7-2: Applying a Hot Soak	*
	275	3	DVD **Practice for Competency** 7-3: Applying a Hot Compress Textbook reference: pp. 239-240	
	281-282		**Evaluation of Competency** 7-3: Applying a Hot Compress	*
	275	3	DVD **Practice for Competency** 7-4: Applying an Ice Bag Textbook reference: pp. 240-241	
	283-284		**Evaluation of Competency** 7-4: Applying an Ice Bag	*
	275	3	DVD **Practice for Competency** 7-5: Applying a Cold Compress Textbook reference: pp. 241-242	
	285-286		**Evaluation of Competency** 7-5: Applying a Cold Compress	*
	275	3	DVD **Practice for Competency** 7-6: Applying a Chemical Pack Textbook reference: pp. 242	
	287-288	3	**Evaluation of Competency** 7-6: Applying a Chemical Pack	*
	275	3	**Practice for Competency** 7-7: Administering an Ultrasound Treatment Textbook reference: pp. 245-246	
	289-290		**Evaluation of Competency** 7-7: Administering an Ultrasound Treatment	*
	275	3	DVD **Practice for Competency** 7-8: Measuring for Axillary Crutches Textbook reference: pp. 255-256	
	291-292		**Evaluation of Competency** 7-8: Measuring for Axillary Crutches	*

Copyright © 2008, 2004, 2000, 1995, 1990 by Saunders, an imprint of Elsevier Inc. All rights reserved.

√ When Assigned By Your Instructor	Study Guide Page(s)	Practices Required	LABORATORY ASSIGNMENTS (Procedure Number and Name)	*Score
	275	3 x for each gait	DVD **Practice for Competency** 7-9: Instructing a Patient in Crutch Gaits Textbook reference: pp. 257-259	
	293-295		**Evaluation of Competency** 7-9: Instructing a Patient in Crutch Gaits	*
	275	Cane: 3 Walker: 3	DVD **Practice for Competency** 7-10 and 7-11: Instructing a Patient in the Use of a Cane and Walker Textbook reference: pp. 259-260	
	297-298		**Evaluation of Competency** 7-10 and 7-11: Instructing a Patient in the Use of a Cane and Walker	*
			ADDITIONAL ASSIGNMENTS	

Copyright © 2008, 2004, 2000, 1995, 1990 by Saunders, an imprint of Elsevier Inc. All rights reserved.

Name ______________________________ Date ______________

PRETEST

True or False

_____ 1. A hot compress is an example of moist heat.

_____ 2. Erythema is redness of the skin caused by dilation of superficial blood vessels.

_____ 3. The local application of cold may be used to relieve muscle spasms.

_____ 4. Therapeutic ultrasound consists of a shortwave electrical current.

_____ 5. An orthodontist is a physician who specializes in the diagnosis and treatment of disorders of the musculoskeletal system.

_____ 6. The most frequent reason for applying a cast is to aid in the nonsurgical correction of a deformity.

_____ 7. Numbness of the fingers or toes may indicate that a cast is too tight.

_____ 8. A coat hanger can be used to scratch under a cast if itching occurs.

_____ 9. Ambulation refers to the inability to walk.

_____ 10. A patient using crutches should be instructed to support his or her weight against the axilla.

POSTTEST

True or False

_____ 1. The recommended time for the application of heat is 15 to 30 minutes.

_____ 2. The local application of heat results in constriction of blood vessels in the area to which it is applied.

_____ 3. The most frequent cause of low back pain is poor posture.

_____ 4. Therapeutic ultrasound produces a superficial heating of the skin.

_____ 5. During an ultrasound treatment, the applicator head must be moved continuously to prevent hot spots.

_____ 6. A wet cast can cause a pressure area to occur.

_____ 7. Synthetic casts dry more quickly and weigh less than plaster casts.

_____ 8. It usually takes 10 to 12 weeks for a fracture to heal.

_____ 9. Incorrectly fitted crutches may cause crutch palsy.

_____ 10. A cane should be held on the strong side of the body.

Copyright © 2008, 2004, 2000, 1995, 1990 by Saunders, an imprint of Elsevier Inc. All rights reserved.

KEY TERM ASSESSMENT

Directions: Match each medical term with its definition.

_______ 1. Ambulation

_______ 2. Brace

_______ 3. Compress

_______ 4. Edema

_______ 5. Erythema

_______ 6. Exudate

_______ 7. Long arm cast

_______ 8. Maceration

_______ 9. Orthopedist

_______ 10. Short leg cast

_______ 11. Soak

_______ 12. Splint

_______ 13. Sprain

_______ 14. Strain

_______ 15. Suppuration

A. A discharge produced by the body's tissues
B. An overstretching of a muscle caused by trauma
C. A soft, moist, absorbent cloth that is folded in several layers and applied to a part of the body in the local application of heat or cold
D. Walking or moving from one place to another
E. The direct immersion of a body part in water or a medicated solution
F. The retention of fluid in the tissues, resulting in swelling
G. An orthopedic device used to support and hold a part of the body in the correct position to allow functioning and healing
H. A cast that extends from the axilla to the fingers
I. Redness of the skin caused by congestion of capillaries in the lower layers of skin
J. Trauma to a joint that causes injury to the ligaments
K. The process of pus formation
L. A physician who specializes in the diagnosis and treatment of disorders of the musculoskeletal system
M. The softening and breaking down of the skin as a result of prolonged exposure to water
N. A cast that begins just below the knee and extends to the toes
O. An orthopedic device used to immobilize, restrain, or support a part of the body

Copyright © 2008, 2004, 2000, 1995, 1990 by Saunders, an imprint of Elsevier Inc. All rights reserved.

Notes

Copyright © 2008, 2004, 2000, 1995, 1990 by Saunders, an imprint of Elsevier Inc. All rights reserved.

EVALUATION OF LEARNING

Directions: Fill in each blank with the correct answer.

1. State whether the following is an example of dry heat, moist heat, dry cold, or moist cold.
   a. Hot compress

   ____

   b. Ice bag

   ____

   c. Heating pad

   ____

   d. Chemical hot pack

   ____

   e. Cold compress

   ____

2. List three factors that must be taken into consideration when applying heat or cold.

   ____

   ____

3. How does the local application of heat to an affected area for a short period of time influence the following?
   a. The diameter of the blood vessels in the affected area

   ____

   b. The blood supply to the affected area

   ____

   c. Tissue metabolism in the affected area

   ____

4. What happens to the diameter of blood vessels if heat is applied for a prolonged period of time (more than 1 hour)?

   ____

   ____

5. List three reasons for applying heat locally.

   ____

   ____

   ____

6. How does the local application of cold for a short period of time to an affected area influence the following?
   a. The diameter of the blood vessels in the affected area

   ____

   ____

   b. The blood supply to the affected area

   ____

   ____

Copyright © 2008, 2004, 2000, 1995, 1990 by Saunders, an imprint of Elsevier Inc. All rights reserved.

c. Tissue metabolism in the affected area

____

____

7. List two reasons for applying cold locally.

____

____

8. Describe the general use of therapeutic ultrasound.

____

____

9. What is the purpose of the ultrasound coupling agent?

____

10. List two instances when the underwater ultrasound method is advocated.

____

____

11. What is the purpose of continuously moving the applicator head during the ultrasound treatment?

____

____

12. Why should the applicator head not be removed from the patient's skin and held up in the air?

____

____

13. List two instances in which the medical assistant should immediately stop the ultrasound treatment.

____

____

____

14. What are three reasons for applying a cast?

____

____

____

15. What causes a pressure area?

____

____

16. What are the symptoms of a pressure area?

____

17. What are the complications of a pressure ulcer?

____

____

Copyright © 2008, 2004, 2000, 1995, 1990 by Saunders, an imprint of Elsevier Inc. All rights reserved.

18. What are the advantages and disadvantages of a synthetic cast as compared with a plaster cast?

____

____

19. What is the purpose of covering the body part with a stockinette before applying a cast?

____

____

20. What is the purpose of applying cast padding during cast application?

____

____

21. Why should each of the following precautions be taken when applying a synthetic cast?
    a. Not covering a wet cast with plastic

    ____

    b. Removing synthetic casting particles using an alcohol swab

    ____

    c. Checking the circulation, sensation, and movement of the extremity

    ____

22. Why is it important to dry a synthetic cast as soon as possible after it gets wet?

____

23. What symptoms may indicate that a cast is too tight and an infection is developing?

____

24. How is a cast removed?

____

____

25. What will the affected extremity look like after a cast has been removed?

____

26. List two examples of conditions for which a splint might be applied.

____

____

27. List one example of a condition for which a brace might be applied.

____

____

28. What factors does the physician take into consideration when prescribing an ambulatory assistive device?

____

____

29. Describe one advantage of the forearm crutch.

____

Copyright © 2008, 2004, 2000, 1995, 1990 by Saunders, an imprint of Elsevier Inc. All rights reserved.

30. What may occur if axillary crutches are not fitted properly?

31. List eight guidelines that must be followed during crutch use to ensure safety.

32. List one use of each of the following crutch gaits:
    a. Four-point gait
    b. Three-point gait
    c. Swing-to gait

33. List and describe the three types of canes.

34. List two reasons for prescribing a cane.

35. List two reasons for prescribing a walker.

CRITICAL THINKING ACTIVITIES

A. DEAR GABBY

Gabby was called out of town unexpectedly and wants you to fill in for her. In the space provided, respond to the following letter.

Dear Gabby:

I am 15 years old and in the 10th grade. I need your help. I have a backpack; my dad weighed it and said it was 40 pounds. I only weigh 105 pounds. My back and neck hurt from lugging it around. I have to walk almost half a mile to the bus stop. I do not have time to use my locker between classes because it is down a flight of stairs and at the end of the hall. Once, when I started using my locker, my science teacher got mad at me because I was late getting to class. Gabby, what should I do?

Signed, Pain in the Neck

Copyright © 2008, 2004, 2000, 1995, 1990 by Saunders, an imprint of Elsevier Inc. All rights reserved.

B. FRACTURES AND SPRAINS

Complete an interactive tutorial on fractures and sprains by following these directions: Go to www.nlm.nih.gov/medlineplus/fractures.html. Under General/Overviews, click on Fractures and Sprains Interactive Tutorial. To start the tutorial, click on Go to Module. Answer the following questions relating to the tutorial:

1. What are the names of the bones in the lower leg?

2. What are the names of the bones that join the wrist to the fingers?

3. What are the names of the bones that join the ankle to the toes?

4. How many phalanges does each finger have? How many does the thumb have?

5. What holds bones together?

6. What is a pneumatic brace?

7. How can itching be relieved when wearing a cast?

8. What is atrophy and how does it occur?

9. What complications can occur from a cast or splint?

10. What might cause a cast to become loose? What should the patient do if this occurs?

11. What symptoms are present when a blood clot occurs in the leg?

Copyright © 2008, 2004, 2000, 1995, 1990 by Saunders, an imprint of Elsevier Inc. All rights reserved.

12. What complication can occur if a blood clot in the leg dislodges?

____

____

C. CAST CARE

1. You are employed by a pediatric orthopedic surgeon. She is concerned because many of her school-age patients do not follow proper guidelines for the care of their fiberglass casts, even with their parent's constant reminder. She asks you to develop a creative and colorful instruction sheet in the shape of a cast that presents cast care instructions at a level that can be understood by this age group (ages 6-12). Use the illustration of the cast on the following page to design your instruction sheet.
2. After developing your instruction sheet, get into a group of 3 to 4 students and share your sheets. Have the group decide if the instructions on each sheet are appropriate for a school-age child and if the sheet would be visually appealing to this age group.

Copyright © 2008, 2004, 2000, 1995, 1990 by Saunders, an imprint of Elsevier Inc. All rights reserved.

Notes

Copyright © 2008, 2004, 2000, 1995, 1990 by Saunders, an imprint of Elsevier Inc. All rights reserved.

C. INSTRUCTION SHEET FOR CAST CARE

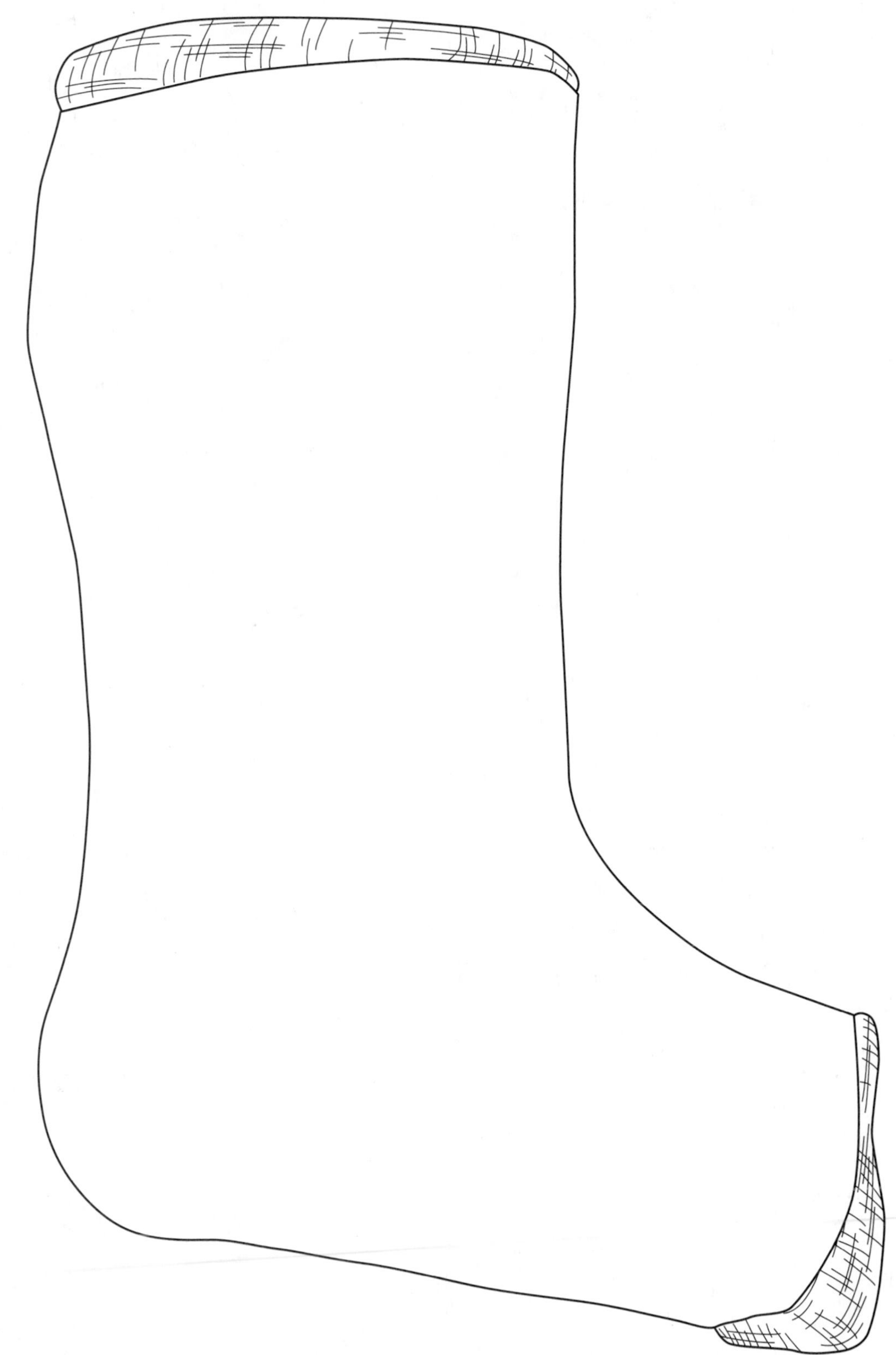

Copyright © 2008, 2004, 2000, 1995, 1990 by Saunders, an imprint of Elsevier Inc. All rights reserved.

D. CRUTCH GUIDELINES

Each of the following patients is wearing a long leg cast because of a broken tibia and is using wooden axillary crutches to ambulate. Evaluate the crutch technique being practiced by each patient. Write **C** if the technique is **correct** and **I** if the technique is **incorrect**. If the technique is **correct**, explain why it should be performed this way. If **incorrect**, indicate what might happen from performing the technique in this manner.

1. Andy Morris wears Nike sports shoes when ambulating with his crutches.

   ____

   ____

2. Juliet Wright does not stand up straight when using her crutches.

   ____

   ____

3. Miguel Saldivia puts his weight on the axilla when getting around on his crutches.

   ____

   ____

4. Lindy Campbell has a lot of decorative throw rugs in her house and she does not want to remove them.

   ____

   ____

5. Andrew Spence likes to move quickly on his crutches so he advances them forward about 20 inches with each step when using the swing-through gait.

   ____

   ____

6. Hanna Romes has tingling in her hands but thinks it is just part of what happens when one uses crutches.

   ____

   ____

7. Tamra Hetrick pads both the shoulder rests and the handgrips of her crutches.

   ____

   ____

8. Erica Anderson's crutch tips get wet but she does not take the time to dry them before going into a shopping mall.

   ____

   ____

Copyright © 2008, 2004, 2000, 1995, 1990 by Saunders, an imprint of Elsevier Inc. All rights reserved.

E. ACCESSIBILITY FOR PHYSICAL DISABILITIES

Next to each of the following facilities, list the features you have observed which facilitate accessibility of individuals with a physical disability.

1. Schools

___

___

2. Grocery stores

___

___

3. Shopping malls

___

___

4. Movie theaters

___

___

5. Restaurants

___

___

6. Doctors' offices

___

___

7. Community parks

___

___

Copyright © 2008, 2004, 2000, 1995, 1990 by Saunders, an imprint of Elsevier Inc. All rights reserved.

F. CROSSWORD PUZZLE

Physical Agents To Promote Tissue Healing

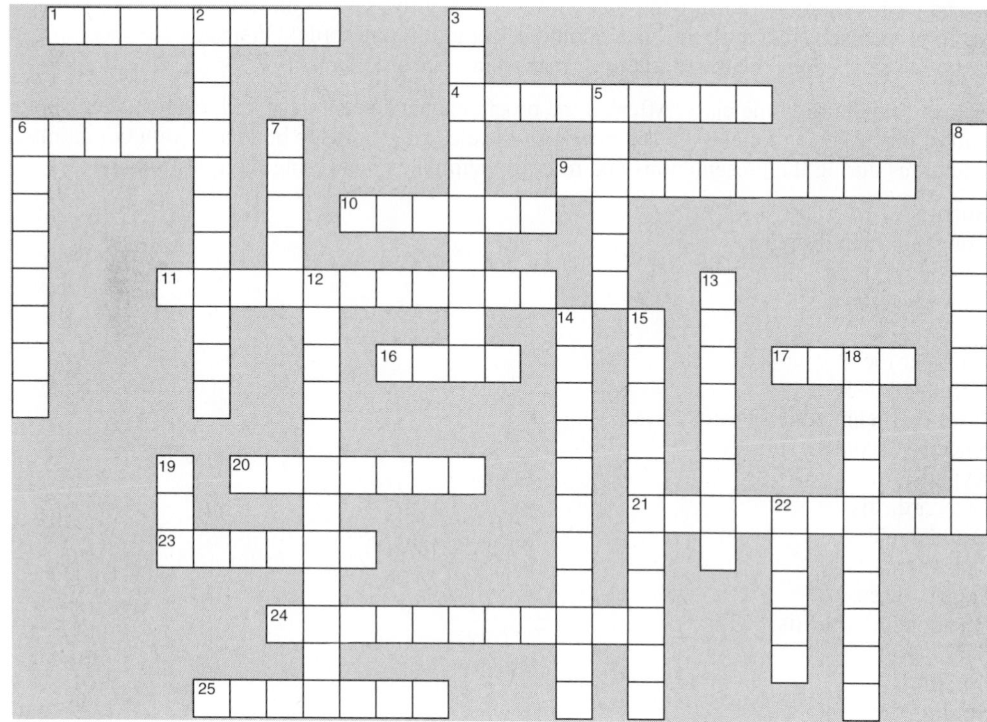

Directions: Complete the crossword puzzle using the clues presented below.

ACROSS

1 Transfers weight from legs to arms
4 Cold blood vessels do this
6 Removable immobilizer
9 Popular synthetic cast
10 Warm blood vessels do this
11 Prevents pressure areas
16 Examples: standard, tripod or quad
17 Takes 4 to 6 weeks for fracture to do this
20 Discharge
21 Purpose of a cast
23 Needed after knee replacement
24 Bone doctor
25 Cuts cast in half

DOWN

2 "Too long" crutches may cause this
3 Soft and broken down skin
5 Maximum minutes for heat application
6 Elevate cast to prevent this
7 Do not bend here to lift!
8 Prevents LBP
12 Cast is rubbing against the skin
13 Red skin
14 Pus formation
15 Located between skin and cast padding
18 Walking
19 Blow-dry a cast on this setting
22 Holds body part in correct position

Copyright © 2008, 2004, 2000, 1995, 1990 by Saunders, an imprint of Elsevier Inc. All rights reserved.

G. BONE AND JOINT CONDITIONS

1. It is National Bone and Joint Week. The mayor has asked you and your classmates to develop informative, creative, and colorful brochures for the community relating to bone and joint conditions. Choose a condition below and design a brochure using the blank FAQ (Frequently Asked Questions) brochure provided on the following page. Each student in the class should select a different topic. On a separate sheet of paper, write three true/false questions relating to the information in your brochure.
2. Present your brochure to the class. After all the brochures have been presented, each student should ask their three questions to the entire class to see how well the class understands bone and joint conditions. (Note: You can take notes during the presentations and refer to them when answering the questions.)

    1. Bursitis
    2. Congenital hip dysplasia
    3. Epicondylitis
    4. Fibromyalgia
    5. Gout
    6. Hammer toe
    7. Herniated disk
    8. Juvenile rheumatoid arthritis
    9. Knee-replacement surgery
    10. Kyphosis
    11. Osteoarthritis
    12. Osteomyelitis
    13. Osteoporosis
    14. Paget's disease
    15. Rheumatoid arthritis
    16. Scoliosis
    17. Sprain
    18. Strain
    19. Tendonitis

Copyright © 2008, 2004, 2000, 1995, 1990 by Saunders, an imprint of Elsevier Inc. All rights reserved.

FAQ on:

Q: A:

Q: A:

Q: A:

Q: A:

Copyright © 2008, 2004, 2000, 1995, 1990 by Saunders, an imprint of Elsevier Inc. All rights reserved.

Q:

A:

Q:

A:

Illustration

Q:

A:

Q:

A:

Copyright © 2008, 2004, 2000, 1995, 1990 by Saunders, an imprint of Elsevier Inc. All rights reserved.

PRACTICE FOR COMPETENCY

Local Application of Heat and Cold

Procedures 7-1, 7-2, and 7-3: Application of Heat. Apply the following heat treatments and record the procedure in the chart provided: Heating Pad, Hot Soak, Hot Compress, and Chemical Hot Pack.

Procedures 7-4, 7-5, and 7-6: Application of Cold. Apply the following cold treatments and record the results in the chart provided: Ice Bag, Cold Compress, and Chemical Cold Pack.

Therapeutic Ultrasound

Procedure 7-7: Ultrasound Therapy. Administer an ultrasound treatment and record the procedure in the chart provided.

Ambulatory Aids

Procedure 7-8: Axillary Crutch Measurement. Measure an individual for axillary crutches and record the procedure in the chart provided.

Procedure 7-9: Crutch Gaits. Instruct an individual in mastering the following crutch gaits: four-point, two-point, three-point, swing-to, and swing-through. Record the procedure in the chart provided.

Procedure 7-10: Cane. Instruct an individual in the use of a cane and record the procedure in the chart provided.

Procedure 7-11 Walker. Instruct an individual in the use of a walker and record the procedure in the chart provided.

CHART	
Date	

Copyright © 2008, 2004, 2000, 1995, 1990 by Saunders, an imprint of Elsevier Inc. All rights reserved.

Chart	
Date	

Copyright © 2008, 2004, 2000, 1995, 1990 by Saunders, an imprint of Elsevier Inc. All rights reserved.

EVALUATION OF COMPETENCY

Procedure 7-1: Applying a Heating Pad

Name: ______________________________ Date: ____________

Evaluated By: ______________________________ Score: ____________

Performance Objective

Outcome:	Apply a heating pad.	
Conditions:	Given a heating pad with a protective covering.	
Standards:	Time: 5 minutes.	Student completed procedure in ____ minutes.
	Accuracy: Satisfactory score on the Performance Evaluation Checklist.	

Performance Evaluation Checklist

Trial 1	Trial 2	Point Value	*Performance Standards*
		•	Sanitized hands.
		•	Assembled equipment.
		•	Greeted the patient and introduced yourself.
		•	Identified the patient and explained the procedure.
		•	Placed the heating pad in protective covering.
		•	Connected the plug to electrical outlet and set selector switch to the proper setting.
		•	Placed heating pad on patient's affected body area and asked how the temperature felt.
		•	Instructed patient not to lie on the pad or turn the temperature setting higher.
		▷	Stated why patient should be instructed not to lie on heating pad.
		▷	Explained why patient may want to increase the temperature.
		•	Checked patient's skin periodically.
		•	Administered treatment for the proper length of time as designated by physician.
		•	Sanitized hands.
		•	Charted the procedure correctly.
		•	Properly cared for and returned equipment to its storage place.
		*	Completed the procedure within 5 minutes.
			TOTALS

Copyright © 2008, 2004, 2000, 1995, 1990 by Saunders, an imprint of Elsevier Inc. All rights reserved.

CHART	
Date	

Evaluation of Student Performance

EVALUATION CRITERIA			COMMENTS
Symbol	Category	Point Value	
✶	Critical Step	16 points	
●	Essential Step	6 points	
▷	Theory Question	2 points	
Score calculation: 100 points – ____ points missed ____ Score Satisfactory score: 85 or above			

AAMA/CAAHEP Competency Achieved:

☑ III. C. 3. b. (4) (f): Prepare patient for and assist with procedures, treatments, and minor office surgeries.

Copyright © 2008, 2004, 2000, 1995, 1990 by Saunders, an imprint of Elsevier Inc. All rights reserved.

EVALUATION OF COMPETENCY

Procedure 7-2: Applying a Hot Soak

Name: ______________________________ Date: ______________

Evaluated By: ______________________________ Score: ______________

Performance Objective

Outcome:	Apply a hot soak.
Conditions:	Given the following: soaking solution, bath thermometer, basin, and bath towels.
Standards:	Time: 10 minutes. Student completed procedure in ____ minutes.
	Accuracy: Satisfactory score on the Performance Evaluation Checklist.

Performance Evaluation Checklist

Trial 1	*Trial 2*	*Point Value*	*Performance Standards*
		•	Sanitized hands.
		•	Assembled equipment.
		•	Check the label on the solution container.
		•	Warmed the soaking solution.
		•	Greeted the patient and introduced yourself.
		•	Identified the patient and explained the procedure.
		•	Filled basin one-half to two-thirds full with the warmed soaking solution.
		•	Checked temperature of the solution with a bath thermometer.
		▷	Stated the safe temperature range that should be used for an adult patient (105° F to 110° F).
		•	Assisted patient in a comfortable position and padded side of the basin with towel.
		•	Slowly and gradually immersed affected body part into the solution and asked patient how the temperature felt.
		•	Kept the solution at a constant temperature by removing cooler solution and adding hot solution.
		•	Placed a hand between patient and solution when adding more solution.
		•	Stirred the solution with your hand while pouring it.
		•	Checked patient's skin periodically.
		•	Applied hot soak for the proper length of time as designated by physician.
		•	Completely dried affected part.
		•	Sanitized hands.

Copyright © 2008, 2004, 2000, 1995, 1990 by Saunders, an imprint of Elsevier Inc. All rights reserved.

		•	Charted the procedure correctly.
		•	Properly cared for and returned equipment to its storage place.
		✶	Completed the procedure within 10 minutes.
			TOTALS

CHART	
Date	

Evaluation of Student Performance

EVALUATION CRITERIA			COMMENTS
Symbol	Category	Point Value	
✶	Critical Step	16 points	
•	Essential Step	6 points	
▷	Theory Question	2 points	
Score calculation: 100 points – ____ points missed ____ Score Satisfactory score: 85 or above			

AAMA/CAAHEP Competency Achieved:

☑ III. C. 3. b. (4) (f): Prepare patient for and assist with procedures, treatments, and minor office surgeries.

Copyright © 2008, 2004, 2000, 1995, 1990 by Saunders, an imprint of Elsevier Inc. All rights reserved.

EVALUATION OF COMPETENCY

Procedure 7-3: Applying a Hot Compress

Name: ______________________ Date: __________

Evaluated By: ______________________ Score: __________

Performance Objective

Outcome: Apply a hot compress.

Conditions: Given the following: solution for the compresses, bath thermometer, basin, washcloths and a towel.

Standards: Time: 10 minutes. Student completed procedure in ____ minutes.

Accuracy: Satisfactory score on the Performance Evaluation Checklist.

Performance Evaluation Checklist

Trial 1	*Trial 2*	*Point Value*	*Performance Standards*
		•	Sanitized hands.
		•	Assembled equipment.
		•	Checked the label on the solution container.
		•	Warmed the soaking solution.
		•	Greeted the patient and introduced yourself.
		•	Identified the patient and explained the procedure.
		•	Filled basin half full with the warmed solution.
		•	Checked temperature of the solution with a bath thermometer.
		▷	Stated the safe temperature range that should be used for an adult patient (105° F to 110° F).
		•	Completely immersed the compress in the solution.
		•	Squeezed excess solution from compress.
		•	Applied compress to affected body part and asked patient how the temperature felt.
		•	Placed additional compresses in the solution.
		•	Repeated the application every 2 to 3 minutes for the duration of time specified by physician.
		•	Checked patient's skin periodically.
		•	Checked temperature of the solution periodically, removed cooler fluid, and added hot fluid if needed.
		•	Administered treatment for proper length of time as designated by a physician.
		•	Thoroughly dried affected part.
		•	Sanitized hands.

Copyright © 2008, 2004, 2000, 1995, 1990 by Saunders, an imprint of Elsevier Inc. All rights reserved.

Trial 1	Trial 2	Point Value	Performance Standards
		•	Charted the procedure correctly.
		•	Properly cared for and returned equipment to its storage place.
		✶	Completed the procedure within 10 minutes.
			TOTALS

CHART	
Date	

Evaluation of Student Performance

EVALUATION CRITERIA			COMMENTS
Symbol	Category	Point Value	
✶	Critical Step	16 points	
•	Essential Step	6 points	
▷	Theory Question	2 points	
Score calculation: 100 points – _____ points missed _____ Score Satisfactory score: 85 or above			

AAMA/CAAHEP Competency Achieved:

☑ III. C. 3. b. (4) (f): Prepare patient for and assist with procedures, treatments, and minor office surgeries.

Copyright © 2008, 2004, 2000, 1995, 1990 by Saunders, an imprint of Elsevier Inc. All rights reserved.

EVALUATION OF COMPETENCY

Procedure 7-4: Applying an Ice Bag

Name: ______________________________ Date: ______________

Evaluated By: ______________________________ Score: ______________

Performance Objective

Outcome:	Apply an ice bag.
Conditions:	Given the following: ice bag and protective covering, and small pieces of ice.
Standards:	Time: 10 minutes. Student completed procedure in ____ minutes.
	Accuracy: Satisfactory score on the Performance Evaluation Checklist.

Performance Evaluation Checklist

Trial 1	*Trial 2*	*Point Value*	*Performance Standards*
		•	Sanitized hands.
		•	Assembled equipment.
		•	Greeted the patient and introduced yourself.
		•	Identified the patient and explained the procedure.
		•	Checked ice bag for leakage.
		•	Filled bag one-half to two-thirds full with small pieces of ice.
		▷	Explained why small pieces of ice are used.
		•	Expelled air from bag.
		▷	Explained the reason for expelling air from bag.
		•	Placed the bag in protective covering.
		▷	Stated the purpose of placing bag in protective covering.
		•	Placed bag on affected body area and asked patient how the temperature felt.
		•	Checked patient's skin periodically.
		▷	Listed skin changes that would warrant removal of bag.
		•	Refilled bag with ice and changed protective covering when needed.
		•	Administered treatment for the proper length of time as designated by physician.
		•	Sanitized hands.
		•	Charted the procedure correctly.
		•	Properly cared for and returned equipment to its storage place.
		*	Completed the procedure within 10 minutes.
			TOTALS

Copyright © 2008, 2004, 2000, 1995, 1990 by Saunders, an imprint of Elsevier Inc. All rights reserved.

Chart	
Date	

Evaluation of Student Performance

EVALUATION CRITERIA			COMMENTS
Symbol	Category	Point Value	
✶	Critical Step	16 points	
●	Essential Step	6 points	
▷	Theory Question	2 points	
Score calculation: 100 points − ____ points missed ____ Score Satisfactory score: 85 or above			

AAMA/CAAHEP Competency Achieved:

☑ III. C. 3. b. (4) (f): Prepare patient for and assist with procedures, treatments, and minor office surgeries.

Copyright © 2008, 2004, 2000, 1995, 1990 by Saunders, an imprint of Elsevier Inc. All rights reserved.

EVALUATION OF COMPETENCY

Procedure 7-5: Applying a Cold Compress

Name: ______________________________ Date: ______________

Evaluated By: ______________________________ Score: ______________

Performance Objective

Outcome: Apply a cold compress.

Conditions: Given the following: ice cubes, a basin, and washcloths.

Standards: Time: 10 minutes. Student completed procedure in ____ minutes.

Accuracy: Satisfactory score on the Performance Evaluation Checklist.

Performance Evaluation Checklist

Trial 1	*Trial 2*	*Point Value*	*Performance Standards*
		•	Sanitized hands.
		•	Assembled equipment.
		•	Checked the label on the solution.
		•	Greeted the patient and introduced yourself.
		•	Identified the patient and explained the procedure.
		•	Placed large ice cubes in basin and added the solution until the basin is half full.
		▷	Explained why larger pieces of ice are used.
		•	Completely immersed the compress in the solution.
		•	Squeezed excess solution from compress.
		•	Applied compress to affected body part and asked patient how the temperature felt.
		•	Placed additional compresses in the solution.
		•	Repeated the application every 2 to 3 minutes for the duration of time specified by physician.
		•	Checked patient's skin periodically.
		•	Added ice if needed to keep the solution cold.
		•	Administered treatment for proper length of time as designated by physician.
		•	Thoroughly dried affected part.
		•	Sanitized hands.
		•	Charted the procedure correctly.
		•	Properly cared for and returned equipment to its storage place.
		*	Completed the procedure within 10 minutes.
			TOTALS

Copyright © 2008, 2004, 2000, 1995, 1990 by Saunders, an imprint of Elsevier Inc. All rights reserved.

CHART	
Date	

Evaluation of Student Performance

EVALUATION CRITERIA			COMMENTS
Symbol	Category	Point Value	
✶	Critical Step	16 points	
●	Essential Step	6 points	
▷	Theory Question	2 points	
Score calculation: 100 points – ______ points missed ____ Score Satisfactory score: 85 or above			

AAMA/CAAHEP Competency Achieved:

☑ III. C. 3. b. (4) (f): Prepare patient for and assist with procedures, treatments, and minor office surgeries.

Copyright © 2008, 2004, 2000, 1995, 1990 by Saunders, an imprint of Elsevier Inc. All rights reserved.

EVALUATION OF COMPETENCY

Procedure 7-6: Applying a Chemical Pack

Name: ______________________ Date: __________

Evaluated By: ______________________ Score: __________

Performance Objective

Outcome:	Apply a chemical cold and hot pack.
Conditions:	Given a chemical cold and hot pack.
Standards:	Time: 5 minutes. Student completed procedure in ____ minutes.
	Accuracy: Satisfactory score on the Performance Evaluation Checklist.

Performance Evaluation Checklist

Trial 1	*Trial 2*	*Point Value*	*Performance Standards*
		•	Sanitized hands.
		•	Assembled equipment.
		•	Greeted the patient and introduced yourself.
		•	Identified the patient and explained the procedure.
		•	Shook the crystals to the bottom of bag.
		•	Squeezed bag firmly to break inner water bag.
		•	Shook bag vigorously to mix the contents.
		•	Covered bag with a protective covering.
		•	Applied bag to affected area.
		•	Checked the patient's skin periodically.
		•	Administered treatment for the proper length of time.
		•	Discarded bag in an appropriate receptacle.
		•	Sanitized hands.
		•	Charted the procedure correctly.
		*	Completed the procedure within 5 minutes.
			TOTALS

CHART	
Date	

Copyright © 2008, 2004, 2000, 1995, 1990 by Saunders, an imprint of Elsevier Inc. All rights reserved.

Evaluation of Student Performance

EVALUATION CRITERIA			COMMENTS
Symbol	**Category**	**Point Value**	
✶	Critical Step	16 points	
●	Essential Step	6 points	
▷	Theory Question	2 points	
Score calculation: 100 points – ____ points missed ____ Score			
Satisfactory score: 85 or above			

AAMA/CAAHEP Competency Achieved:

☑ III. C. 3. b. (4) (f): Prepare patient for and assist with procedures, treatments, and minor office surgeries.

Copyright © 2008, 2004, 2000, 1995, 1990 by Saunders, an imprint of Elsevier Inc. All rights reserved.

EVALUATION OF COMPETENCY

Procedure 7-7: Administering an Ultrasound Treatment

Name: ______________________ Date: ____________

Evaluated By: ______________________ Score: ____________

Performance Objective

Outcome:	Administer an ultrasound treatment.
Conditions:	Using an ultrasound machine.
Standards:	Time: 15 minutes. Student completed procedure in ____ minutes.
	Accuracy: Satisfactory score on the Performance Evaluation Checklist.

Performance Evaluation Checklist

Trial 1	*Trial 2*	*Point Value*	*Performance Standards*
		•	Sanitized hands.
		•	Assembled equipment.
		•	Greeted the patient and introduced yourself.
		•	Identified the patient and explained the procedure.
		•	Instructed patient to report any pain or discomfort experienced during the treatment.
		•	Asked patient to remove appropriate clothing.
		•	Positioned patient for the treatment.
		•	Applied coupling agent liberally to patient's skin.
		▷	Explained why coupling agent should be at room temperature.
		•	Placed the intensity control at the minimum position.
		•	Set timer to the specified amount of time.
		•	Checked to make sure that the intensity was at zero.
		•	Advanced the intensity control to the treatment level specified by physician.
		•	Placed applicator head into coupling medium in the treatment area.
		•	Moved applicator head in a back-and-forth stroking motion or in a circular motion at rate of 1 to 2 inches per second.
		▷	Explained why the applicator head should be moved continuously.
		•	Continued the treatment until the timer went off.
		•	Moved applicator head continuously during the treatment.
		•	Did not remove applicator head from the skin and hold it up in the air during the treatment.

Copyright © 2008, 2004, 2000, 1995, 1990 by Saunders, an imprint of Elsevier Inc. All rights reserved.

Trial 1	Trial 2	Point Value	*Performance Standards*
		▷	Explained why applicator head should not be held up in the air.
		•	Stopped the treatment immediately if patient complained of any pain or discomfort.
		•	Removed applicator head from patient's skin when timer went off.
		•	Wiped coupling medium from applicator head.
		•	Wiped excess coupling medium from patient's skin with paper towel and instructed patient to get dressed.
		•	Sanitized hands.
		•	Charted the procedure correctly.
		*	Completed the procedure within 15 minutes.
			TOTALS

CHART	
Date	

Evaluation of Student Performance

EVALUATION CRITERIA			COMMENTS
Symbol	Category	Point Value	
*	Critical Step	16 points	
•	Essential Step	6 points	
▷	Theory Question	2 points	
Score calculation: 100 points – ______ points missed ____ Score Satisfactory score: 85 or above			

AAMA/CAAHEP Competency Achieved:

☑ III. C. 3. b. (4) (d): Prepare and maintain examination and treatment areas.
☑ III. C. 3. b. (4) (f): Prepare patient for and assist with procedures, treatments, and minor office surgeries.

Copyright © 2008, 2004, 2000, 1995, 1990 by Saunders, an imprint of Elsevier Inc. All rights reserved.

EVALUATION OF COMPETENCY

Procedure 7-8: Measuring for Axillary Crutches

Name: ____________________ Date: __________

Evaluated By: ____________________ Score: __________

Performance Objective

Outcome:	Measure a patient for axillary crutches.
Conditions:	Given the following: axillary crutches and a tape measure.
Standards:	Time: 10 minutes. Student completed procedure in ____ minutes.
	Accuracy: Satisfactory score on the Performance Evaluation Checklist.

Performance Evaluation Checklist

Trial 1	*Trial 2*	*Point Value*	*Performance Standards*
		•	Asked patient to stand erect.
		•	Positioned crutches with the tips at a distance of 2 inches in front of, and 4 to 6 inches to the side of each foot.
		•	Adjusted crutch length so that the shoulder rests were approximately 1½ to 2 inches below the axilla.
		•	Asked the patient to support his or her weight by the handgrips.
		•	Adjusted the handgrips so that patient's elbow was flexed approximately 30 degrees.
		•	Checked the fit of the crutches by placing two fingers between the top of crutch and patient's axilla.
		•	Charted the procedure correctly.
		*	Completed the procedure within 10 minutes.
			TOTALS

CHART	
Date	

Copyright © 2008, 2004, 2000, 1995, 1990 by Saunders, an imprint of Elsevier Inc. All rights reserved.

Evaluation of Student Performance

EVALUATION CRITERIA			COMMENTS
Symbol	**Category**	**Point Value**	
✶	Critical Step	16 points	
●	Essential Step	6 points	
▷	Theory Question	2 points	
Score calculation: 100 points – ______ points missed _____ Score Satisfactory score: 85 or above			

AAMA/CAAHEP Competency Achieved: Include competency number

☑ III. C. 3. b. (4) (f): Prepare patient for and assist with procedures, treatments, and minor office surgeries.

Copyright © 2008, 2004, 2000, 1995, 1990 by Saunders, an imprint of Elsevier Inc. All rights reserved.

EVALUATION OF COMPETENCY

Procedure 7-9: Instructing a Patient in Crutch Gaits

Name: ______________________________ Date: ____________

Evaluated By: ______________________________ Score: ____________

Performance Objective

Outcome: Instruct an individual in the following crutch gaits: four-point, two-point, three-point, swing-to, and swing-through.

Conditions: Given axillary crutches.

Standards: Time: 15 minutes. Student completed procedure in ____ minutes.

Accuracy: Satisfactory score on the Performance Evaluation Checklist.

Performance Evaluation Checklist

Trial 1	Trial 2	Point Value	*Performance Standards*
			TRIPOD POSITION
			Instructed the patient to:
		•	Stand erect and face straight ahead.
		•	Place the tips of crutches 4 to 6 inches in front of, and 4 to 6 inches to side of each foot.
		▷	Stated one use of the tripod position.
			FOUR-POINT GAIT
			Instructed the patient to:
		•	Begin in the tripod position.
		•	Move the right crutch forward.
		•	Move the left foot forward to the level of the left crutch.
		•	Move the left crutch forward.
		•	Move the right foot forward to the level of the right crutch.
		•	Repeat the above sequence.
		▷	Stated one use of the four-point gait.
			TWO-POINT GAIT
			Instructed the patient to:
		•	Begin in the tripod position.
		•	Move the left crutch and the right foot forward at the same time.
		•	Move the right crutch and left foot forward at the same time.
		•	Repeat the above sequence.

Copyright © 2008, 2004, 2000, 1995, 1990 by Saunders, an imprint of Elsevier Inc. All rights reserved.

Trial 1	Trial 2	Point Value	*Performance Standards*
		▷	Stated one use of the two-point gait.
			THREE-POINT GAIT
			Instructed the patient to:
		•	Begin in the tripod position.
		•	Move both crutches and the affected leg forward.
		•	Move the unaffected leg forward while balancing weight on both crutches.
		•	Repeat the above sequence.
		▷	Stated two uses of the three-point gait.
			SWING-TO GAIT
			Instructed patient to:
		•	Begin in the tripod position.
		•	Move both crutches forward together.
		•	Lift and swing body to the crutches.
		•	Repeat the above sequence.
		▷	Stated one use of the swing-to gait.
			SWING-THROUGH GAIT
			Instructed patient to:
		•	Begin in the tripod position.
		•	Move both crutches forward together.
		•	Lift and swing body past the crutches.
		•	Repeat the above sequence.
		▷	Stated one use of the swing-through gait.
		*	Completed the procedure within 15 minutes.
			TOTALS

Copyright © 2008, 2004, 2000, 1995, 1990 by Saunders, an imprint of Elsevier Inc. All rights reserved.

Evaluation of Student Performance

EVALUATION CRITERIA			COMMENTS
Symbol	**Category**	**Point Value**	
✶	Critical Step	16 points	
•	Essential Step	6 points	
▷	Theory Question	2 points	
Score calculation: 100 points – ______ points missed ____ Score Satisfactory score: 85 or above			

AAMA/CAAHEP Competency Achieved:

☑ III. C. 3. b. (4) (f): Prepare patient for and assist with procedures, treatments, and minor office surgeries.
☑ III. C. 3. c. (3) (b): Instruct individuals according to their needs.

Copyright © 2008, 2004, 2000, 1995, 1990 by Saunders, an imprint of Elsevier Inc. All rights reserved.

Notes

Copyright © 2008, 2004, 2000, 1995, 1990 by Saunders, an imprint of Elsevier Inc. All rights reserved.

EVALUATION OF COMPETENCY

Procedures 7-10 and 7-11: Instructing a Patient in Use of a Cane and Walker

Name: ______________________________ Date: ______________

Evaluated By: ______________________________ Score: ______________

Performance Objective

Outcome: Instruct an individual in the use of a cane and walker.

Conditions: Given the following: a cane and a walker.

Standards: Time: 10 minutes. Student completed procedure in ____ minutes.

Accuracy: Satisfactory score on the Performance Evaluation Checklist.

Performance Evaluation Checklist

Trial 1	*Trial 2*	*Point Value*	*Performance Standards*
			CANE
			Instructed the patient to:
		•	Hold the cane on the strong side of body.
		•	Place tip of the cane 4 to 6 inches to the side of foot.
		•	Move the cane forward approximately 12 inches.
		•	Move the affected leg forward to the level of the cane.
		•	Move strong leg forward and ahead of the cane and weak leg.
		•	Repeat the above sequence.
		▷	Stated one condition for which a cane is used.
			WALKER
			Instructed the patient to:
		•	Pick up the walker and move it forward approximately 6 inches.
		•	Move the right foot and then the left foot up to the walker.
		•	Repeat the above sequence.
		▷	Stated one condition for which a walker is used.
		*	Completed the procedure within 10 minutes.
			TOTALS

Copyright © 2008, 2004, 2000, 1995, 1990 by Saunders, an imprint of Elsevier Inc. All rights reserved.

Evaluation of Student Performance

EVALUATION CRITERIA			COMMENTS
Symbol	Category	Point Value	
*	Critical Step	16 points	
•	Essential Step	6 points	
▷	Theory Question	2 points	
Score calculation: 100 points – ______ points missed ______ Score Satisfactory score: 85 or above			

AAMA/CAAHEP Competency Achieved:

☑ III. C. 3. b. (4) (f): Prepare patient for and assist with procedures, treatments, and minor office surgeries.

Copyright © 2008, 2004, 2000, 1995, 1990 by Saunders, an imprint of Elsevier Inc. All rights reserved.

8

The Gynecological Examination and Prenatal Care

CHAPTER ASSIGNMENTS

√ After Completing	Date Due	Textbook Page(s)	TEXTBOOK ASSIGNMENTS	Possible Points	Points You Earned
		265-317	Read Chapter 8: The Gynecological Examination and Prenatal Care		
		268 311	Read Case Study 1 Case Study 1 questions	5	
		288 311-312	Read Case Study 2 Case Study 2 questions	5	
		298 312	Read Case Study 3 Case Study 3 questions	5	
		302 312	Read Case Study 4 Case Study 4 questions	5	
		312-314	Apply Your Knowledge questions	15	
			TOTAL POINTS		

√ After Completing	Date Due	Study Guide Page(s)	STUDY GUIDE ASSIGNMENTS (CTA: Critical Thinking Activity)	Possible Points	Points You Earned
		303	Pretest	10	
		304-305	Key Term Assessment	53	
		306-313	Evaluation of Learning questions	56	
		313-314	CTA A: Breast Cancer (5 pts/question)	15	
			CD Activity: Chapter 8 What's on your Tray? (Record points earned)		
		314-317	CTA B: Methods of Contraception (3 pts/each method)	42	

Copyright © 2008, 2004, 2000, 1995, 1990 by Saunders, an imprint of Elsevier Inc. All rights reserved.

√ After Completing	Date Due	Study Guide Page(s)	STUDY GUIDE ASSIGNMENTS (CTA: Critical Thinking Activity)	Possible Points	Points You Earned
		317-322	CTA C: Herpes and HPV (40 pts/brochure)	80	
		323	CTA D: Signs and Symptoms of Pregnancy	16	
		323	CTA E: Calculation of the EDD	5	
		324	CTA F: Recording Gravidity and Parity	4	
		324-325	CTA G: Nutrition During Pregnancy	8	
		326	CTA H: Minor Discomforts of Pregnancy	10	
		327	CTA I: Health Promotion During Pregnancy	7	
		327-328	CTA J: Breast-Feeding	8	
		328	CTA K: Prenatal Ultrasound	5	
		329	CTA L: Crossword Puzzle	31	
		330	CTA M: Road to Recovery Game OB/GYN Terminology (Team Players) (Record points earned)		
			CD Activity: Chapter 8 Road to Recovery Game OB/GYN Terminology (Individual Player) (Record points earned)		
			CD Activity: Chapter 8 Animations	20	
		303	Posttest	10	
			ADDITIONAL ASSIGNMENTS		
			TOTAL POINTS		

Copyright © 2008, 2004, 2000, 1995, 1990 by Saunders, an imprint of Elsevier Inc. All rights reserved.

√ When Assigned By Your Instructor	Study Guide Page(s)	Practices Required	LABORATORY ASSIGNMENTS (Procedure Number and Name)	*Score
	339	5	**Practice for Competency** 8-1: Breast Self-Examination Instructions Textbook reference: pp. 278-280	
	349-351		**Evaluation of Competency** 8-1: Breast Self-Examination Instructions	*
	341	5	**Practice for Competency** 8-2: Assisting with a Gynecologic Examination Textbook reference: pp. 280-284	
	353-356		**Evaluation of Competency** 8-2: Assisting with a Gynecologic Examination	*
	343	5	**Practice for Competency** 8-3: Assisting with a Return Prenatal Examination Textbook reference: pp. 307-309	
	357-359		**Evaluation of Competency** 8-3: Assisting with a Return Prenatal Examination	*
			ADDITIONAL ASSIGNMENTS	

Copyright © 2008, 2004, 2000, 1995, 1990 by Saunders, an imprint of Elsevier Inc. All rights reserved.

Notes

Copyright © 2008, 2004, 2000, 1995, 1990 by Saunders, an imprint of Elsevier Inc. All rights reserved.

Name ______________________________ Date ______________

PRETEST

True or False

_____ 1. A complete gynecologic examination consists of a breast examination and a pelvic examination.

_____ 2. The American Cancer Society recommends that a woman perform a breast self-examination weekly.

_____ 3. The purpose of the Pap test is for the early detection of cervical cancer.

_____ 4. The patient should be instructed to douche before having a Pap test.

_____ 5. Trichomoniasis produces a profuse, frothy vaginal discharge.

_____ 6. Another name for candidiasis is a yeast infection.

_____ 7. Prenatal refers to the care of the pregnant woman before delivery of the infant.

_____ 8. During each return prenatal visit, the mother's urine is tested for glucose and protein.

_____ 9. The normal range for the fetal pulse rate is between 120 and 160 beats per minute.

_____ 10. Amniocentesis can be used to diagnose certain genetically transmitted conditions.

POSTTEST

True or False

_____ 1. The patient position for a breast examination is the lithotomy position.

_____ 2. Most breast lumps are discovered by the physician.

_____ 3. Trichomoniasis is caused by a virus.

_____ 4. Chlamydia often occurs in association with syphilis.

_____ 5. In the absence of complications, the first prenatal visit should be scheduled after a woman misses her first period.

_____ 6. True labor pains are referred to as Braxton Hicks contractions.

_____ 7. The purpose of measuring fundal height is to determine the degree of cervical dilation and effacement.

_____ 8. The fetal heart tones can first be detected between 4 and 6 weeks of gestation using a Doppler fetal pulse detector.

_____ 9. The mother must fast for 12 hours before having an obstetric ultrasound scan.

_____ 10. The perineum is the period of time in which the body systems are returning to their prepregnant state.

Copyright © 2008, 2004, 2000, 1995, 1990 by Saunders, an imprint of Elsevier Inc. All rights reserved.

KEY TERM ASSESSMENT

The Gynecologic Examination

Directions: Match each medical term with its definition.

_______ 1. Adnexal
_______ 2. Amenorrhea
_______ 3. Atypical
_______ 4. Cervix
_______ 5. Colposcopy
_______ 6. Cytology
_______ 7. Dysmenorrhea
_______ 8. Dyspareunia
_______ 9. Dysplasia
_______ 10. Endocervix
_______ 11. External os
_______ 12. Gynecology
_______ 13. Internal os
_______ 14. Menopause
_______ 15. Menorrhagia
_______ 16. Metrorrhagia
_______ 17. Perimenopause
_______ 18. Perineum
_______ 19. Risk factor
_______ 20. Vulva

A. The opening of the cervical canal of the uterus into the vagina
B. The mucous membrane lining the cervical canal
C. Deviation from the normal
D. The external region between the vaginal orifice and the anus in a female and between the scrotum and the anus in a male
E. Adjacent
F. The absence or cessation of the menstrual period
G. The region of the external genital organs in the female
H. The science that deals with the study of cells, including their origin, structure, function, and pathology
I. The branch of medicine that deals with the diseases of the reproductive organs of women
J. The internal opening of the cervical canal into the uterus
K. Anything that increases an individual's chance of developing a disease
L. The growth of abnormal cells
M. Before the onset of menopause, the phase during which the woman with regular periods changes to irregular cycles and increased periods of amenorrhea
N. Pain in the vagina or pelvis experienced by a woman during sexual intercourse
O. Examination of the cervix using a lighted instrument with a magnifying lens
P. Bleeding between menstrual periods
Q. Excessive bleeding during a menstrual period
R. The lower narrow end of the uterus that opens into the vagina
S. Pain associated with the menstrual period
T. The permanent cessation of menstruation

Prenatal Care

Directions: Match each medical term with its definition.

_______ 1. Abortion
_______ 2. Braxton Hicks contractions
_______ 3. Dilation (of the cervix)
_______ 4. EDD
_______ 5. Effacement
_______ 6. Embryo
_______ 7. Engagement
_______ 8. Fetal heart tones
_______ 9. Fetus

A. A woman who has completed two or more pregnancies to the age of viability regardless of whether they ended in live infants or stillbirths
B. The entrance of the fetal head or the presenting part into the pelvic inlet
C. Before birth
D. Three months, or one third, of the gestational period of pregnancy
E. The condition of having borne offspring regardless of the outcome
F. The period of time, usually 4 to 6 weeks, in which the uterus and the body systems are returning to normal delivery
G. The termination of the pregnancy before the fetus reached the age of viability (20 Weeks)
H. The dome-shaped upper portion of the uterus between the fallopian tubes

Copyright © 2008, 2004, 2000, 1995, 1990 by Saunders, an imprint of Elsevier Inc. All rights reserved.

_______ 10. Fundus

_______ 11. Gestation

_______ 12. Gestational age

_______ 13. Gravidity

_______ 14. High-risk

_______ 15. Infant

_______ 16. Lochia

_______ 17. Multigravida

_______ 18. Multipara

_______ 19. Nullipara

_______ 20. Obstetrics

_______ 21. Parity

_______ 22. Pelvimetry

_______ 23. Postpartum

_______ 24. Preeclampsia

_______ 25. Prenatal

_______ 26. Presentation

_______ 27. Preterm birth

_______ 28. Primigravida

_______ 29. Primipara

_______ 30. Puerperium

_______ 31. Quickening

_______ 32. Term birth

_______ 33. Toxemia

I. Having an increased possibility of suffering harm, damage, or death

J. The first movements of the fetus in utero as felt by the mother

K. The child in utero, from the third month after conception to birth

L. A woman who has been pregnant more than once

M. Expected date of delivery, or due date

N. A woman who has carried a pregnancy to viability for the first time, regardless of whether the infant was stillborn or alive at birth

O. The stretching of the external os from an opening a few millimeters wide to an opening large enough to allow the passage of an infant (approximately 10 cm)

P. The period of intrauterine development from conception to birth

Q. A discharge from the uterus after delivery consisting of blood, tissue, white blood cells, and some bacteria

R. The thinning and shortening of the cervical canal from its normal length of 1 to 2 cm to a structure with paper-thin edges in which there is no canal at all

S. The total number of pregnancies a woman has had regardless of duration, including a current pregnancy

T. A woman who has not carried a pregnancy to the point of viability (20 weeks of gestation)

U. The branch of medicine concerned with the care of the woman during pregnancy, childbirth, and the postpartal period

V. A woman who is pregnant for the first time

W. Occurring after childbirth

X. Intermittent and irregular painless uterine contractions that occur throughout pregnancy

Y. Measurement of the capacity and diameter of the maternal pelvis

Z. The heartbeat of the fetus as heard through the mother's abdominal wall

AA. A child from birth to 12 months of age

BB. The child in utero from the time of conception to the beginning of the first trimester

CC. The age of the fetus between conception and birth

DD. A major complication of pregnancy characterized by increasing hypertension, albuminuria, and edema

EE. Indication of the part of the fetus that is closest to the cervix and will be delivered first

FF. Delivery occurring between 20 and 37 weeks regardless of whether the child was born alive or stillborn

GG. Delivery occurring after 37 weeks regardless of whether the child was born alive or stillborn

HH. A condition occurring in pregnant women that includes preeclampsia and eclampsia

Copyright © 2008, 2004, 2000, 1995, 1990 by Saunders, an imprint of Elsevier Inc. All rights reserved.

EVALUATION OF LEARNING

The Gynecological Examination

Directions: Fill in each blank with the correct answer.

1. What is the purpose of the gynecological examination?

____

____

____

2. What is the purpose of performing a breast examination?

____

____

____

3. How often should a woman perform a breast self-examination at home? When should it be performed in relation to the menstrual cycle and why?

____

____

____

4. What are the components of the pelvic examination?

____

____

5. What position is generally used for the pelvic examination?

____

6. How can the medical assistant help the patient to relax during the pelvic examination?

____

____

7. What is the function of a vaginal speculum?

____

____

8. Describe how you would lubricate the vaginal speculum when the physician performs the following:

   a. A Pap test using the direct-smear method: ______________________________

   ____

   b. A Pap test using the liquid-based method: ______________________________

   ____

9. What is the purpose of performing a visual examination of the vagina and the cervix?

____

____

Copyright © 2008, 2004, 2000, 1995, 1990 by Saunders, an imprint of Elsevier Inc. All rights reserved.

10. What is the purpose of performing a Pap test?

11. Describe the schedule for having a Pap test recommended by the American Cancer Society.

12. Why should a specimen for a Pap test not be taken from a woman during her menstrual period?

13. Why should the medical assistant instruct the patient not to douche or insert vaginal medications for 2 days before coming to the medical office to have a Pap test?

14. What are the three types of specimens that may be obtained for a Pap test? Where is each collected?

15. Why must the slides be fixed immediately after collection of a specimen for the direct-smear Pap test method?

16. What are the advantages of using the liquid-based Pap test method?

17. List three conditions that the maturation index can help to evaluate.

18. Why is the Bethesda system recommended for reporting the results of the Pap test?

Copyright © 2008, 2004, 2000, 1995, 1990 by Saunders, an imprint of Elsevier Inc. All rights reserved.

19. Describe the information included in each of the following categories of a cytology report:
    a. Specimen type
    b. Satisfactory for evaluation
    c. Unsatisfactory for evaluation
    d. Negative for intraepithelial lesion or malignancy
    e. Epithelial cell abnormality
    f. Interpretation/result
    g. Automated review
    h. Ancillary testing

20. What is the purpose of performing the bimanual pelvic examination?

21. What is the purpose of the rectal-vaginal examination?

22. Describe the laboratory procedure that can be used to identify *Trichomonas vaginalis* in the medical office.

23. What medication is used to treat trichomoniasis? Why must the patient's sexual partner also be treated?

Copyright © 2008, 2004, 2000, 1995, 1990 by Saunders, an imprint of Elsevier Inc. All rights reserved.

24. Describe the laboratory procedure that can be used to identify *Candida albicans* in the medical office.

25. What medications are used to treat candidiasis?

26. What are the symptoms of PID? What complications can occur from PID?

27. How are chlamydia and gonorrhea usually diagnosed?

28. List the symptoms of each of the following sexually transmitted diseases:
    a. Trichomoniasis in the female

    b. Candidiasis in the female

    c. Chlamydia
        a. Female:

        b. Male:

    d. Gonorrhea
        a. Female:

        b. Male:

Copyright © 2008, 2004, 2000, 1995, 1990 by Saunders, an imprint of Elsevier Inc. All rights reserved.

Prenatal Care

Directions: Fill in each blank with the correct answer.

1. List the three categories of medical office visits for provision of prenatal and postnatal care to the pregnant woman.

___

___

___

2. List the four components of the first prenatal visit.

___

___

___

___

3. What is the purpose of the prenatal record?

___

___

4. List two types of information included in the past medical history (of the prenatal record).

___

___

___

5. List three types of information included in the present pregnancy history.

___

___

___

6. What are the warning signs of a spontaneous abortion?

___

___

7. What is the purpose of the interval prenatal history?

___

___

8. Explain the importance of performing a physical examination on the prenatal patient.

___

___

___

Copyright © 2008, 2004, 2000, 1995, 1990 by Saunders, an imprint of Elsevier Inc. All rights reserved.

9. List the procedures generally included in the initial prenatal examination and, next to each procedure, list the purpose for performing each.

10. What is the importance of making sure a pregnant woman does not have gonorrhea before delivery of the infant?

11. Why is a pregnant woman tested for group B streptococcus (GBS)? When is the woman tested for GBS?

12. What is the purpose of performing a hemoglobin and hematocrit evaluation on a prenatal patient?

13. What is the importance of assessing the Rh factor and ABO blood type of a pregnant woman?

14. What is the purpose of performing a glucose challenge test on a pregnant woman?

15. What is the purpose of performing a rubella titer test on a pregnant woman?

16. Why does the CDC recommend that pregnant women have a blood test to screen for exposure to the hepatitis B virus?

17. What is the purpose of the return prenatal visit? List the usual schedule for return prenatal visits.

Copyright © 2008, 2004, 2000, 1995, 1990 by Saunders, an imprint of Elsevier Inc. All rights reserved.

18. What tests are performed on the patient's urine specimen at each return visit and why is each of these performed?

19. List two purposes of measuring the fundal height.

20. What is the normal range for the fetal heart rate?

21. What is the purpose of performing a vaginal examination as the patient nears term?

22. What is the purpose for performing each of the following special tests and procedures?
    a. Triple screen test
    b. Obstetric ultrasound scan
    c. Amniocentesis
    d. Fetal heart rate monitoring

23. What type of patient preparation is required for transabdominal ultrasound scan?

24. What conditions might warrant performing an amniocentesis?

25. What is the difference between the following fetal heart rate monitoring tests: nonstress test and contraction stress test?

26. What occurs during the puerperium?

Copyright © 2008, 2004, 2000, 1995, 1990 by Saunders, an imprint of Elsevier Inc. All rights reserved.

27. Explain the changes in the lochia that should normally occur during the puerperium.

28. List the procedures generally included in the 6-week postpartum examination.

CRITICAL THINKING ACTIVITIES

A. BREAST CANCER

Select three of the following questions that interest you the most. Using the following Internet sites, answer these questions in the space provided.

National Cancer Institute: www.cancer.gov

American Cancer Society: www.cancer.org

Cancer Facts: www.cancerfacts.com

1. Can a male develop breast cancer? Elaborate on your answer.
2. How does tamoxifen work in treating breast cancer?
3. What are the pros and cons of being tested for the breast cancer gene?
4. What methods are used to reconstruct the breast following a mastectomy?
5. What new diagnostic methods are currently being explored to detect breast cancer?
6. What complementary and alternative therapies are being used in the treatment of breast cancer?

Question # __________

Question # __________

Copyright © 2008, 2004, 2000, 1995, 1990 by Saunders, an imprint of Elsevier Inc. All rights reserved.

Question # ______________________________

____

____

____

____

____

B. METHODS OF CONTRACEPTION

Patients coming to the medical office for gynecological examinations frequently ask the medical assistant questions regarding methods of contraception. The medical assistant should have knowledge of the various types of contraceptives, how they work to prevent pregnancy, and the advantages and disadvantages of each. A list of common contraceptive methods is presented on the next page. List the information requested for each in the spaces provided. The contraceptive Internet sites listed under **On the Web** at the end of Chapter 8 in your textbook can be used to complete this activity.

Contraceptive Method	Mode of Action	Advantages	Disadvantages
Oral contraceptives			
Contraceptive injections			
Contraceptive patch			

Copyright © 2008, 2004, 2000, 1995, 1990 by Saunders, an imprint of Elsevier Inc. All rights reserved.

Contraceptive Method	Mode of Action	Advantages	Disadvantages
Male condom			
Female condom			
Spermicide			
Diaphragm			

Copyright © 2008, 2004, 2000, 1995, 1990 by Saunders, an imprint of Elsevier Inc. All rights reserved.

Contraceptive Method	Mode of Action	Advantages	Disadvantages
Cervical cap			
Vaginal sponge			
Vaginal ring			
IUD			

Copyright © 2008, 2004, 2000, 1995, 1990 by Saunders, an imprint of Elsevier Inc. All rights reserved.

Contraceptive Method	Mode of Action	Advantages	Disadvantages
Natural family planning			
Surgical sterilization			
Emergency contraception			

C. HERPES AND HPV

You are working for an OB/GYN office. Your physician is concerned about the increase in the number of patients contracting herpes and HPV. He asks you to design a colorful, creative, and informative brochure on herpes and HPV using the brochures provided on the following pages. These brochures will be published and placed in the waiting room to educate patients about these sexually transmitted diseases. The STD Internet sites listed under **On the Web** at the end of Chapter 8 in your textbook can be used to complete this activity.

Copyright © 2008, 2004, 2000, 1995, 1990 by Saunders, an imprint of Elsevier Inc. All rights reserved.

Notes

Copyright © 2008, 2004, 2000, 1995, 1990 by Saunders, an imprint of Elsevier Inc. All rights reserved.

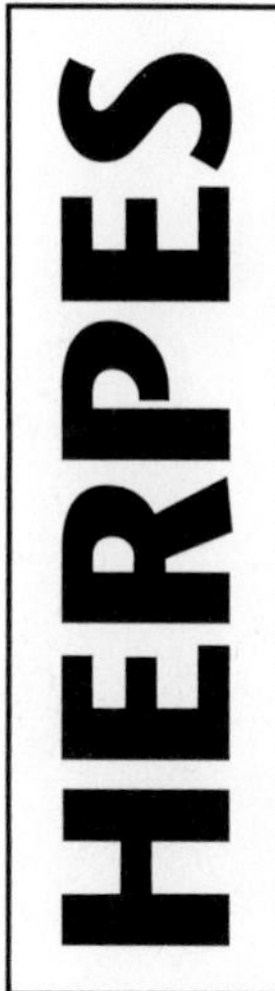

How common is herpes?

How can herpes be prevented?

Copyright © 2008, 2004, 2000, 1995, 1990 by Saunders, an imprint of Elsevier Inc. All rights reserved.

What is herpes?

What are the symptoms?

How do you get herpes?

What causes herpes to recur?

How is herpes diagnosed?

How is herpes treated?

Copyright © 2008, 2004, 2000, 1995, 1990 by Saunders, an imprint of Elsevier Inc. All rights reserved.

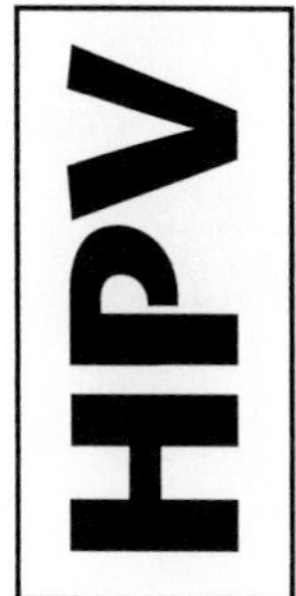

How common is HPV?

What are the complications of HPV?

Copyright © 2008, 2004, 2000, 1995, 1990 by Saunders, an imprint of Elsevier Inc. All rights reserved.

What is HPV?

What are the symptoms?

How do you get HPV?

How is HPV diagnosed?

How is HPV tested?

How can HPV be prevented?

Copyright © 2008, 2004, 2000, 1995, 1990 by Saunders, an imprint of Elsevier Inc. All rights reserved.

D. SIGNS AND SYMPTOMS OF PREGNANCY

Listed here are common signs and symptoms of pregnancy. Define each of them and, if possible, explain what causes the sign or symptom to occur. The pregnancy and childbirth Internet sites listed under **On the Web** at the end of Chapter 8 in your textbook can be used to obtain information to complete this activity.

1. Amenorrhea

____

____

2. Fatigue

____

____

3. Urinary frequency ____

____

4. Quickening

____

____

5. Goodell's sign ____

____

6. Hegar's sign

____

____

7. Braxton Hicks contractions

____

____

8. Skin changes: striae gravidarum, chloasma, linea nigra

____

____

____

____

E. CALCULATION OF THE EDD

Calculate the EDD of the following patients using Nägele's rule. The first day of each patient's last menstrual period (LMP) is listed here:

1. February 10, 2008 ____
2. April 28, 2008 ____
3. July 20, 2008 ____
4. October 2, 2008 ____
5. December22, 2008 ____

Copyright © 2008, 2004, 2000, 1995, 1990 by Saunders, an imprint of Elsevier Inc. All rights reserved.

F. RECORDING GRAVIDITY AND PARITY

The following patients are in your medical office for their first prenatal visit. In the space provided, record the following information in terms of gravidity and parity.

1. Melissa Turner is pregnant for the third time. Her first pregnancy resulted in the birth of a baby boy, now alive and well. She lost her second pregnancy at 16 weeks gestation.

   G: _________ T: _________ P: _________ A: _________ L: _________

2. Amanda Schuster is pregnant for the third time. Her first pregnancy resulted in the birth of twin girls, now alive and well. Her second pregnancy resulted in the birth of a baby girl, now alive and well.

   G: _________ T: _________ P: _________ A: _________ L: _________

3. Leah Morrow is pregnant for the fourth time. She lost her first pregnancy at 2 month's gestation. Her second pregnancy was carried to term, but resulted in the birth of a stillborn. Her third pregnancy resulted in the birth of a baby girl, now alive and well.

   G: _________ T: _________ P: _________ A: _________ L: _________

4. Rose Samson is pregnant for the fifth time. She carried her first pregnancy to 24 weeks and delivered a stillborn baby. Her second pregnancy resulted in the birth of a baby girl, now alive and well. She lost her third pregnancy at 12 weeks gestation. Her fourth pregnancy resulted in the birth of a baby boy, now alive and well.

   G: _________ T: _________ P: _________ A: _________ L: _________

G. NUTRITION DURING PREGNANCY

1. Brianna Flint is in your medical office for her first prenatal visit. This is her first pregnancy, and she is concerned about adequate nutrition during her pregnancy. Explain why the following nutrients are of particular importance during pregnancy and provide good food sources of each. The pregnancy and childbirth Internet sites listed under **On the Web** at the end of Chapter 8 in your textbook can be used to obtain information to complete this activity.
2. In a classroom situation, select a partner. In a role-playing situation, one student takes the role of the medical assistant and the other plays the role of the patient. Explain to the patient the importance of these nutrients and list good food sources of each.

Copyright © 2008, 2004, 2000, 1995, 1990 by Saunders, an imprint of Elsevier Inc. All rights reserved.

Nutrient	Importance during Pregnancy	Food Sources
Iron		
Calcium		
Protein		
Folic acid		

Copyright © 2008, 2004, 2000, 1995, 1990 by Saunders, an imprint of Elsevier Inc. All rights reserved.

H. MINOR DISCOMFORTS OF PREGNANCY

1. Listed here are the minor discomforts that a prenatal patient may experience during pregnancy. Indicate measures the patient can take to help prevent or relieve each discomfort. The pregnancy and childbirth Internet sites listed under **On the Web** at the end of Chapter 8 in your textbook can be used to obtain information to complete this activity.
2. In a classroom situation, select a partner. In a role-playing situation, one student takes the role of the medical assistant and the other plays the role of the patient. The patient should indicate that they have a problem with each of these discomforts, and the medical assistant should respond by describing measures the patient can take to help prevent or relive each problem.

   a. Nausea (morning sickness)

   ______

   ______

   b. Heartburn

   ______

   ______

   c. Fatigue

   ______

   ______

   d. Constipation

   ______

   ______

   e. Backache

   ______

   ______

   f. Breathing difficulties

   ______

   ______

   g. Varicose veins

   ______

   ______

   h. Hemorrhoids

   ______

   ______

   i. Leg cramps

   ______

   ______

   j. Swelling of the lower legs and feet

   ______

   ______

Copyright © 2008, 2004, 2000, 1995, 1990 by Saunders, an imprint of Elsevier Inc. All rights reserved.

I. HEALTH PROMOTION DURING PREGNANCY

1. Obtain a prenatal guidebook and list the information included in it regarding guidelines the patient should follow with respect to each of the areas presented below. The pregnancy and childbirth Internet sites listed under **On the Web** at the end of Chapter 8 in your textbook can also be used to obtain information to complete this activity.
2. In a classroom situation, select a partner. In a role-playing situation, one student takes the role of the medical assistant and the other plays the role of the patient. The patient should ask for guidance regarding each of these areas, and the medical assistant should respond with appropriate information.

   a. Nutrition ____________________

   ____

   b. Employment

   ____

   ____

   c. Exercise

   ____

   ____

   d. Travel

   ____

   ____

   e. Smoking

   ____

   ____

   f. Alcohol

   ____

   ____

   g. Medication

   ____

   ____

J. BREAST-FEEDING

1. Lucy Clark asks you for information regarding the advantages and disadvantages of both breast-feeding and bottle-feeding. List these in the following chart. The pregnancy and childbirth Internet sites listed under **On the Web** at the end of Chapter 8 in your textbook can also be used to obtain information to complete this activity.
2. In a classroom situation, select a partner. In a role-playing situation, one student takes the role of the medical assistant and the other plays the role of the patient. The patient should ask for information regarding the advantages and disadvantages of both methods, and the medical assistant should respond with appropriate information.

Copyright © 2008, 2004, 2000, 1995, 1990 by Saunders, an imprint of Elsevier Inc. All rights reserved.

Bottle-feeding	
Advantages	*Disadvantages*
Breast-feeding	
Advantages	*Disadvantages*

K. PRENATAL ULTRASOUND

View obstetric ultrasound scans at the following Internet site: www.ob-ultrasound.net/frames.htm. The following scans can be viewed at this site:

1. Gestational sac
2. Fetus at various gestational ages
3. Fetal measurements
4. Fetal organs
5. 3-D images of the fetus

Copyright © 2008, 2004, 2000, 1995, 1990 by Saunders, an imprint of Elsevier Inc. All rights reserved.

L. CROSSWORD PUZZLE
Gynecology and Obstetrics

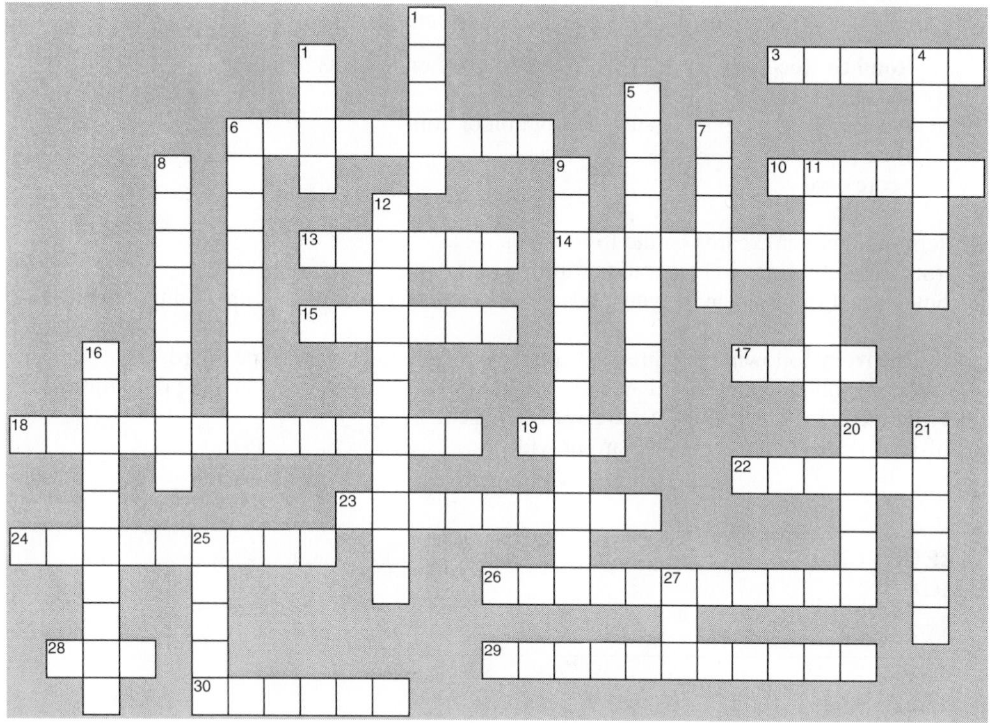

Directions: Complete the crossword puzzle using the clues presented below.

ACROSS

3 STD preventer
6 Breast radiograph
10 Malignant or benign?
13 What most breast lumps are
14 May not occur with STD, especially females
15 Age to begin BSE
17 Definite minor Pap changes
18 Abnormal reported as normal
19 Screening test for GDM
22 Breast exam position
23 Pelvic exam position
24 STD symptom
26 Freezes the cervix
28 Cervical cancer risk factor
29 Spread of cancer

DOWN

1 Birth size of macrosomia baby
2 Warning sign of breast cancer
4 Risk factor for GDM
5 Antibiotics cure this STD
6 Menstrual cycle ceases
7 HPV symptom
8 What all STDs can be
9 Cervical cancer surgery
11 What a GDM mother might need
12 Serious STD complication
16 Examination of the cervix
20 Breast cancer increases (age)
21 A viral STD
25 Slightly abnormal Pap cells
27 Long-term use increases breast cancer risk
30 How cervical cancer develops

Copyright © 2008, 2004, 2000, 1995, 1990 by Saunders, an imprint of Elsevier Inc. All rights reserved.

M. ROAD TO RECOVERY
OB/GYN Terminology

Object: The object of the game is to lead your "patient" to recovery by correctly providing the definition to medical terms relating to gynecology and obstetrics.

Needed: **Road to Recovery** game board (located at the end of this manual)
Game cards
A token for each player (such as a button or coin)
Dice (1)
Score card

Directions:

1. Cut out the terminology game cards on the following pages.
2. Study the terms and definitions in preparation for the game.
3. Place one complete set of terms on the game board with the definitions facing up (and the medical terms facing down).
4. Play **Road to Recovery** following the directions on the reverse side of the game board.
5. Place the set of cards on the game board again with the medical terms face up and the definitions face down; continue playing the game until all the cards have been used.
6. Keep track of your points using the score card provided.

ROAD TO RECOVERY
SCORE CARD

Name: ______________________________

Recording Points:
Using the Game Card Points box, cross off a number each time you answer a game card correctly (starting with 5 and continuing in sequence). Your total game card points will be equal to the last number you crossed off. Record this number in the space provided (1). Record any extra points you were awarded during the game (2), and any points that were deducted (3). To determine your total points, add (1) and (2) together and deduct (3). Record this number in the Total Points Earned space provided. Compare your score with the other players and determine where you placed. Place a check mark next to the level of recovery your patient attained.

Game Card Points:

5	75	145	215
10	80	150	220
15	85	155	225
20	90	160	230
25	95	165	235
30	100	170	240
35	105	175	245
40	110	180	250
45	115	185	255
50	120	190	260
55	125	195	265
60	130	200	270
65	135	205	275
70	140	210	280

Calculation of Points:

(1) Total Game Card Points: ________

(2) Additional Points Awarded: ________

(3) Deducted Points: ________

TOTAL POINTS EARNED: ________

LEVEL OF RECOVERY:

Patient's Name: ______________________

☐ First Place: **Fully Recovered**
☐ Second Place: **Almost Recovered**
☐ Third Place: **Still Recovering**
☐ Fourth Place: **Gasping for Air**

Copyright © 2008, 2004, 2000, 1995, 1990 by Saunders, an imprint of Elsevier Inc. All rights reserved.

Abortion	Adnexal	Amenorrhea	Atypical
Braxton Hicks contractions	Cervix	Colposcopy	Cytology
Dilation (of the cervix)	Dysmenorrhea	Dyspareunia	Dysplasia
EDD	Effacement	Embryo	Endocervix

Deviation from normal	The absence, or cessation, of a normal menstrual period	Adjacent	Termination of the pregnancy before the fetus reaches the age of viability (20 weeks)
The science that deals with the study of cells	Examination of the cervix using a lighted instrument with a magnifying lens	The lower narrow end of the uterus that opens into the vagina	Intermittent and irregularpainless uterine contractions that occur throughout pregnancy
The growth of abnormal cells	Pain in the vagina or pelvis during sexual intercourse	Pain associated with the menstrual period	The stretching of the external os to an opening large enough to allow the passage of an infant
The mucous membrane lining the cervical canal	The child in utero from the time of conception to the beginning of the first trimester	The thinning and shortening of the cervical canal to no canal at all	Expected date of delivery

Engagement	External Os	Fetal heart rate	Fetal heart tones
Fetus	Fundus	Gestation	Gestational age
Gravidity	Gynecology	Infant	Internal os
Lochia	Menopause	Menorrhagia	Metrorrhagia

The heart beat of the fetus as heard through the mother's abdominal wall	The number of times the fetal heart beats per minute	The opening of the cervical canal of the uterus into the vagina	The entrance of the fetal head into the pelvic in let
The age of the fetus between conception and birth	The period of intrauterine development from conception to birth	The dome-shaped upper portion of the uterus between the fallopian tubes	The child in utero from the third month after conception to birth
The internal opening of the cervical canal into the uterus	A child from birth to 1 year of age	The branch of medicine that deals with diseases of the reproductive organs of women	The total number of pregnancies a woman has had
Bleeding between menstrual periods	Excessive bleeding during a menstrual period	The permanent cessation of menstruation	A discharge from the uterus after delivery

Multigravida	**Multipara**	**Nullipara**	**Obstetrics**
Ectocervix	**Perimenopause**	**Perineum**	**Position**
Postpartum	**Preeclampsia**	**Prenatal**	**Presentation**
Preterm birth	**Primigravida**	**Primipara**	**Puerperium**

The branch of medicine concerned with the care of the woman during pregnancy, childbirth, and the postpartal period

A woman who has not carried a pregnancy to the point of viability

A woman who has completed two or more pregnancies to the age of viability

A woman who has been pregnant more than once

The relationship of the presenting part of the fetus to the maternal pelvis

The external region between the vaginal orifice and the anus in a female

The phase prior to the onset of menopause

The part of the cervix that projects into the vagina

The part of the fetus that is closest to the cervix and will be delivered first

Before birth

A major complication of pregnancy of unknown cause, characterized by increasing hypertension, albuminuria, and edema

Occurring after child birth

The period of time in which the uterus and body systems are returning to normal following delivery

A woman who has carried a pregnancy to viability for the first time

A woman who is pregnant for the first time

Delivery occurring between 20 and 37 weeks

Quickening	Risk factor	Term birth	Toxemia
Trimester	Vulva		

A condition occurring in pregnant women that includes preeclampsia and eclampsia	Delivery occurring after 37 weeks	Anything that increases an individual's chance of developing a disease	The first movements of the fetus as felt by the mother
		The region of the external genital organs in the female	Three months or one third of the gestational period of pregnancy

PRACTICE FOR COMPETENCY

Procedure 8-1: Breast Self-Examination. Instruct an individual about the procedure for performing a breast self-examination and record the procedure in the chart provided.

CHART	
Date	

Copyright © 2008, 2004, 2000, 1995, 1990 by Saunders, an imprint of Elsevier Inc. All rights reserved.

Chart	
Date	

Copyright © 2008, 2004, 2000, 1995, 1990 by Saunders, an imprint of Elsevier Inc. All rights reserved.

Procedure 8-2: Gynecological Examination

1. Complete the cytology request form provided using a female classmate as the patient.
2. Practice the procedure for assisting with a gynecological examination. Record the vital signs and height and weight in the chart provided.

CHART	
Date	

Copyright © 2008, 2004, 2000, 1995, 1990 by Saunders, an imprint of Elsevier Inc. All rights reserved.

GYN CYTOLOGY REQUISITION

THOMAS WOODSIDE, MD
501 MAIN ST
ST. LOUIS, MO 63146
(314) 883–0093

PATIENT INFO

Patient's Name (Last)	(First)	(MI)	Date of Birth MO | DAY | YR	Collection Time : AM PM	Collection Date MO | DAY | YR	Patient's ID #

Patient's Address	Phone	
City	State	ZIP

RESP. PARTY

Name of Responsible Party (if different from patient)		
Address of Responsible Party	APT #	
City	State	ZIP

INSURANCE

Patient's Relationship to Responsible Party: 1. Self 2. Spouse 3. Child 4. Other

Insurance Comany Name	Plan	Carrier Code
Subscriber/Member #	Location	Group #
Insurance Address	Physician's Provider #	
City	State	ZIP
Employer's Name or Number	Insured SSN	

Diagnosis/Signs/Symptoms in ICD-9 Format (Highest Specificity)

REQUIRED

ICD-9 codes are the internationally accepted method of describing the clinical picture of the patient. All diagnoses should be provided by the ordering physician or his or her authorized designee. The following is a partial list of of common diagnoses in ICD-9 format. Most third party payers require an ICD-9 code to indicate the medical necessity of the test(s) and or profile(s) ordered. For a complete list of all ICD-9 codes, please refer to a current ICD-9 manual.

V76.2	Routine Cervical Pap Smear	616.0	Cervicitis	626.8	Abnormal Bleeding
V15.89	High Risk Cervical Screening	616.10	Vaginitis	627.1	Postmenopausal Bleeding
V22.2	Pregnancy	617.0	Endometriosis, Uterus	627.3	Atrophic Vaginitis
079.4	Human Papillomavirus	622.1	Dysplasia, Cervix	795.0	Abnormal Cervical Pap Smear
180.0	Malignant Neoplasm, Cervix	623.0	Dysplasia, Vagina		

COLLECTION METHOD

Liquid Based Prep

192055 ☐ Thin Prep Pap Test

192039 ☐ Thin Prep Pap Test w/reflex to HPV Hybrid Capture when ASC-US or SIL

192047 ☐ Thin Prep Pap Test w/reflex to high-risk only HPV Hybrid Capture when ASC-US

Pap Smear

009100 ☐ 1 Slide 009191 ☐ 2 Slides

Pap Smear and Maturation Index

009209 ☐ 1 Slide 190074 ☐ 2 Slides

SOURCE OF SPECIMEN

☐ **Cervical**
☐ **Endocervical**
☐ **Vaginal**

Date LMP

____/____/____
Mo Day Year

COLLECTION TECHNIQUE

☐ **Spatula**
☐ **Brush**
☐ **Broom**
☐ **Other**
____

PATIENT HISTORY

☐ **Pregnant**
☐ **Lactating**
☐ **Oral Contraceptives**
☐ **Postmenopausal**
☐ **Hormone Replacement Therapy**
☐ **PMP Bleeding**
☐ **Postpartum**
☐ **IUD**
☐ **Postcoital Bleeding**
☐ **DES Exposure**
☐ **Previous Abnormal Pap Test**
☐ **Other** ____________

PREVIOUS TREATMENT — Date/Results

☐ **None**
☐ **Colposcopy and Bx** ____________
☐ **Cryosurgery** ____________
☐ **LEEP** ____________
☐ **Laser Vaporization** ____________
☐ **Conization** ____________
☐ **Hysterectomy** ____________
☐ **Radiation** ____________
☐ **Chemotherapy** ____________

Copyright © 2008, 2004, 2000, 1995, 1990 by Saunders, an imprint of Elsevier Inc. All rights reserved.

Procedure 8-3: Return Prenatal Examination

1. Complete the prenatal health history form provided using a female classmate as the patient.
2. Prepare the patient and assist with a return prenatal examination. Record the results of procedures you performed on the chart provided.

CHART	
Date	

Copyright © 2008, 2004, 2000, 1995, 1990 by Saunders, an imprint of Elsevier Inc. All rights reserved.

Chart	
Date	

Copyright © 2008, 2004, 2000, 1995, 1990 by Saunders, an imprint of Elsevier Inc. All rights reserved.

PRENATAL HEALTH HISTORY

PATIENT INFORMATION

Date: ______________ EDD: ______________ Referred By: ______________
Name: ______________ Phone (home): ______________
LAST FIRST MIDDLE
Phone (work): ______________
Address: ______________ Emergency Contact: ______________
Phone: ______________
CITY STATE ZIP

Date of Birth: ___/___/___ Age: ___ Marital Status: ______________
Occupation: ______________
Education: ☐ High School ☐ College ☐ Post-graduate

PAST MEDICAL HISTORY

	O Neg + Pos	DETAIL POSITIVE REMARKS INCLUDE DATE AND TREATMENT			O Neg + Pos	DETAIL POSITIVE REMARKS INCLUDE DATE AND TREATMENT
1. DIABETES				16. D (Rh) SENSITIZED		
2. HYPERTENSION				17. PULMONARY (TB, ASTHMA)		
3. HEART DISEASE				18. RHEUMATIC FEVER		
4. AUTOIMMUNE DISORDER				19. BLEEDING TENDENCY		
5. KIDNEY DISEASE/UTI				20. GYN SURGERY		
6. NEUROLOGIC/EPILEPSY						
7. PSYCHIATRIC				21. OPERATIONS/HOSPITALIZATIONS (YEAR AND REASON)		
8. HEPATITIS/LIVER DISEASE						
9. VARICOSITIES/PHLEBITIS						
10. THYROID DYSFUNCTION				22. ANESTHETIC COMPLICATIONS		
11. TRAUMA/DOMESTIC VIOLENCE				23. HISTORY OF ABNORMAL PAP		
12. BLOOD TRANSFUSION				24. UTERINE ANOMALY/DES		
	AMT/DAY PREPREG.	AMT/DAY PREG.	# YEARS USE	25. INFERTILITY		
13. TOBACCO				26. SEXUALLY TRANSMITTED DISEASE		
14. ALCOHOL						
15. STREET DRUGS				27. OTHER		

IMMUNIZATIONS:

Mark an X next to those you have had.

☐ Influenza ☐ Chickenpox
☐ Hepatitis B ☐ Pneumococcal
☐ Hib ☐ Tuberculin Test
☐ Polio ☐ Tetanus Booster
☐ MMR

ALLERGIES:

List all allergies (foods, drugs, environment). ☐ None

____
____
____
____
____
____

MENSTRUAL HISTORY

Menarche: Age of Onset ______________ GYN Disorders (List): ______________
Frequency: Q ______ Days
Duration: ______ Days
Amount of Flow: ☐ Small ☐ Moderate ☐ Large
On contraceptive at conception? ☐ Yes ☐ No

Copyright © 2008, 2004, 2000, 1995, 1990 by Saunders, an imprint of Elsevier Inc. All rights reserved.

OBSTETRIC HISTORY

G ________ T ________ P ________ A ________ L ________
(Total Pregnancies) (Term) (Preterm) (Abortions) (Living Children)

PREVIOUS PREGNANCIES:

DATE MONTH/ YEAR	WEEKS GEST.	LENGTH OF LABOR	BIRTH WEIGHT	SEX M/F	TYPE DELIVERY	ANES.	MATERNAL COMPLICATIONS	INFANT COMPLICATIONS

PRESENT PREGNANCY HISTORY

NAUSEA			ABDOMINAL PAIN		
VOMITING			URINARY COMPLAINTS		
FATIGUE			VAGINAL BLEEDING		
BREAST CHANGES			VAGINAL DISCHARGE		
INDIGESTION			PRURITIS		
CONSTIPATION			ACCIDENTS		
PERSISTENT HEADACHES			SURGERY		
DIZZINESS			X-RAYS		
VISUAL DISTURBANCE			RUBELLA EXPOSURE		
EDEMA (SPECIFY AREA)			OTHER VIRAL INFECTIONS		

LMP _____/_____/_____
Mo Day Year

Amount of Flow: ☐ **Small** ☐ **Moderate** ☐ **Large**

CURRENT MEDICATIONS: (Include prescription, OTC, herbal, and vitamins). ☐ **None**

Medication **Frequency**

____

____

____

INITIAL PHYSICAL EXAMINATION

DATE ___/___/___

1. HEENT	☐ NORMAL	☐ ABNORMAL	12. VULVA	☐ NORMAL	☐ CONDYLOMA	☐ LESIONS
2. FUNDI	☐ NORMAL	☐ ABNORMAL	13. VAGINA	☐ NORMAL	☐ INFLAMMATION	☐ DISCHARGE
3. TEETH	☐ NORMAL	☐ ABNORMAL	14. CERVIX	☐ NORMAL	☐ INFLAMMATION	☐ LESIONS
4. THYROID	☐ NORMAL	☐ ABNORMAL	15. UTERUS SIZE	______ WEEKS		☐ FIBROIDS
5. BREASTS	☐ NORMAL	☐ ABNORMAL	16. ADNEXA	☐ NORMAL	☐ MASS	
6. LUNGS	☐ NORMAL	☐ ABNORMAL	17. RECTUM	☐ NORMAL	☐ ABNORMAL	
7. HEART	☐ NORMAL	☐ ABNORMAL	18. DIAGONAL CONJUGATE	☐ REACHED	☐ NO	______ CM
8. ABDOMEN	☐ NORMAL	☐ ABNORMAL	19. SPINES	☐ AVERAGE	☐ PROMINENT	☐ BLUNT
9. EXTREMITIES	☐ NORMAL	☐ ABNORMAL	20. SACRUM	☐ CONCAVE	☐ STRAIGHT	☐ ANTERIOR
10. SKIN	☐ NORMAL	☐ ABNORMAL	21. SUBPUBIC ARCH	☐ NORMAL	☐ WIDE	☐ NARROW
11. LYMPH NODES	☐ NORMAL	☐ ABNORMAL	22. GYNECOID PELVIC TYPE	☐ YES	☐ NO	

COMMENTS (Number and explain abnormals): ______________________________

____

____

______________________ **EXAM BY** ______________________

Copyright © 2008, 2004, 2000, 1995, 1990 by Saunders, an imprint of Elsevier Inc. All rights reserved.

PATIENT'S NAME ____________________

INTERVAL PRENATAL HISTORY

Date 20__	Weeks Gestation	Height of Fundus (cm)	Weight	B/P	Urine Glucose	Urine Protein	FHT	Vaginal Examination	Presentation	Edema	Discharge	Bleeding	Contractions	Fetal Activity	NST	Next Appt.	Initials
				/													
				/													
				/													
				/													
				/													
				/													
				/													
				/													
				/													
				/													
				/													
				/													
				/													
				/													

PLANS/EDUCATION (COUNSELED ☑)

- ☐ ANESTHESIA PLANS ____________
- ☐ TOXOPLASMOSIS PRECAUTIONS (CATS/RAW MEAT) ____________
- ☐ CHILDBIRTH CLASSES ____________
- ☐ PHYSICAL/SEXUAL ACTIVITY ____________
- ☐ LABOR SIGNS ____________
- ☐ NUTRITION COUNSELING ____________
- ☐ BREAST OR BOTTLE FEEDING ____________
- ☐ NEWBORN CAR SEAT ____________
- ☐ POSTPARTUM BIRTH CONTROL ____________
- ☐ ENVIRONMENTAL/WORK HAZARDS ____________
- ☐ TUBAL STERILIZATION ____________
- ☐ VBAC COUNSELING ____________
- ☐ CIRCUMCISION ____________
- ☐ TRAVEL ____________
- ☐ LIFESTYLE, TOBACCO, ALCOHOL ____________

REQUESTS ____________

TUBAL STERILIZATION CONSENT SIGNED **DATE** __/__/__ **INITIALS** ____________

Copyright © 2008, 2004, 2000, 1995, 1990 by Saunders, an imprint of Elsevier Inc. All rights reserved.

LABORATORY		PATIENT'S NAME ______		
INITIAL LABS	**DATE**	**RESULTS**	**REVIEWED**	**COMMENTS**
BLOOD TYPE	/ /	A B AB O		
Rh FACTOR	/ /	☐ Pos ☐ Neg		
Rh ANTIBODY SCREEN	/ /	☐ Pos ☐ Neg		
HCT/HGB	/ /	____% ____ g/dL		
RUBELLA ANTIBODY TITER	/ /	Immune Nonimmune		
VDRL	/ /	☐ NR ☐ R		
HBsAg (HEPATITIS B)	/ /	☐ Pos ☐ Neg		
HIV	/ /	☐ Pos ☐ Neg ☐ Declined		
URINE CULTURE/SCREEN	/ /			
PAP TEST	/ /	☐ Normal ☐ Abnormal		
CHLAMYDIA (DNA PROBE)	/ /	☐ Pos ☐ Neg		
GONORRHEA (DNA PROBE)	/ /	☐ Pos ☐ Neg		
7–20 WEEK LABS (WHEN INDICATED/ELECTED)	**DATE**	**RESULTS**	**REVIEWED**	**COMMENTS**
ULTRASOUND #1 (7–13 WEEKS)	/ /	EDD:		
ULTRASOUND #2 (18–20 WEEKS)	/ /	EFW:		
TRIPLE SCREEN (15–20 WEEKS)	/ /			
CVS	/ /			
AMNIOCENTESIS	/ /			
24–28 WEEK LABS (WHEN INDICATED)	**DATE**	**RESULTS**	**REVIEWED**	**COMMENTS**
HCT/HGB	/ /	____ % ____ g/dL		
GCT (24–28 WKS)	/ /	1 Hour ______		
GTT (IF SCREEN ABNORMAL)	/ /	____ FBS ____ 1 Hour ____ 2 Hour ____ 3 Hour		
D (Rh) ANTIBODY SCREEN	/ /			
D IMMUNE GLOBULIN (RhIG) GIVEN (28 WKS)	/ /	SIGNATURE		
32–36 WEEK LABS	**DATE**	**RESULTS**	**REVIEWED**	**COMMENTS**
HCT/HGB (32 WKS)	/ /	____ % ____ g/dL		
ULTRASOUND #3 (34 WKS)	/ /	EFW:		
GROUP B STREP (35–37 WKS)	/ /	☐ Pos ☐ Neg		
ADDITIONAL LAB TESTS	**DATE**	**RESULTS**	**REVIEWED**	**COMMENTS**
	/ /			
	/ /			
	/ /			
	/ /			
	/ /			

Copyright © 2008, 2004, 2000, 1995, 1990 by Saunders, an imprint of Elsevier Inc. All rights reserved.

EVALUATION OF COMPETENCY

Procedure 8-1: Breast Self-Examination Instructions

Name: ______________________________ Date: ____________

Evaluated By: ______________________________ Score: ____________

Performance Objective

Outcome:	Instruct an individual in the procedure for performing a breast self-examination.
Conditions:	Small pillow.
Standards:	Time: 10 minutes. Student completed procedure in ____ minutes.
	Accuracy: Satisfactory score on the Performance Evaluation Checklist.

Performance Evaluation Checklist

Trial 1	*Trial 2*	*Point Value*	*Performance Standards*
		•	Greeted the patient and introduced yourself.
		•	Identified patient and explained that you will be instructing the patient in a BSE.
		▷	Explained the purpose of the exam, when to perform it, and the three methods of examination.
		▷	Explained why three methods are used to examine the breasts.
			INSTRUCTED THE PATIENT AS FOLLOWS:
			1. Before a Mirror
		•	Remove clothing from the waist up.
			Place arms at sides and inspect the breasts.
		•	Inspect for a change in size or shape; swelling, puckering, or dimpling; change in skin texture; nipple retraction; change in nipple size or position compared to other breast.
		▷	Described what might cause puckering or dimpling of the skin.
		•	Slowly raise arms over head and inspect the breasts.
		▷	Stated what should normally occur when the arms are moved at the same time.
		•	Rest palms on hips, press down firmly, and inspect the breasts.
		▷	Stated the purpose of flexing the chest muscles.
		•	Gently squeeze each nipple and look for a discharge.
			2. Lying Down
		•	Place a pillow (or folded towel) under right shoulder.
		•	Place right hand behind head.
		▷	Stated the purpose of the pillow and hand placement.

Copyright © 2008, 2004, 2000, 1995, 1990 by Saunders, an imprint of Elsevier Inc. All rights reserved.

Trial 1	Trial 2	Point Value	*Performance Standards*
		•	Use the finger pads of the middle three fingers of the left hand.
		▷	Explained why the finger pads should be used.
		•	Use small rotating motions and continuous firm pressure.
		•	Use one of the following patterns to move around the breast: circular, vertical strip, or wedge.
		▷	Stated why a pattern is used.
			Circular:
		•	Visualize breast as a clock face.
		•	Start at outside edge of breast.
		•	Proceed clockwise until you return to starting point.
		•	Move in 1 inch and repeat the circle.
		•	Continue until nipple is reached.
			Vertical Strip:
		•	Divide breast into strips.
		•	Start at underarm.
		•	Slowly move fingers down until they are below the breast.
		•	Move fingers 1 inch toward middle and move back up.
		•	Repeat until entire breast has been examined.
			Wedge:
		•	Divide breasts into wedges.
		•	Start at outer edge of breast.
		•	Move fingers toward the nipple and back to edge of breast.
		•	Repeat until entire breast has been examined.
			Use the following techniques during the exam:
		•	Press firmly enough to feel the different breast tissues.
		▷	Explained how to perform each pattern.
		•	Palpate for lumps, hard knots, or thickening.
		▷	Explained how normal breast tissue feels.
		•	Examine the entire chest area from your collarbone to the base of a properly fitted bra and from the breastbone to the underarm.
		•	Pay special attention to the area between the breast and underarm including the underarm itself.
		▷	Explained why the underarm should be examined.
		•	Continue the examination until every part of the right breast has been examined, including the nipple.
		•	Repeat the procedure on the left breast, with a pillow or rolled towel under the left shoulder, the left hand behind the head, and using the right hand to palpate.

Copyright © 2008, 2004, 2000, 1995, 1990 by Saunders, an imprint of Elsevier Inc. All rights reserved.

Trial 1	Trial 2	Point Value	Performance Standards
			3. In the Shower
		●	Gently lather each breast.
		▷	Explained why the breasts should be examined in the shower.
		●	Place right hand behind head.
		●	Use the finger pads of the middle three fingers of the left hand.
		●	Use small rotating motions and continuous firm pressure.
		●	Use your preferred pattern to thoroughly examine the right breast and underarm for lumps, hard knots, or thickening.
		●	Repeat the procedure on the left breast using the pads of your right fingers.
		●	Instructed the patient to report any lumps or changes to the physician immediately.
		▷	Explained why it is important to report changes immediately.
		●	Charted the procedure correctly.
		*	Completed the procedure within 10 minutes.
			TOTALS

CHART	
Date	

Evaluation of Student Performance

EVALUATION CRITERIA			COMMENTS
Symbol	Category	Point Value	
*	Critical Step	16 points	
●	Essential Step	6 points	
▷	Theory Question	2 points	
Score calculation: 100 points – ______ points missed _____ Score Satisfactory score: 85 or above			

AAMA/CAAHEP Competency Achieved:

☑ III. C. 3. c. (3) (c): Provide instruction for health maintenance and disease prevention.

Copyright © 2008, 2004, 2000, 1995, 1990 by Saunders, an imprint of Elsevier Inc. All rights reserved.

Notes

Copyright © 2008, 2004, 2000, 1995, 1990 by Saunders, an imprint of Elsevier Inc. All rights reserved.

EVALUATION OF COMPETENCY

Procedure 8-2: Assisting with a Gynecological Examination

Name: ______________________________ Date: ____________

Evaluated By: ______________________________ Score: ____________

Performance Objective

Outcome: Assist with a gynecologic examination.

Conditions: Using an examining table.

Given the following: disposable gloves, examining gown and drape, disposable vaginal speculum, lubricant, gauze pads, Hemoccult slide and developing solution, tissues, biohazard waste container, cytology request form, biohazard specimen transport bag.

Direct Smear Method: ThinPrep Vial, plastic spatula and endocervical brush or cytology broom.

Liquid-Prep Method: ThinPrep Vial, plastic spatula and endocervical brush or cytology broom.

Standards: Time: 15 minutes. Student completed procedure in ____ minutes.

Accuracy: Satisfactory score on the Performance Evaluation Checklist.

Performance Evaluation Checklist

Trial 1	Trial 2	Point Value	*Performance Standards*
		•	Sanitized hands.
		•	Assembled equipment.
		•	Completed as much of the cytology request form as possible.
			Prepared the collection materials:
		•	***Pap Smear Method:*** Identified the slides on the frosted edge.
		•	***Liquid-Prep Method:*** Checked the expiration date and labeled the vial.
		•	Greeted the patient and introduced yourself.
		•	Identified the patient and explained the procedure.
		•	Escorted the patient to the examining room.
		•	Asked patient if she has any problems or concerns and chart the informaton.
		•	Completed the cytology request by asking necessary questions.

Copyright © 2008, 2004, 2000, 1995, 1990 by Saunders, an imprint of Elsevier Inc. All rights reserved.

Trial 1	Trial 2	Point Value	*Performance Standards*
		•	Measured vital signs and height and weight and charted the results correctly.
			Prepared patient for the examination:
		•	Asked patient if she needs to empty bladder.
		▷	Explained why the bladder should be empty for the examination.
		•	Instructed the patient to undress and put on the examining gown with opening in front.
		•	Informed patient that physician would be in soon.
		•	Left the room to provide patient privacy.
			Made medical record available for review by the physician.
		•	Checked to make sure patient is ready.
		•	Informed physician that the patient was ready.
			Assisted the physician:
		•	Positioned and draped patient in a supine position for the breast examination.
		•	Positioned and draped patient in the lithotomy position for the pelvic examination.
		•	Prepared the vaginal speculum and handed it to the physician.
		▷	Explained how to prepare the speculum for the Pap smear method and the liquid-prep method.
		•	Prepared the light for physician.
		•	Handed vaginal speculum to physician.
		•	Reassured patient and helped her to relax during the examination.
		▷	Explained why patient should be relaxed during the examination.
			Assisted with collection of the Pap specimen:
		•	Applied gloves.
			1. *Direct Smear Method*
		•	Held each slide for the physician to smear the specimen on it.
		•	Immediately fixed the slides.
		•	Allowed slides to dry and placed them in a slide container.
			2(a). ThinPrep Spatula and Brush Method
		•	Held the vial to receive the collection device from the physician.
		•	Correctly rinsed each collection device in the liquid preservative.
		▷	Explained why the collection device should be swirled vigorously.
		•	Discarded each collection device in a biohazard waste container.
		•	Tightened the cap on the vial.
			2(b). Thin Prep Broom Method
		•	Held the vial to receive the broom from the physician.
		•	Correctly rinsed the broom in the liquid preservative.
		•	Discarded the broom in a biohazard waste container.
		•	Tightened the cap on the vial.
			3. SurePath Spatula and Brush Method

Copyright © 2008, 2004, 2000, 1995, 1990 by Saunders, an imprint of Elsevier Inc. All rights reserved.

Trial 1	Trial 2	Point Value	Performance Standards
		•	Held the vial to receive each collection device from the physician.
		•	Broke off or disconnected tip of each collection device.
		•	Discarded each handle in a regular waste container.
		•	Tightened cap on the vial.
			Assisted with the remainder of the examination:
		•	Removed light source.
		•	Discarded vaginal speculum in a biohazard waste container.
		•	Provided the physician with lubricant for the bimanual and rectal-vaginal examinations.
		•	Assisted as required with the collection of the fecal occult blood specimen.
		•	Assisted the patient into a sitting position and allowed her to rest.
		▷	Explained why the patient should be allowed to rest.
		•	Offered the patient tissues to remove lubricant from the perineum.
		•	Assisted patient from the examining table.
		•	Instructed patient to get dressed.
		•	Informed patient of the method used by the medical office to relay test results.
		•	Tested the fecal occult blood specimen and charted the results.
		•	Prepared Pap specimen for transport to the laboratory.
		•	Placed specimen in a biohazard specimen bag and sealed the bag.
		•	Inserted the cytology requisition into the outside pocket of bag.
		•	Placed bag in appropriate location for pickup by the laboratory.
		•	Charted the transport of the Pap specimen to an outside laboratory.
		•	Cleaned the examining room.
		*	Completed the procedure within 15 minutes.
			TOTALS

CHART	
Date	

Evaluation of Student Performance

EVALUATION CRITERIA			COMMENTS
Symbol	Category	Point Value	
*	Critical Step	16 points	
•	Essential Step	6 points	
▷	Theory Question	2 points	
Score calculation: 100 points – ____ points missed ____ Score Satisfactory score: 85 or above			

Copyright © 2008, 2004, 2000, 1995, 1990 by Saunders, an imprint of Elsevier Inc. All rights reserved.

AAMA/CAAHEP Competency Achieved:

☑ III. C. 3. b. (4) (d): Prepare and maintain examination and treatment areas.
☑ III. C. 3. b. (4) (e): Prepare patient for and assist with routine and specialty examinations.
☑ III. C. 3. c. (3) (b): Instruct individuals according to their needs.

GYN CYTOLOGY REQUISITION

THOMAS WOODSIDE, MD
501 MAIN ST
ST. LOUIS, MO 63146
(314) 883–0093

PATIENT INFO

Patient's Name (Last)	(First)	(MI)	Date of Birth MO | DAY | YR	Collection Time : AM PM	Collection Date MO | DAY | YR	Patient's ID #

Patient's Address	Phone	
City	State	ZIP

RESP. PARTY

Name of Responsible Party (if different from patient)		
Address of Responsible Party	APT #	
City	State	ZIP

INSURANCE

Patient's Relationship to Responsible Party ☐ 1. Self ☐ 2. Spouse ☐ 3. Child ☐ 4. Other

Insurance Comany Name	Plan	Carrier Code
Subscriber/Member #	Location	Group #
Insurance Address		Physician's Provider #
City	State	ZIP
Employer's Name or Number		Insured SSN

Diagnosis/Signs/Symptoms in ICD-9 Format (Highest Specificity)

REQUIRED

ICD-9 codes are the internationally accepted method of describing the clinical picture of the patient. All diagnoses should be provided by the ordering physician or his or her authorized designee. The following is a partial list of of common diagnoses in ICD-9 format. Most third party payers require an ICD-9 code to indicate the medical necessity of the test(s) and or profile(s) ordered. For a complete list of all ICD-9 codes, please refer to a current ICD-9 manual.

V76.2	Routine Cervical Pap Smear	616.0	Cervicitis	626.8	Abnormal Bleeding
V15.89	High Risk Cervical Screening	616.10	Vaginitis	627.1	Postmenopausal Bleeding
V22.2	Pregnancy	617.0	Endometriosis, Uterus	627.3	Atrophic Vaginitis
079.4	Human Papillomavirus	622.1	Dysplasia, Cervix	795.0	Abnormal Cervical Pap Smear
180.0	Malignant Neoplasm, Cervix	623.0	Dysplasia, Vagina		

COLLECTION METHOD

Liquid Based Prep
192055 ☐ Thin Prep Pap Test
192039 ☐ Thin Prep Pap Test w/reflex to HPV Hybrid Capture when ASC-US or SIL
192047 ☐ Thin Prep Pap Test w/reflex to high-risk only HPV Hybrid Capture when ASC-US

Pap Smear
009100 ☐ 1 Slide **009191** ☐ 2 Slides

Pap Smear and Maturation Index
009209 ☐ 1 Slide **190074** ☐ 2 Slides

SOURCE OF SPECIMEN

☐ **Cervical**
☐ **Endocervical**
☐ **Vaginal**

Date LMP

___/___/___
Mo Day Year

COLLECTION TECHNIQUE

☐ **Spatula**
☐ **Brush**
☐ **Broom**
☐ **Other** ________

PATIENT HISTORY

☐ **Pregnant**
☐ **Lactating**
☐ **Oral Contraceptives**
☐ **Postmenopausal**
☐ **Hormone Replacement Therapy**
☐ **PMP Bleeding**
☐ **Postpartum**
☐ **IUD**
☐ **Postcoital Bleeding**
☐ **DES Exposure**
☐ **Previous Abnormal Pap Test**
☐ **Other** ________

PREVIOUS TREATMENT	Date/Results
☐ None	
☐ Colposcopy and Bx	________
☐ Cryosurgery	________
☐ LEEP	________
☐ Laser Vaporization	________
☐ Conization	________
☐ Hysterectomy	________
☐ Radiation	________
☐ Chemotherapy	________

Copyright © 2008, 2004, 2000, 1995, 1990 by Saunders, an imprint of Elsevier Inc. All rights reserved.

EVALUATION OF COMPETENCY

Procedure 8-3: Assisting with a Return Prenatal Examination

Name: ______________________ Date: __________

Evaluated By: ______________________ Score: __________

Performance Objective

Outcome:	Prepare the patient and assist with a return prenatal examination.
Conditions:	Using an examining table.
	Given the following: centimeter tape measure, Doppler fetal pulse detector, ultrasound coupling agent, paper towel, disposable vaginal speculum, disposable gloves, lubricant, gauze pads, examining gown and drape, and a biohazard waste container.
Standards:	Time: 15 minutes. Student completed procedure in ____ minutes.
	Accuracy: Satisfactory score on the Performance Evaluation Checklist.

Performance Evaluation Checklist

Trial 1	*Trial 2*	*Point Value*	*Performance Standards*
		•	Sanitized hands.
		•	Set up the tray for the prenatal examination.
		•	Greeted the patient and introduced yourself.
		•	Identified patient and explained the procedure.
		•	Asked the patient to obtain a urine specimen.
		•	Escorted the patient to the examining room and asked her to be seated.
		•	Asked the patient if she has experienced any problems since her last visit and recorded information in the prenatal record.
		•	Measured patient's blood pressure and charted the results correctly.
		•	Weighed the patient and charted the results correctly.
		▷	Stated the importance of weighing the patient.
		•	Instructed and prepared patient for the examination.
		•	Left room to provide patient with privacy.
		•	Made medical record available for review by the physician.
		•	Tested the urine specimen for glucose and protein and charted the results correctly.
		•	Checked to make sure the patient is ready to be seen by physician.
		•	Informed physician that patient is ready.
		•	Stated how the physician can be informed that the patient is ready.
		•	Assisted patient into a supine position and properly draped her.

Copyright © 2008, 2004, 2000, 1995, 1990 by Saunders, an imprint of Elsevier Inc. All rights reserved.

Trial 1	Trial 2	Point Value	*Performance Standards*
			Assisted physician during the examination:
		•	Handed physician the tape measure for determination of fundal height.
		•	Applied coupling gel to the patient's abdomen and handed physician Doppler device.
		•	Removed gel from patient's abdomen.
		•	Cleaned the probe head of the Doppler device.
		•	Assisted patient into the lithotomy position if a vaginal specimen is to be obtained or if vaginal examination is to be performed.
		•	***After completion of the examination:*** Assisted patient into a sitting position and allowed her to rest.
		•	Assisted patient from examining table.
		•	Provided patient teaching and explanation of physician's instructions as required.
		•	Escorted patient to the reception area.
		•	Cleaned the examining room in preparation for the next patient.
		•	Prepared any specimens collected for transport to an outside laboratory.
		*	Completed the procedure within 15 minutes.
			TOTALS

CHART	
Date	

Evaluation of Student Performance

EVALUATION CRITERIA			COMMENTS
Symbol	Category	Point Value	
*	Critical Step	16 points	
•	Essential Step	6 points	
▷	Theory Question	2 points	
Score calculation: 100 points – ____ points missed ____ Score Satisfactory score: 85 or above			

Copyright © 2008, 2004, 2000, 1995, 1990 by Saunders, an imprint of Elsevier Inc. All rights reserved.

AAMA/CAAHEP Competency Achieved:

☑ III. C. 3. b. (4) (c): Obtain and record patient history.
☑ III. C. 3. b. (4) (d): Prepare and maintain examination and treatment areas.
☑ III. C. 3. b. (4) (e): Prepare patient for and assist with routine and specialty examinations.
☑ III. C. 3. c. (1) (a): Respond to and initiate written communications.
☑ III. C. 3. c. (1) (b): Recognize and respond to verbal communications.
☑ III. C. 3. c. (1) (c): Recognize and respond to nonverbal communications.
☑ III. C. 3. c. (3) (c): Provide instruction for health maintenance and disease prevention.

PATIENT'S NAME ____

INTERVAL PRENATAL HISTORY

Date 20__	Weeks Gestation	Height of Fundus (cm)	Weight	B/P	Urine Glucose	Urine Protein	FHT	Vaginal Examination	Presentation	Edema	Discharge	Bleeding	Contractions	Fetal Activity	NST	Next Appt.	Initials
				/													
				/													
				/													
				/													
				/													
				/													
				/													
				/													
				/													
				/													
				/													
				/													
				/													
				/													

Copyright © 2008, 2004, 2000, 1995, 1990 by Saunders, an imprint of Elsevier Inc. All rights reserved.

Notes

Copyright © 2008, 2004, 2000, 1995, 1990 by Saunders, an imprint of Elsevier Inc. All rights reserved.

9

The Pediatric Examination

CHAPTER ASSIGNMENTS

√ After Completing	Date Due	Textbook Page(s)	TEXTBOOK ASSIGNMENTS	Possible Points	Points You Earned
		318-360	Read Chapter 9: The Pediatric Examination		
		327 357	Read Case Study 1 Case Study 1 questions	5	
		342 357	Read Case Study 2 Case Study 2 questions	5	
		346 357	Read Case Study 3 Case Study 3 questions	5	
		358-359	Apply Your Knowledge questions	10	
			TOTAL POINTS		

√ After Completing	Date Due	Study Guide Page(s)	STUDY GUIDE ASSIGNMENTS (CTA: Critical Thinking Activity)	Possible Points	Points You Earned
		365	Pretest	10	
		366	Key Term Assessment	12	
		368-370	Evaluation of Learning questions	30	
		371	CTA A: Pediatric Weight	7	
			CD Activity: Chapter 9 Pounds and Ounces (Record points earned)		
		371	CTA B: Pediatric Length	8	
			CD Activity: Chapter 9 Inch by Inch (Record points earned)		
		371	CTA C: Growth Charts	18	
		372-374	CTA D: Motor and Social Development (5 pts/each category)	65	

Copyright © 2008, 2004, 2000, 1995, 1990 by Saunders, an imprint of Elsevier Inc. All rights reserved.

√ After Completing	Date Due	Study Guide Page(s)	STUDY GUIDE ASSIGNMENTS (CTA: Critical Thinking Activity)	Possible Points	Points You Earned
		375	CTA E: Intramuscular Injection	15	
		375-376	CTA F: Vaccine Information Statement	10	
		376	CTA G: Locating and Interpreting a VIS	20	
		377	CTA H: Crossword Puzzle	30	
		379	CTA I: Choose-a-Clue Game (Record points earned)		
		365	Posttest	10	
			ADDITIONAL ASSIGNMENTS		
			TOTAL POINTS		

Copyright © 2008, 2004, 2000, 1995, 1990 by Saunders, an imprint of Elsevier Inc. All rights reserved.

√ When Assigned By Your Instructor	Study Guide Page(s)	Practices Required	LABORATORY ASSIGNMENTS (Procedure Number and Name)	*Score
	385	3	**Practice for Competency** 9-A: Carrying an Infant Textbook reference: pp. 328-330	
	391-392		**Evaluation of Competency** Carrying an Infant	*
	386	5	**Practice for Competency** 9-1: Measuring the Weight and Length of an Infant Textbook reference: pp. 332-333	
	393-394		**Evaluation of Competency** 9-1: Measuring the Weight and Length of an Infant	*
	387	5	**Practice for Competency** 9-2: Measuring Head and Chest Circumference of an Infant Textbook reference: pp. 333-334	
	395-396		**Evaluation of Competency** 9-2: Measuring Head and Chest Circumference of an Infant	*
	386	5	**Practice for Competency** 9-3: Calculating Growth Percentiles Textbook reference: pp. 334-340	
	397-398		**Evaluation of Competency** 9-3: Calculating Growth Percentiles	*
	388	5	**Practice for Competency** 9-4: Applying a Pediatric Urine Collector Textbook reference: pp. 343-344	
	399-401		**Evaluation of Competency** 9-4: Applying a Pediatric Urine Collector	*
	389	5	**Practice for Competency** 9-5: Newborn Screening Test Textbook reference: pp. 354-356	
	403-405		**Evaluation of Competency** 9-5: Newborn Screening Test	*
			ADDITIONAL ASSIGNMENTS	

Copyright © 2008, 2004, 2000, 1995, 1990 by Saunders, an imprint of Elsevier Inc. All rights reserved.

Notes

Copyright © 2008, 2004, 2000, 1995, 1990 by Saunders, an imprint of Elsevier Inc. All rights reserved.

Name ______________________________ Date ______________

PRETEST

True or False

_____ 1. A pediatrician is a medical doctor who specializes in the diagnosis and treatment of disease in children.

_____ 2. The first well-child visit is usually scheduled 1 week after birth.

_____ 3. Length is measured with the child standing with his or her back to the measuring device.

_____ 4. Blood pressure should be taken on a child starting at 8 years of age.

_____ 5. It is best not to tell a child that an immunization will hurt.

_____ 6. The vastus lateralis muscle site is recommended for administering an injection to an infant.

_____ 7. An MMR injection includes the following immunizations: measles, meningitis, and rubella.

_____ 8. A Vaccine Information Statement explains the benefits and risks of a vaccine in lay terminology.

_____ 9. The hepatitis B vaccine can be given to a newborn.

_____ 10. The blood specimen for a newborn screening test is obtained from the infant's earlobe.

POSTTEST

True or False

_____ 1. A well-child visit is also referred to as a health maintenance visit.

_____ 2. A reason for weighing a child is to determine proper medication dosage.

_____ 3. Growth charts can be used to identify children with growth abnormalities.

_____ 4. Measuring pediatric blood pressure helps to identify children at risk for developing Type 1 diabetes.

_____ 5. Using a blood pressure cuff that is too large for the child can result in a falsely low reading.

_____ 6. The length of the needle used for a pediatric IM injection depends on the amount of medication being administered.

_____ 7. The resistance of the body to pathogenic microorganisms or their toxins is known as inflammation.

_____ 8. The recommended route of administration for an MMR is subcutaneous.

_____ 9. Before administering a pediatric immunization, the NCVIA requires that the parent sign a consent form.

_____ 10. If PKU is left untreated, it can lead to malnutrition.

Copyright © 2008, 2004, 2000, 1995, 1990 by Saunders, an imprint of Elsevier Inc. All rights reserved.

KEY TERM ASSESSMENT

Directions: Match each medical term with its definition.

_____ 1. Immunity

_____ 2. Immunization

_____ 3. Infant

_____ 4. Length

_____ 5. Pediatrician

_____ 6. Pediatrics

_____ 7. Preschooler

_____ 8. School-age child

_____ 9. Toddler

_____ 10. Toxoid

_____ 11. Vaccine

_____ 12. Vertex

A. A medical doctor who specializes in the care and development of children and the diagnosis and treatment of children's diseases
B. A child from 1 to 3 years of age
C. The summit, or top, especially the top of the head
D. The resistance of the body to the effects of a harmful agent such as a pathogenic microorganism or its toxins
E. The branch of medicine that deals with the care and development of children and the diagnosis and treatment of children's diseases
F. A suspension of attenuated or killed microorganisms administered to an individual to prevent an infectious disease
G. The process of becoming immune or of rendering an individual immune through the use of a vaccine or toxoid
H. The measurement from the vertex of the head to the heel of the foot in a supine position
I. A toxin that has been treated by heat or chemicals to destroy its harmful properties
J. A child from birth to 12 months of age
K. A child from 3 to 6 years of age
L. A child from 6 to 12 years of age

Copyright © 2008, 2004, 2000, 1995, 1990 by Saunders, an imprint of Elsevier Inc. All rights reserved.

Notes

Copyright © 2008, 2004, 2000, 1995, 1990 by Saunders, an imprint of Elsevier Inc. All rights reserved.

EVALUATION OF LEARNING

Directions: Fill in each blank with the correct answer.

1. What are the components of the well-child visit?

2. What is the usual schedule for well-child visits?

3. What is the purpose of the sick-child visit?

4. What procedures are often performed by the medical assistant during pediatric office visits?

5. Why is it important for the medical assistant to develop a rapport with the pediatric patient?

6. List the two positions that can be used to safely carry an infant.

7. Why is it important to measure the growth (weight and height or length) of the child during each office visit?

8. What is the difference between height and length?

9. What is the purpose of measuring head circumference?

10. What is the primary use of growth charts?

11. What is the primary cause of childhood obesity?

Copyright © 2008, 2004, 2000, 1995, 1990 by Saunders, an imprint of Elsevier Inc. All rights reserved.

12. What problems are associated with childhood obesity?

13. List five guidelines for preventing childhood obesity.

14. According to the American Academy of Pediatrics, at what age and how often should blood pressure be measured in children?

15. What is the importance of measuring blood pressure in children?

16. What criteria must be followed to determine the correct cuff size for a child?

17. What occurs if the blood pressure cuff is too small or too large?

18. What three factors must be taken into consideration when determining if a child has hypertension?

19. List three reasons for collecting a urine specimen from a child.

20. Why should the child's genitalia be cleansed before applying a pediatric urine collector?

21. What gauge and length (range) of needle are recommended for giving an intramuscular injection to a child?

22. Why is the dorsogluteal site not recommended for use as an intramuscular injection site in infants and young children?

Copyright © 2008, 2004, 2000, 1995, 1990 by Saunders, an imprint of Elsevier Inc. All rights reserved.

23. Why is the vastus lateralis muscle recommended as a good site for giving an intramuscular injection to an infant or young child?

24. What is the difference between a vaccine and a toxoid?

25. According to the American Academy of Pediatrics, what immunizations are recommended for each of the following pediatric patients?
   a. 2-month-old infant
   b. 6-month-old infant
   c. 12-month-old infant
   d. 5-year-old child

26. What information must be provided to parents as required by the National Childhood Vaccine Injury Act?

27. According to the NCVIA, what information must be recorded in the patient's medical record after a pediatric immunization has been administered?

28. The newborn screening test screens for which metabolic diseases?

29. What are the symptoms of PKU, if left untreated?

30. Why can the PKU screening test be performed earlier on infants on formula as compared with breast-fed babies?

Copyright © 2008, 2004, 2000, 1995, 1990 by Saunders, an imprint of Elsevier Inc. All rights reserved.

CRITICAL THINKING ACTIVITIES

A. PEDIATRIC WEIGHT

Locate the following weight values on your pediatric scale. Place a check mark next to each one after it has been correctly located.

1. 7 pounds, 9 ounces _______
2. 8 pounds, 5 ounces _______
3. 12 pounds, 10 ounces _______
4. 15 pounds, 11 ounces _______
5. 19 pounds, 7 ounces _______
6. 23 pounds, 6 ounces _______
7. 25 pounds, 3 ounces _______

B. PEDIATRIC LENGTH

Locate the following length values on your pediatric measuring device. Place a check mark next to each after it has been correctly located.

1. 20 ½ inches _______
2. 22 ½ inches _______
3. 24 inches _______
4. 25 ¾ inches _______
5. 28 ½ inches _______
6. 31 inches _______
7. 33 ¼ inches _______
8. 36 ½ inches _______

C. GROWTH CHARTS

Matthew Williams, age 2 years (24 months), has had health maintenance visits at the intervals listed below. His length and weight measurements were taken during each visit and are recorded here. Plot these on the growth chart on p. 337 of your textbook. You can also print out a growth chart from your computer by going to the following website: **www.cdc.gov/growthcharts** (Choose "Clinical Growth Charts: Set 1"). Calculate the percentile for each and record it in the space provided. (Note: His birth weight was 7 pounds, 8 ounces, and his length was 20 inches.)

		Well-Child Visit		
AGE	WEIGHT	PERCENTILE	LENGTH	PERCENTILE
1 month	9 lb,10 oz	__________	22 in	__________
2 months	12 lb, 4 oz	__________	23 ½ in	__________
4 months	16 lb, 5 oz	__________	25 ¼ in	__________
6 months	18 lb, 8 oz	__________	27 in	__________
9 months	22 lb, 4 oz	__________	29 ¼ in	__________
12 months	24 lb, 4 oz	__________	30 ½ in	__________
15 months	26 lb, 8 oz	__________	31 ½ in	__________
18 months	27 lb	__________	32 ½ in	__________
24 months	28 lb	__________	35 ¾ in	__________

Copyright © 2008, 2004, 2000, 1995, 1990 by Saunders, an imprint of Elsevier Inc. All rights reserved.

D. MOTOR AND SOCIAL DEVELOPMENT

Using a reference source, describe the motor and social development of the age groups listed here. The first one is done for you.

AGE	MOTOR AND SOCIAL DEVELOPMENT
Birth to 3 months	Raises head but not stable, can turn head from side to side, activities are limited to reflexes, cries when hungry, responsive social smile, coos, eyes can focus on an object and follow a moving object 180 degrees.
4 to 6 months	
7 to 9 months	
10 to 12 months	

Copyright © 2008, 2004, 2000, 1995, 1990 by Saunders, an imprint of Elsevier Inc. All rights reserved.

AGE	MOTOR AND SOCIAL DEVELOPMENT
1 year	
2 years	
3 years	
4 years	
5 years	

Copyright © 2008, 2004, 2000, 1995, 1990 by Saunders, an imprint of Elsevier Inc. All rights reserved.

AGE	MOTOR AND SOCIAL DEVELOPMENT
6 years	
7 years	
8 to 10 years	
Preadolescent	
Adolescent	

Copyright © 2008, 2004, 2000, 1995, 1990 by Saunders, an imprint of Elsevier Inc. All rights reserved.

E. INTRAMUSCULAR INJECTION

How would you prepare the following children for an intramuscular injection of penicillin in order to reduce apprehension and fear? Table 9-4, Techniques for Interacting with Children, on page 329 of your textbook can be used as a reference for this activity.

a. Katie Waugh, age 5:

____

____

____

b. Patrick Williams, age 8:

____

____

____

c. Julie Anderson, age 15:

____

____

____

F. VACCINE INFORMATION STATEMENT

Refer to the Diphtheria, Tetanus, and Pertussis VIS in your textbook (pp. 350 and 351) and answer the following questions:

1. How does an individual contract tetanus?

____

____

2. What are the symptoms of:

   a. Diphtheria ______________________________

   b. Tetanus ______________________________

   c. Pertussis ______________________________

3. Why is DTaP now used instead of DTP?

____

____

4. What is the immunization schedule for DTaP?

____

____

5. Who should not get a DTaP immunization?

____

____

6. Do adults need a DTaP booster?

____

____

7. What mild problems may occur from a DTaP vaccine?

____

____

Copyright © 2008, 2004, 2000, 1995, 1990 by Saunders, an imprint of Elsevier Inc. All rights reserved.

8. What moderate problems may occur from a DTaP vaccine?

____

____

9. What should be done if the patient develops fever and pain after receiving a DTaP?

____

____

10. What should be done if a moderate or severe reaction occurs with a DTaP immunization?

____

____

G. LOCATING AND INTERPRETING A VIS

Obtain a Vaccine Information Statement for a vaccine that you would like to know more about (other than the DTaP vaccine already included in your textbook). List the information that would be important for a parent to know before this immunization is administered to his or her child. The following Internet sites can be used to obtain Vaccine Information Statements:

www.cdc.gov/nip/publications/vis
www.immunize.org/vis

Name of Immunization: ____

Publication Date: ____

Information to Relay to a Parent:

____

____

____

____

____

____

____

____

____

____

Copyright © 2008, 2004, 2000, 1995, 1990 by Saunders, an imprint of Elsevier Inc. All rights reserved.

H. CROSSWORD PUZZLE
Pediatrics

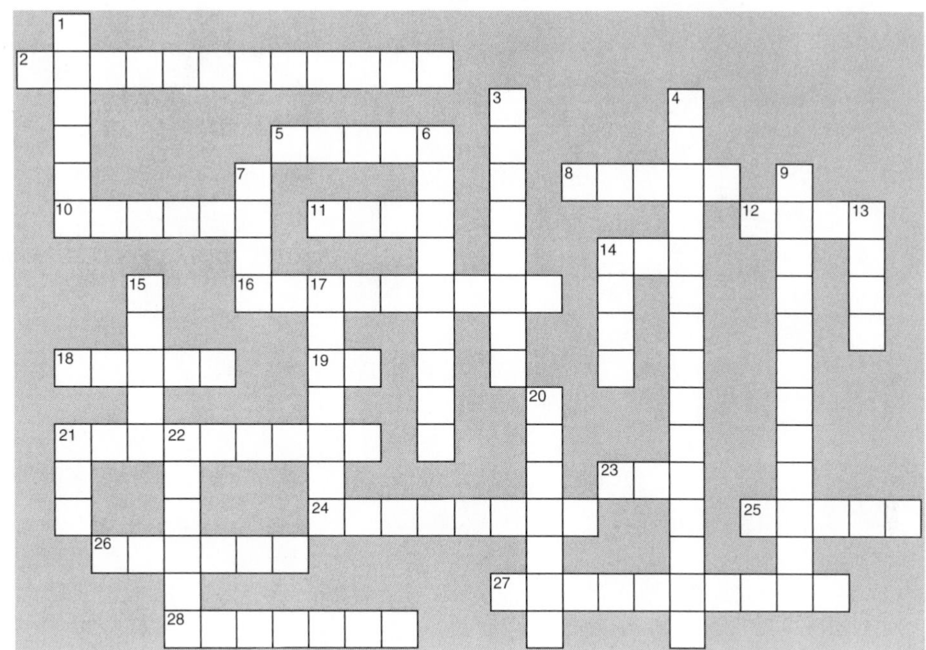

Directions: Complete the crossword puzzle using the clues presented below.

ACROSS

2 Baby doctor
5 Causes a lot of crying
8 BMI over 30
10 Stand up straight
11 PKU puncture site
12 Right size for kid's B/P?
14 No phenylalanine enzyme
16 Whooping cough
18 Kid's vaccine act
19 Begin at 3
21 Not caused by chickens
23 Not for pregnant women
24 Fights with an MO
25 Not given po anymore
26 Hold-me position
27 Can give at birth vaccine
28 Can lock your jaw

DOWN

1 Vertex to heel
3 Resistance to MOs
4 Injection site for babies
6 First breast milk
7 3 in 1 vaccine
9 MMR administration route
13 Not a kid reward
14 Child's work
15 Common immunization side effect
17 German measles
20 From 1 to 3
21 Immunization explainer
22 Title expires at 1 year

Copyright © 2008, 2004, 2000, 1995, 1990 by Saunders, an imprint of Elsevier Inc. All rights reserved.

Notes

Copyright © 2008, 2004, 2000, 1995, 1990 by Saunders, an imprint of Elsevier Inc. All rights reserved.

I. CHOOSE-A-CLUE GAME

Object: The object of the game is to become familiar with childhood diseases.

Directions:

1. Cut out the game cards on the following pages.
2. List three clues for each condition specified on the reverse of the card. Your clues should include information on symptoms, prevention, and treatment.The name of the disease *must not* be written on this side of the card.
3. Use the game cards as flash cards to study the diseases.
4. Get into a group of 3 students.
5. Place your game cards on the table in front of you with the clues facing up.
6. One of the players should name the first disease on the list presented below.
7. Each player places the appropriate game card on the table with the clues facing upward.
8. When all players have placed a card on the table, turn the cards over.
9. Award yourself 5 points if you have correctly determined the disease.
10. Review the information each player listed on his or her game card.
11. Keep track of your points on the score card provided.
12. Continue playing until all the diseases have been identified.

Good Internet reference sources to help you find clues include:

www.kidshealth.org

www.merck.com

Childhood Diseases

1. Conjunctivitis
2. Fifth disease
3. Head lice
4. Impetigo
5. Influenza
6. Meningococcal meningitis
7. Methicillin resistant staphylococcal aureus (MRSA)
8. Otitis media
9. Pertussis
10. Pinworms
11. Roseola
12. Respiratory synctial virus (RSV)
13. Scarlet fever
14. Strep throat
15. Urinary tract infection
16. Varicella (chickenpox)

Copyright © 2008, 2004, 2000, 1995, 1990 by Saunders, an imprint of Elsevier Inc. All rights reserved.

CHOOSE-A-CLUE
SCORE CARD

Name: ____

Recording Points:
Cross off a number each time you properly identify a disease (starting with 5 and continuing in sequence). Your total points will be equal to the last number you crossed off. Record this number in the space provided and place a check-mark next to the level you achieved.

Points:	
5	75
10	80
15	85
20	90
25	95
30	100
35	105
40	110
45	115
50	120
55	125
60	130
65	135
70	140

TOTAL POINTS: ________

LEVEL:

- ☐ 75 points and above: **Free from Infection**
- ☐ 65 to 70 points: **Putting Up a Good Fight**
- ☐ 55 to 60 points: **Susceptible**
- ☐ 50 points and under: **Infected**

Copyright © 2008, 2004, 2000, 1995, 1990 by Saunders, an imprint of Elsevier Inc. All rights reserved.

Conjunctivitis

Fifth disease

Head lice

Impetigo

Influenza

Meningococcal meningitis

Otitis media

Pertussis

Sym:

Prev:

Tx:

Sym:

Prev:

Tx:

Sym:

Prev:

Tx:

Sym:

Prev:

Tx:

Sym:

Prev:

Tx:

Sym:

Prev:

Tx:

Sym:

Prev:

Tx:

Sym:

Prev:

Tx:

Pinworms

MRSA

Roseola

Respiratory synctial virus (RSV)

Scarlet fever

Strep throat

Urinary tract infection

Varicella (chicken pox)

Sym:

Prev:

Tx:

Sym:

Prev:

Tx:

Sym:

Prev:

Tx:

Sym:

Prev:

Tx:

Sym:

Prev:

Tx:

Sym:

Prev:

Tx:

Sym:

Prev:

Tx:

Sym:

Prev:

Tx:

PRACTICE FOR COMPETENCY

Procedure 9-A: Carrying an Infant

Practice the procedure for carrying an infant, using a pediatric training mannequin in the following positions: cradle and upright.

CARRYING POSITION	NUMBER OF PRACTICES

Copyright © 2008, 2004, 2000, 1995, 1990 by Saunders, an imprint of Elsevier Inc. All rights reserved.

Procedures 9-1 and 9-3: Weight, Length, and Growth Charts

1. **Weight and Length.** Measure the weight of an infant using a pediatric training mannequin. Record the results in the chart provided.
2. **Growth Charts**. Calculate growth percentiles on a growth chart using the values presented below. Assume these values were taken from the same (female) child over the course of her first year of life.

Age	Weight	Length
2 months	9 pounds	21 inches
4 months	11 pounds, 8 ounces	23 ½ inches
6 months	14 pounds, 8 ounces	25 ¼ inches
9 months	18 pounds, 8 ounces	27 ¼ inches
12 months	21 pounds, 6 ounces	28 ¾ inches

CHART	
Date	

Copyright © 2008, 2004, 2000, 1995, 1990 by Saunders, an imprint of Elsevier Inc. All rights reserved.

Procedure 9-2: Head and Chest Circumference. Measure the head and chest circumference of an infant using a pediatric training mannequin. Record the results in the chart provided.

Chart	
Date	

Copyright © 2008, 2004, 2000, 1995, 1990 by Saunders, an imprint of Elsevier Inc. All rights reserved.

Procedure 9-4: Pediatric Urine Collector. Practice the procedure for applying a pediatric urine collector, using a pediatric training mannequin. Record the procedure in the chart provided.

CHART	
Date	

Copyright © 2008, 2004, 2000, 1995, 1990 by Saunders, an imprint of Elsevier Inc. All rights reserved.

Procedure 9-5: Newborn Screening Test

1. Complete the information section of the Newborn Screening Test Card provided for you on the following page.
2. Practice the procedure for specimen collection for the newborn screening test using a pediatric training mannequin. Record the procedure in the chart provided.

CHART	
Date	

Copyright © 2008, 2004, 2000, 1995, 1990 by Saunders, an imprint of Elsevier Inc. All rights reserved.

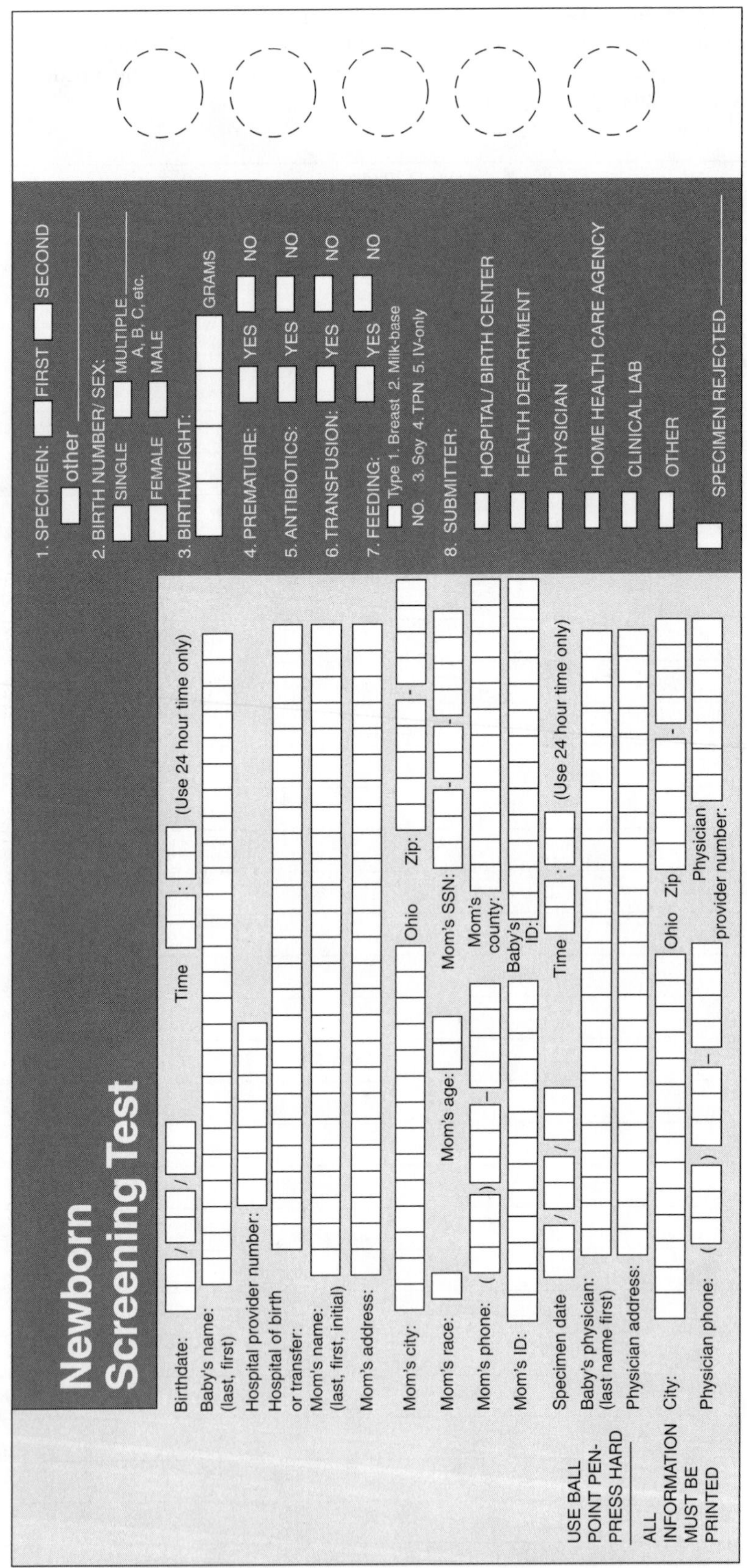

Newborn Screening Test

USE BALL POINT PEN-PRESS HARD

ALL INFORMATION MUST BE PRINTED

Birthdate: ___ / ___ / ___ Time ___ : ___ (Use 24 hour time only)

Baby's name: (last, first)

Hospital provider number:

Hospital of birth or transfer:

Mom's name: (last, first, initial)

Mom's address:

Mom's city: Ohio Zip: ___ - ___

Mom's race: Mom's age: Mom's SSN: ___ - ___ - ___

Mom's phone: (___) ___ - ___ Mom's county:

Mom's ID: Baby's ID:

Specimen date ___ / ___ / ___ Time ___ : ___ (Use 24 hour time only)

Baby's physician: (last name first)

Physician address:

City: Ohio Zip ___ - ___

Physician phone: (___) ___ - ___ Physician provider number:

1. SPECIMEN: ☐ FIRST ☐ SECOND ☐ other ______
2. BIRTH NUMBER/ SEX: ☐ SINGLE ☐ MULTIPLE ______ A, B, C, etc. ☐ FEMALE ☐ MALE
3. BIRTHWEIGHT: ___ GRAMS
4. PREMATURE: ☐ YES ☐ NO
5. ANTIBIOTICS: ☐ YES ☐ NO
6. TRANSFUSION: ☐ YES ☐ NO
7. FEEDING: ☐ Type 1. Breast 2. Milk-base NO. 3. Soy 4. TPN 5. IV-only ☐ YES ☐ NO
8. SUBMITTER:
   - ☐ HOSPITAL/ BIRTH CENTER
   - ☐ HEALTH DEPARTMENT
   - ☐ PHYSICIAN
   - ☐ HOME HEALTH CARE AGENCY
   - ☐ CLINICAL LAB
   - ☐ OTHER

☐ SPECIMEN REJECTED ______

Copyright © 2008, 2004, 2000, 1995, 1990 by Saunders, an imprint of Elsevier Inc. All rights reserved.

EVALUATION OF COMPETENCY

Procedure 9-A: Carrying an Infant

Name: ______________________________ Date: ______________

Evaluated By: ______________________________ Score: ______________

Performance Objective

Outcome:	Carry an infant in the following positions: cradle and upright.	
Conditions:	Given a pediatric training mannequin.	
Standards:	Time: 5 minutes.	Student completed procedure in ____ minutes.
	Accuracy: Satisfactory score on the Performance Evaluation Checklist.	

Performance Evaluation Checklist

Trial 1	*Trial 2*	*Point Value*	*Performance Standards*
			Cradle Position
		•	Slid the left hand and arm under infant's back.
		•	Grasped infant's upper arm from behind.
		•	Encircled infant's upper arm with the thumb and fingers.
		•	Supported infant's head, shoulders, and back on your arm.
		•	Slipped the right arm up and under the infant's buttocks.
		•	Cradled infant in your arms with the infant's body resting against your chest.
			Upright Position
		•	Slipped the right hand under infant's head and shoulders.
		•	Spread the fingers apart to support infant's head and neck.
		•	Slipped the left forearm under infant's buttocks.
		•	Allowed infant to rest against your chest.
		*	Completed the procedure within 5 minutes.
			TOTALS

Chart	
Date	

Copyright © 2008, 2004, 2000, 1995, 1990 by Saunders, an imprint of Elsevier Inc. All rights reserved.

Evaluation of Student Performance

EVALUATION CRITERIA			COMMENTS
Symbol	**Category**	**Point Value**	
✶	Critical Step	16 points	
●	Essential Step	6 points	
▷	Theory Question	2 points	
Score calculation: 100 points – ____ points missed ____ Score Satisfactory score: 85 or above			

AAMA/CAAHEP Competency Achieved:

☑ III. C. 3. b. (4) (e): Prepare patient for and assist with routine and specialty examinations.

Copyright © 2008, 2004, 2000, 1995, 1990 by Saunders, an imprint of Elsevier Inc. All rights reserved.

EVALUATION OF COMPETENCY

Procedure 9-1: Measuring the Weight and Length of an Infant

Name: ______________________________ Date: ______________

Evaluated By: ______________________________ Score: ______________

Performance Objective

Outcome:	Measure the weight and length of an infant.
Conditions:	Using a pediatric training mannequin and a pediatric balance scale (table model). Given a paper protector.
Standards:	Time: 5 minutes. Student completed procedure in ____ minutes. Accuracy: Satisfactory score on the Performance Evaluation Checklist.

Performance Evaluation Checklist

Trial 1	Trial 2	Point Value	*Performance Standards*
			Weight
		•	Sanitized hands.
		•	Greeted the infant's parent and introduced yourself.
		•	Identified the infant.
		•	Explained the procedure to the child's parent.
		•	Based on the medical office policy asked parent to: a. Remove infant's clothing and put on a dry diaper. b. Remove infant's clothing including the diaper.
		▷	Stated why the infant should not be weighed with a wet diaper.
		•	Unlocked pediatric scale and placed a clean paper protector on it.
		▷	Stated the purpose of the paper protector.
		•	Checked the balance scale for accuracy.
		▷	Stated the purpose for balancing the scale.
		•	Gently placed infant on his or her back on the scale.
		•	Placed one hand slightly above infant.
		•	Balanced scale.
		• •	Read results while infant was lying still. Jotted down value or made a mental note of it.
		*	The reading was identical to the evaluator's reading.
		•	Returned balance to its resting position and locked the scale.

Copyright © 2008, 2004, 2000, 1995, 1990 by Saunders, an imprint of Elsevier Inc. All rights reserved.

Trial 1	Trial 2	Point Value	Performance Standards
			Length
		•	Placed the vertex of infant's head against the headboard at the zero mark.
		•	Asked parent to hold infant's head in position.
		•	Straightened infant's knees and placed soles of infant's feet firmly against the upright foot board.
		•	Read infant's length in inches from the measure.
		•	Jotted down value or made a mental note of it.
		*	The reading was identical to the evaluator's reading.
		•	Removed infant from the scale and handed him or her to the parent.
		•	Returned headboard and footboard to their resting positions.
		•	Sanitized hands.
		•	Charted the results correctly.
		*	Completed the procedure within 5 minutes.
			TOTALS

CHART	
Date	

Evaluation of Student Performance

EVALUATION CRITERIA			COMMENTS
Symbol	Category	Point Value	
*	Critical Step	16 points	
•	Essential Step	6 points	
▷	Theory Question	2 points	
Score calculation: 100 points – _____ points missed _____ Score Satisfactory score: 85 or above			

AAMA/CAAHEP Competency Achieved:

☑ III. C. 3. b. (4) (e): Prepare patient for and assist with routine and specialty examinations.

Copyright © 2008, 2004, 2000, 1995, 1990 by Saunders, an imprint of Elsevier Inc. All rights reserved.

EVALUATION OF COMPETENCY

Procedure 9-2: Measuring Head and Chest Circumference of an Infant

Name: ______________________________ Date: ______________

Evaluated By: ______________________________ Score: ______________

Performance Objective

Outline: Measure the head and chest circumference of an infant.

Conditions: Given a flexible nonstretch tape measure (in centimeters).

Standards: Time: 5 minutes. Student completed procedure in ____ minutes.

Accuracy: Satisfactory score on the Performance Evaluation Checklist.

Performance Evaluation Checklist

Trial 1	*Trial 2*	*Point Value*	*Performance Standards*
			Measurement of Head Circumference
		•	Sanitized hands.
		•	Assembled equipment.
		•	Positioned the infant.
		▷	Stated what positions can be used to measure head circumference.
		•	Positioned the measuring device around the infant's head.
		•	The tape measure was placed slightly above the eyebrows and pinna of the ears and around the occipital prominence at the back of the skull.
		•	Read the results in centimeters (or inches).
		•	Jotted down value or made a mental note of it.
		*	The reading was identical to the evaluator's reading.
		•	Sanitized hands.
		•	Charted the results correctly.
			Measurement of Chest Circumference
		•	Positioned the infant on his or her back on the examining table.
		•	Encircled the measuring device around the infant's chest at the nipple line.
		•	Ensured that the measuring device was snug but not too tight.
		•	Read the results in centimeters (or inches).
		•	Jotted down this value or made a mental note of it.

Copyright © 2008, 2004, 2000, 1995, 1990 by Saunders, an imprint of Elsevier Inc. All rights reserved.

		*	The reading was identical to the evaluator's reading.
		•	Charted the results correctly.
		*	Completed the procedure within 5 minutes.
			TOTALS

CHART	
Date	

Evaluation of Student Performance

EVALUATION CRITERIA			COMMENTS
Symbol	Category	Point Value	
*	Critical Step	16 points	
•	Essential Step	6 points	
▷	Theory Question	2 points	
Score calculation: 100 points – ______ points missed ____ Score Satisfactory score: 85 or above			

AAMA/CAAHEP Competency Achieved:

☑ III. C. 3. b. (4) (e): Prepare patient for and assist with routine and specialty examinations.

Copyright © 2008, 2004, 2000, 1995, 1990 by Saunders, an imprint of Elsevier Inc. All rights reserved.

EVALUATION OF COMPETENCY

Procedure 9-3: Calculating Growth Percentiles

Name: ______________________________ Date: ______________

Evaluated By: ______________________________ Score: ______________

Performance Objective

Outcome:	Plot a pediatric growth value on a growth chart.	
Conditions:	Given a pediatric growth chart.	
Standards:	Time: 5 minutes.	Student completed procedure in ____ minutes.
	Accuracy: Satisfactory score on the Performance Evaluation Checklist.	

Performance Evaluation Checklist

Trial 1	*Trial 2*	*Point Value*	*Performance Standards*
		•	Selected the proper growth chart.
		•	Located the child's age in the horizontal column at the bottom of the chart.
		•	Located the growth value in the vertical column under the appropriate category.
		•	Drew a (imaginary) vertical line from the child's age mark and an imaginary horizontal line from the growth mark.
		•	Found the site at which the two lines intersected on the graph.
		•	Placed a dot on this site.
		•	Determined the percentile by following the curved percentile line upward.
		•	Read the value located on the right side of the chart.
		•	Estimated the results if the value did not fall exactly on a percentile line.
		•	Charted the results correctly.
		*	The value was within ±2 percentage points of the evaluator's determination.
		*	Completed the procedure within 5 minutes.
			TOTALS

CHART	
Date	

Copyright © 2008, 2004, 2000, 1995, 1990 by Saunders, an imprint of Elsevier Inc. All rights reserved.

Evaluation of Student Performance

EVALUATION CRITERIA			COMMENTS
Symbol	**Category**	**Point Value**	
✶	Critical Step	16 points	
●	Essential Step	6 points	
▷	Theory Question	2 points	
Score calculation: 100 points – _____ points missed ____ Score Satisfactory score: 85 or above			

AAMA/CAAHEP Competency Achieved:

☑ III. C. 3. b. (4) (e): Prepare patient for and assist with routine and specialty examinations.

Copyright © 2008, 2004, 2000, 1995, 1990 by Saunders, an imprint of Elsevier Inc. All rights reserved.

EVALUATION OF COMPETENCY

Procedure 9-4: Applying a Pediatric Urine Collector

Name: ______________________ Date: __________

Evaluated By: ______________________ Score: __________

Performance Objective

Outcome:	Apply a pediatric urine collector.	
Conditions:	Using a pediatric training mannequin.	
	Given the following: disposable gloves, personal antiseptic wipes, pediatric urine collector bag, urine specimen container and label, and a waste container.	
Standards:	Time: 10 minutes.	Student completed procedure in ____ minutes.
	Accuracy: Satisfactory score on the Performance Evaluation Checklist.	

Performance Evaluation Checklist

Trial 1	Trial 2	Point Value	*Performance Standards*
		•	Sanitized hands.
		•	Assembled equipment.
		•	Greeted the child's parent and introduced yourself.
		•	Identified the child and explained the procedure to the parent.
		•	Applied gloves.
		•	Positioned child on his or her back with legs spread apart.
			Cleanse the area and apply the bag:
			Females
		•	Cleansed each side of the meatus with a separate wipe using a front-to-back motion.
		•	Cleansed directly down the middle with a third wipe.
		•	Discarded each wipe after cleansing.
		▷	Stated the reason for cleansing the urinary meatus.
		•	Allowed the area to dry completely.
		▷	Explained why the area should be allowed to dry.
		•	Removed paper backing from urine collector bag.
		•	Placed the bottom of the adhesive ring on the perinuem and work upward.
		•	Firmly pressed the adhesive surface firmly to the skin surrounding the external genitalia.
		•	Made sure there was no puckering.

Copyright © 2008, 2004, 2000, 1995, 1990 by Saunders, an imprint of Elsevier Inc. All rights reserved.

Trial 1	*Trial 2*	*Point Value*	*Performance Standards*
		•	The opening of the bag was placed directly over the urinary meatus.
		•	The excess length of the bag was positioned toward the feet.
			Males
		•	Retracted the foreskin of the penis if the child is not circumcised.
		•	Cleansed each side of the urethral orifice with a separate wipe.
		•	Cleansed directly over the urethral orifice.
		•	Cleansed the scrotum.
		•	Discarded each wipe after cleansing.
		•	Allowed the area to dry completely.
		•	Removed the paper backing from urine collector bag.
		•	Positioned the bag so that child's penis and scrotum are projected through the opening of the bag.
		•	Firmly pressed the adhesive surface firmly to the skin.
		•	The excess length of the bag was positioned toward the feet.
			Completed the procedure:
		•	Loosely diapered child.
		•	Checked bag every 15 minutes until urine specimen was obtained.
		•	Gently removed collector bag from top to bottom.
		•	Cleansed genital area with a personal antiseptic wipe and rediapered child.
		•	Transferred urine specimen into specimen container and tightly applied the lid.
		•	Applied label to container.
		•	Disposed of collector bag in a regular waste container.
		•	Tested the specimen or prepared it for transfer to an outside laboratory.
		▷	Explained why the urine specimen should not be allowed to stand at room temperature.
		•	Removed gloves and sanitized hands.
		•	Charted the procedure correctly.
		✶	Completed the procedure within 10 minutes.
			TOTALS

CHART	
Date	

Copyright © 2008, 2004, 2000, 1995, 1990 by Saunders, an imprint of Elsevier Inc. All rights reserved.

Evaluation of Student Performance

EVALUATION CRITERIA			COMMENTS
Symbol	Category	Point Value	
*	Critical Step	16 points	
•	Essential Step	6 points	
▷	Theory Question	2 points	
Score calculation: 100 points – ______ points missed ____ Score Satisfactory score: 85 or above			

AAMA/CAAHEP Competency Achieved:

☑ III. C. 3. b. (4) (f): Prepare patient for and assist with procedures, treatments, and minor office surgeries.

Copyright © 2008, 2004, 2000, 1995, 1990 by Saunders, an imprint of Elsevier Inc. All rights reserved.

Notes

Copyright © 2008, 2004, 2000, 1995, 1990 by Saunders, an imprint of Elsevier Inc. All rights reserved.

EVALUATION OF COMPETENCY

Procedure 9-5: Newborn Screening Test

Name: ______________________________ Date: ____________

Evaluated By: ______________________________ Score: ____________

Performance Objective

Outcome:	Collect a capillary blood specimen for a newborn screening test.
Conditions:	Using a pediatric training mannequin.
	Given the following: disposable gloves, sterile lancet, heel warmer or warm compress, antiseptic wipe, newborn testing card, mailing envelope, sterile gauze pad, adhesive bandages, and a biohazard sharps container.
Standards:	Time: 10 minutes. Student completed procedure in ____ minutes.
	Accuracy: Satisfactory score on the Performance Evaluation Checklist.

Performance Evaluation Checklist

Trial 1	*Trial 2*	*Point Value*	*Performance Standards*
		•	Sanitized hands.
		•	Assembled equipment.
		•	Greeted the infant's parent and introduced yourself.
		•	Identified the infant and explained the procedure to the parent.
		•	Completed the information section of the newborn screening card.
		•	Selected an appropriate puncture site.
		•	Identified the sites that can be used for the heel puncture.
		▷	Explained what could occur if a different site is used.
		•	Warmed the puncture site.
		▷	Stated the purpose of warming the site.
		•	Cleaned the puncture site with an antiseptic wipe and allowed it to air dry.
		•	Applied gloves and grasped infant's foot around the puncture site.
		•	Punctured the heel using a sterile lancet, and disposed of the lancet.
		•	Wiped away the first drop of blood with a gauze pad.
		▷	Explained why the first drop of blood should be wiped away.
		•	Encouraged a large drop of blood to form by exerting gentle pressure on the heel.
		•	Did not excessively squeeze the heel.
		▷	Explained why the excessive squeezing should be avoided.

Copyright © 2008, 2004, 2000, 1995, 1990 by Saunders, an imprint of Elsevier Inc. All rights reserved.

Trial 1	Trial 2	Point Value	*Performance Standards*
		•	Touched the drop of blood to the center of the first circle on the test card.
		•	Completely filled the circle on the test card with blood.
		•	Continued until all the circles are completely filled with blood.
		▷	Explained why each circle must be completely filled with blood.
		•	Did not touch the blood specimen with your gloved hand.
		▷	Stated why the specimen should not be touched.
		•	Held a gauze pad over the puncture site and applied pressure.
		•	Remained with infant until bleeding stopped. Applied an adhesive bandage if needed.
		•	Removed gloves and sanitized hands.
		•	Allowed test card to air-dry horizontally for 3 hours at room temperature.
		•	Did not allow the blood specimen to come in contact with any other surface.
		•	Did not place the specimen in a plastic bag.
		▷	Explained what occurs if the specimen is placed in a plastic bag.
		•	Placed test card in its protective envelope.
		•	Mailed card to laboratory within 48 hours.
		▷	Stated why the specimen must be mailed within 48 hours.
		•	Charted the procedure correctly.
		*	Completed the procedure within 10 minutes.
			TOTALS

CHART	
Date	

Evaluation of Student Performance

EVALUATION CRITERIA			COMMENTS
Symbol	Category	Point Value	
*	Critical Step	16 points	
•	Essential Step	6 points	
▷	Theory Question	2 points	

Score calculation: 100 points
– ____ points missed
____ Score

Satisfactory score: 85 or above

AAMA/CAAHEP Competency Achieved:

☑ III. C. 3. b. (4) (f): Prepare patient for and assist with procedures, treatments, and minor office surgeries.

Copyright © 2008, 2004, 2000, 1995, 1990 by Saunders, an imprint of Elsevier Inc. All rights reserved.

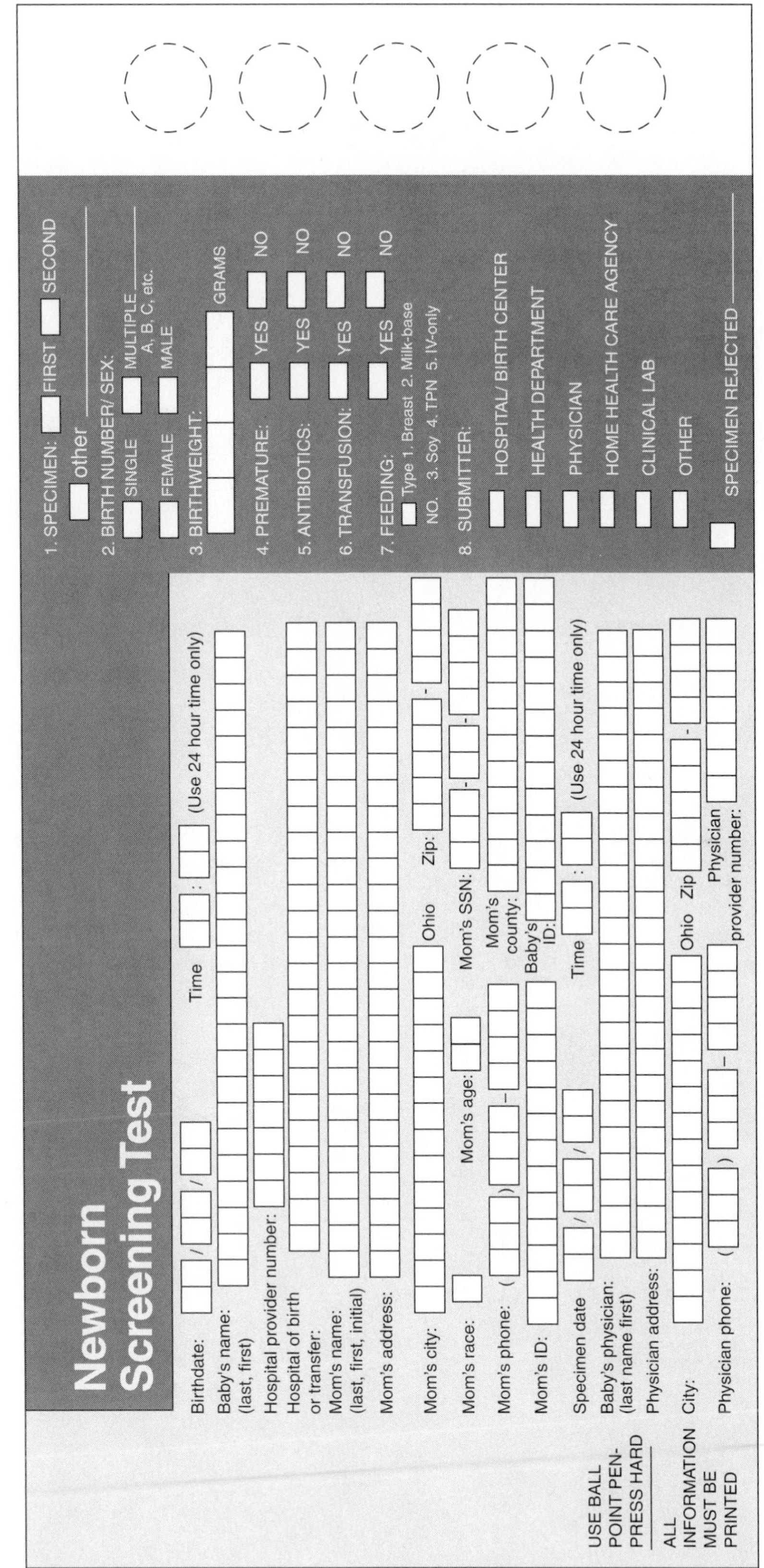

USE BALL POINT PEN- PRESS HARD

ALL INFORMATION MUST BE PRINTED

Newborn Screening Test

Birthdate: / / Time : (Use 24 hour time only)

Baby's name: (last, first)

Hospital provider number:

Hospital of birth or transfer:

Mom's name: (last, first, initial)

Mom's address:

Mom's city: Ohio Zip: -

Mom's race: Mom's age: Mom's SSN: - -

Mom's phone: ( ) - Mom's county:

Mom's ID: Baby's ID:

Specimen date / / Time : (Use 24 hour time only)

Baby's physician: (last name first)

Physician address:

City: Ohio Zip -

Physician phone: ( ) - Physician provider number:

1. SPECIMEN: FIRST SECOND other
2. BIRTH NUMBER/ SEX: SINGLE MULTIPLE A, B, C, etc. FEMALE MALE
3. BIRTHWEIGHT: GRAMS
4. PREMATURE: YES NO
5. ANTIBIOTICS: YES NO
6. TRANSFUSION: YES NO
7. FEEDING: YES NO Type 1. Breast 2. Milk-base NO. 3. Soy 4. TPN 5. IV-only
8. SUBMITTER: HOSPITAL/ BIRTH CENTER HEALTH DEPARTMENT PHYSICIAN HOME HEALTH CARE AGENCY CLINICAL LAB OTHER

SPECIMEN REJECTED

Copyright © 2008, 2004, 2000, 1995, 1990 by Saunders, an imprint of Elsevier Inc. All rights reserved.

Notes

Copyright © 2008, 2004, 2000, 1995, 1990 by Saunders, an imprint of Elsevier Inc. All rights reserved.

10

Minor Office Surgery

CHAPTER ASSIGNMENTS

√ After Completing	Date Due	Textbook Page(s)	TEXTBOOK ASSIGNMENTS	Possible Points	Points You Earned
		361-416	Read Chapter 10: Minor Office Surgery		
		384 411	Read Case Study 1 Case Study 1 questions	5	
		393 412	Read Case Study 2 Case Study 2 questions	5	
		404 412	Read Case Study 3 Case Study 3 questions	5	
		412-413	Apply Your Knowledge questions	10	
			TOTAL POINTS		
√ After Completing	**Date Due**	**Study Guide Page(s)**	**STUDY GUIDE ASSIGNMENTS (CTA: Critical Thinking Activity)**	**Possible Points**	**Points You Earned**
		411	Pretest	10	
		412	Key Term Assessment	25	
		413-416	Evaluation of Learning questions	43	
		416-417	CTA A: Medical and Surgical Asepsis	10	
		418	CTA B: Violation of Surgical Asepsis	10	
		419-421	CTA C: Surgical Instruments (2 points each)	26	
			CD Activity: Chapter 10 It's Instrumental (Record points earned)		
			CD Activity: Chapter 10 Keep It Sterile (Record points earned)		

Copyright © 2008, 2004, 2000, 1995, 1990 by Saunders, an imprint of Elsevier Inc. All rights reserved.

√ After Completing	Date Due	Study Guide Page(s)	STUDY GUIDE ASSIGNMENTS (CTA: Critical Thinking Activity)	Possible Points	Points You Earned
		421	CTA D: Pioneers in Surgical Asepsis (5 points each)	15	
		422	CTA E: Crossword Puzzle	24	
		423-425	CTA F: Patient Instruction Sheet	20	
		427	CTA G: Road to Recovery game (Record points earned)		
		411	Posttest	10	
			ADDITIONAL ASSIGNMENTS		
			TOTAL POINTS		

Copyright © 2008, 2004, 2000, 1995, 1990 by Saunders, an imprint of Elsevier Inc. All rights reserved.

√ When Assigned By Your Instructor	Study Guide Page(s)	Practices Required	LABORATORY ASSIGNMENTS (Procedure Number and Name)	*Score
	431	5	**Practice for Competency** 10-1: Applying and Removing Sterile Gloves Textbook reference: pp. 372-373	
	433-434		**Evaluation of Competency** 10-1: Applying and Removing Sterile Gloves	*
	431	5	**Practice for Competency** 10-2: Opening a Sterile Package Textbook reference: pp. 374-375	
	435-436		**Evaluation of Competency** 10-2: Opening a Sterile Package	*
	431	5	**Practice for Competency** Using Commercially Prepared Sterile Packages Textbook reference: p. 371	
	437-438		**Evaluation of Competency** Using Commercially Prepared Sterile Packages	*
	431	3	**Practice for Competency** 10-3: Pouring a Sterile Solution Textbook reference: p. 375	
	439-440		**Evaluation of Competency** 10-3: Pouring a Sterile Solution	*
	431	5	**Practice for Competency** 10-4: Changing a Sterile Dressing Textbook reference: pp. 378-380	
	441-443		**Evaluation of Competency** 10-4: Changing a Sterile Dressing	*
	431	Sutures: 3 Staples: 3	**Practice for Competency** 10-5: Removing Sutures and Staples Textbook reference: pp. 385-387	
	445-446		**Evaluation of Competency** 10-5: Removing Sutures and Staples	*
	431	3	**Practice for Competency** 10-6: Applying and Removing Adhesive Skin Closures Textbook reference: pp. 388-391	
	447-449		**Evaluation of Competency** 10-6: Applying and Removing Adhesive Skin Closures	*

Copyright © 2008, 2004, 2000, 1995, 1990 by Saunders, an imprint of Elsevier Inc. All rights reserved.

√ When Assigned By Your Instructor	Study Guide Page(s)	Practices Required	LABORATORY ASSIGNMENTS (Procedure Number and Name)	*Score
	431	5	**Practice for Competency** 10-7: Assisting with Minor Office Surgery Textbook reference: pp. 395-399	
	451-453		**Evaluation of Competency** 10-7: Assisting with Minor Office Surgery	*
	431	Each bandage turn: 3	**Practice for Competency** 10-A: Bandage Turns Textbook reference: pp. 406-408	
	455-456		**Evaluation of Competency** 10-A: Bandage Turns	*
	432	3	**Practice for Competency** 10-8: Applying a Tubular Gauze Bandage Textbook reference: pp. 409-411	
	457-458		**Evaluation of Competency** 10-8: Applying a Tubular Gauze Bandage	*
			ADDITIONAL ASSIGNMENTS	

Copyright © 2008, 2004, 2000, 1995, 1990 by Saunders, an imprint of Elsevier Inc. All rights reserved.

Name ______________________________ Date ______________

PRETEST

True or False

_____ 1. Surgical asepsis refers to practices that keep objects and areas free from all microorganism.

_____ 2. Something that is sterile is contaminated if it comes in contact with a pathogen.

_____ 3. Reaching over a sterile field is a violation of sterile technique.

_____ 4. An incision is a jagged tearing of the tissues.

_____ 5. The skin is the first line of defense of the body.

_____ 6. One of the local signs of inflammation is fever.

_____ 7. Sutures approximate the edges of a wound until proper healing occurs.

_____ 8. A biopsy is usually performed to determine if an infection is present.

_____ 9. An ingrown toenail can be caused by shoes that are too tight.

_____ 10. One of the functions of a bandage is to hold a dressing in place.

POSTTEST

True or False

_____ 1. Measuring a patient's temperature requires the use of surgical asepsis.

_____ 2. Hemostatic forceps are used to clamp off blood vessels.

_____ 3. An instrument with a ratchet should be kept in a closed position when not in use.

_____ 4. The physician would be most likely to order a tetanus booster for an abrasion.

_____ 5. Inflammation is the protective response of the body to trauma and the entrance of foreign substances.

_____ 6. A serous exudate is red in color.

_____ 7. Size 4-0 sutures have a smaller diameter than size 3 sutures.

_____ 8. Sebaceous cysts are commonly found on the palms of the hand.

_____ 9. Colposcopy is frequently used to evaluate lesions of the cervix.

_____ 10. Cryosurgery is used in the treatment of cervical cancer.

Copyright © 2008, 2004, 2000, 1995, 1990 by Saunders, an imprint of Elsevier Inc. All rights reserved.

KEY TERM ASSESSMENT

Directions: Match each medical term with its definition.

_____ 1. Abrasion
_____ 2. Abscess
_____ 3. Absorbable suture
_____ 4. Approximation
_____ 5. Bandage
_____ 6. Biopsy
_____ 7. Capillary action
_____ 8. Colposcope
_____ 9. Colposcopy
_____ 10. Contaminate
_____ 11. Contusion
_____ 12. Cryosurgery
_____ 13. Fibroblast
_____ 14. Forceps
_____ 15. Furuncle
_____ 16. Hemostasis
_____ 17. Incision
_____ 18. Infection
_____ 19. Inflammation
_____ 20. Laceration
_____ 21. Nonabsorbable suture
_____ 22. Puncture
_____ 23. Sterile
_____ 24. Surgical asepsis
_____ 25. Wound

A. A protective response of the body to trauma and the entrance of foreign matter
B. To cause a sterile object or surface to become unsterile
C. A wound made by a sharp pointed object piercing the skin
D. The condition in which the body is invaded by a pathogen
E. A collection of pus in a cavity surrounded by inflamed tissue
F. The arrest of bleeding by natural or artificial means
G. Free of all living microorganisms and bacterial spores
H. A wound in which the tissues are torn apart, leaving ragged and irregular edges
I. A lighted instrument with a binocular magnifying lens used to examine the vagina and cervix
J. A localized staphylococcal infection that originates deep within a hair follicle; also known as a boil
K. An injury to the tissues under the skin that causes blood vessels to rupture, allowing blood to seep into the tissues
L. The surgical removal and examination of tissue from the living body
M. A wound in which the outer layers of the skin are damaged
N. The action that causes liquid to rise along a wick, a tube, or a gauze dressing
O. A two-pronged instrument for grasping and squeezing
P. Practices that keep objects and areas sterile or free from microorganisms
Q. A break in the continuity of an external or internal surface caused by physical means
R. The therapeutic use of freezing temperatures to destroy abnormal tissue
S. The visual examination of the vagina and cervix using a lighted instrument with a magnifying lens
T. Suture material that is gradually digested by tissue enzymes and absorbed by the body
U. The process of bringing two parts, such as tissue, together, through the use of sutures or other means
V. A strip of woven material used to wrap or cover a part of the body
W. A clean cut caused by a cutting instrument
X. Suture material that is not absorbed by the body
Y. An immature cell from which connective tissue can develop

Copyright © 2008, 2004, 2000, 1995, 1990 by Saunders, an imprint of Elsevier Inc. All rights reserved.

EVALUATION OF LEARNING

Directions: Fill in each blank with the correct answer.

1. List the responsibilities of the medical assistant during a minor surgical operation.

____

____

____

____

2. What is the function of a speculum?

____

3. List five guidelines that should be followed in caring for instruments.

____

____

____

____

4. What is the difference between a closed and an open wound?

____

____

5. Why does a puncture wound encourage the growth of tetanus bacteria?

____

____

6. What is the purpose of inflammation?

____

7. List the four local signs that occur during inflammation.

____

8. What occurs during the inflammatory phase of wound healing?

____

____

9. What occurs during the granulation phase of wound healing?

____

____

10. What occurs during the maturation phase of wound healing?

____

11. What is an exudate?

____

____

Copyright © 2008, 2004, 2000, 1995, 1990 by Saunders, an imprint of Elsevier Inc. All rights reserved.

12. Define the following types of exudates:
    a. Serous ______
    b. Sanguineous______
    c. Purulent ______

13. List two functions of a sterile dressing.

______

______

14. Listed below are the names and sizes of sutures. In each of the following, circle the suture that has the smaller diameter:
    a. 4-0 surgical silk
       00 surgical silk
    b. 0 chromic gut
       3-0 chromic gut
    c. 2-0 polypropylene
       2 polypropylene

15. List five examples of materials used for nonabsorbable sutures.

______

______

16. What is a swaged needle? List advantages of using a swaged needle.

______

______

17. Why are sutures inserted in the head and neck generally removed sooner than other sutures?

______

______

18. List two advantages of using surgical skin staples to approximate a wound.

______

______

19. List three advantages of adhesive skin closures.

______

______

______

20. What is the purpose of preparing the patient's skin before minor office surgery?

______

21. What is the purpose of a fenestrated drape?

______

______

Copyright © 2008, 2004, 2000, 1995, 1990 by Saunders, an imprint of Elsevier Inc. All rights reserved.

22. List the names of two local anesthetics commonly used in the medical office during minor office surgery.

23. Explain how an instrument should be handed to the physician during minor office surgery.

24. What is a sebaceous cyst, and what causes it to form?

25. What is the purpose of using a rubber Penrose drain after incising a localized infection?

26. What is the purpose of a needle biopsy?

27. What is an ingrown toenail?

28. List three causes of an ingrown toenail.

29. List three reasons for performing a colposcopy.

30. What is the purpose of performing a cervical punch biopsy?

31. List the postoperative instructions that must be relayed to the patient following a cervical punch biopsy.

32. List two uses of cryosurgery.

33. List the postoperative instructions that must be relayed to the patient following cervical cryosurgery.

Copyright © 2008, 2004, 2000, 1995, 1990 by Saunders, an imprint of Elsevier Inc. All rights reserved.

34. List three functions of a bandage.

35. List four guidelines to follow when applying a bandage.

36. List four signs that may indicate a bandage is too tight.

37. Why should the medical assistant be careful when applying an elastic bandage?

38. What is the purpose of reversing the spiral during a spiral-reverse turn?

39. List two uses of the figure-eight bandage turn.

40. What type of bandage turn is used to anchor a bandage?

41. List four examples of body parts to which a tubular bandage can be applied.

42. List two advantages for using a tubular bandage (as compared with a roller bandage).

43. Explain why a tubular bandage cannot be used over an open wound.

CRITICAL THINKING ACTIVITIES

A. MEDICAL AND SURGICAL ASEPSIS

Refer to Chapter 2 and describe the difference between medical asepsis and surgical asepsis.

Copyright © 2008, 2004, 2000, 1995, 1990 by Saunders, an imprint of Elsevier Inc. All rights reserved.

Which technique (medical asepsis or surgical asepsis) would be employed during the following procedures? In those procedures requiring surgical asepsis, indicate which of the following reasons necessitate the use of surgical asepsis: caring for broken skin, penetrating a skin surface, or entering a body cavity that is normally sterile.

1. Administering oral medication

____

____

2. Inserting sutures

____

____

3. Measuring oral temperature

____

____

4. Applying a bandage to the forearm

____

____

5. Performing a needle biopsy

____

____

6. Removing a sebaceous cyst

____

____

7. Obtaining a Pap smear

____

____

8. Inserting a urinary catheter

____

____

9. Incision and drainage of an abscess

____

____

10. Applying a dressing to an open wound

____

____

Copyright © 2008, 2004, 2000, 1995, 1990 by Saunders, an imprint of Elsevier Inc. All rights reserved.

B. VIOLATION OF SURGICAL ASEPSIS

In the situations that follow, the principles of surgical asepsis have been violated. In the space provided, explain why the techniques should not be performed in this manner.

1. Not checking the sterilization indicator on a sterile package before opening it

2. Wearing rings during the application of sterile gloves

3. Talking over a sterile field

4. Reaching over a sterile field

5. Holding sterile gauze below waist level

6. Not palming the label when pouring an antiseptic solution

7. Spilling an antiseptic solution on the sterile field

8. Passing a soiled dressing over the sterile field

9. Placing a vial of Xylocaine on the sterile field

10. Using bare hands to arrange articles on the sterile field

Copyright © 2008, 2004, 2000, 1995, 1990 by Saunders, an imprint of Elsevier Inc. All rights reserved.

C. SURGICAL INSTRUMENTS

In the space provided, state the name and use of each of the following types of surgical instruments. Identify any of the following parts present on each instrument by labeling the instrument: box lock, spring handle, ratchets, serrations, cutting edge, and teeth.

(Courtesy of Elmed Incorporated, Addison, IL.)

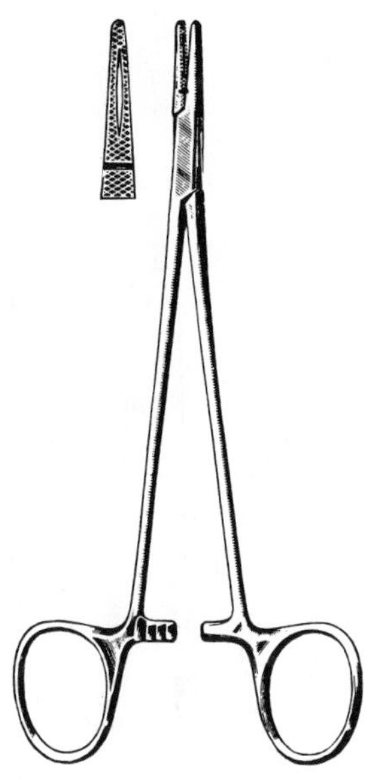

1. Name: ____________________

Use: ____________________

____

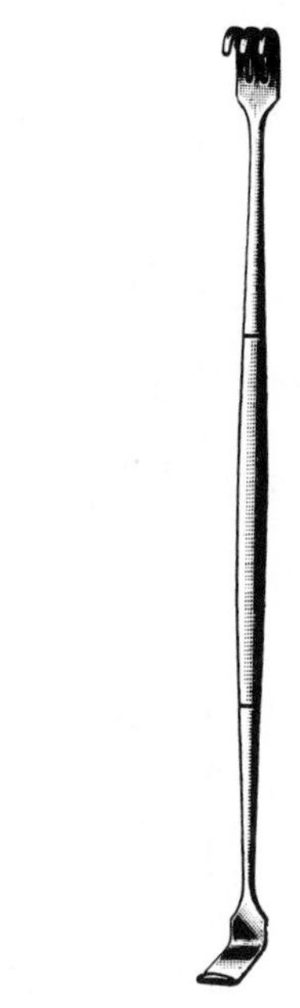

2. Name: ____________________

Use: ____________________

____

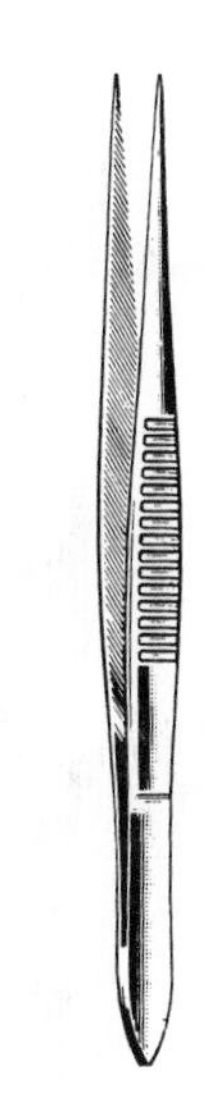

3. Name: ____________________

Use: ____________________

____

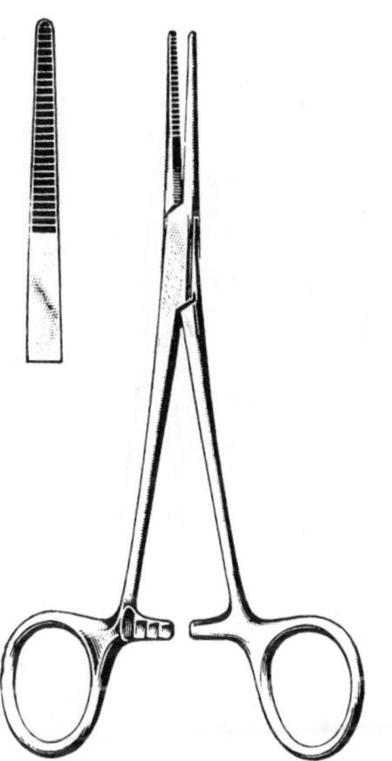

4. Name: ____________________

Use: ____________________

____

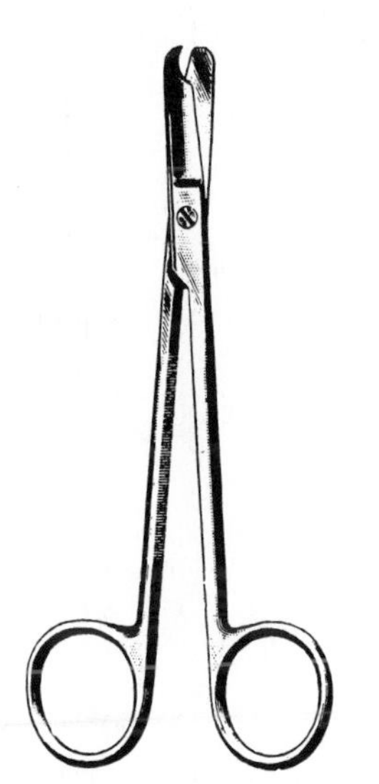

5. Name: ____________________

Use: ____________________

____

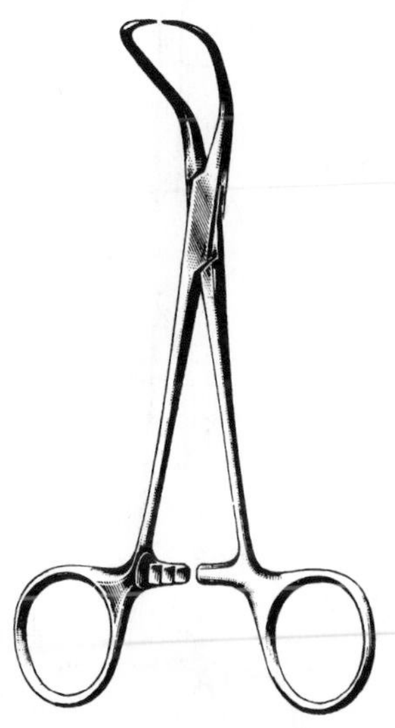

6. Name: ____________________

Use: ____________________

____

(Courtesy of Elmed Incorporated, Addison, IL.)

Copyright © 2008, 2004, 2000, 1995, 1990 by Saunders, an imprint of Elsevier Inc. All rights reserved.

(Courtesy of Elmed Incorporated, Addison, IL.)

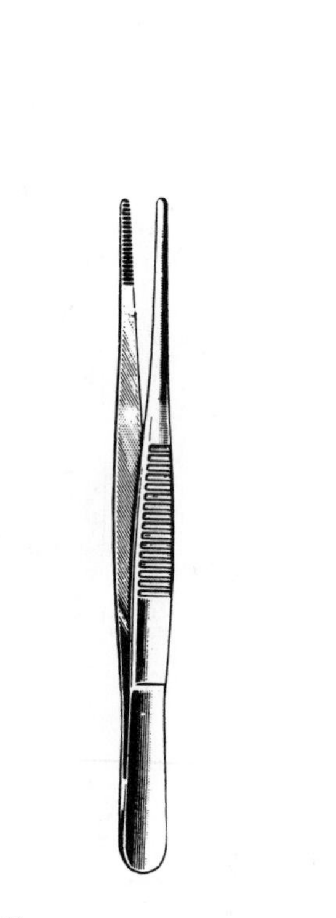

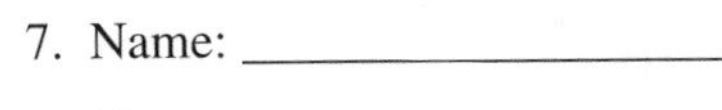

7. Name: ______________________
   Use: ______________________
   ____

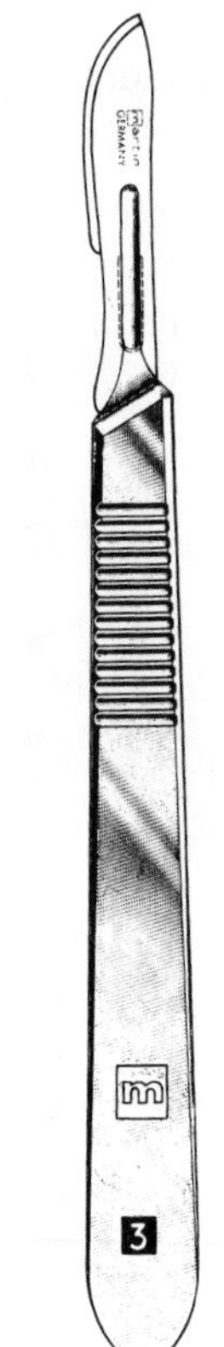

8. Name: ______________________
   Use: ______________________
   ____

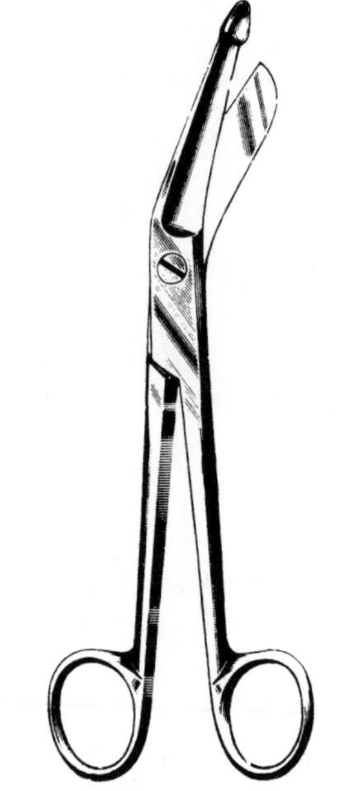

9. Name: ______________________
   Use: ______________________
   ____

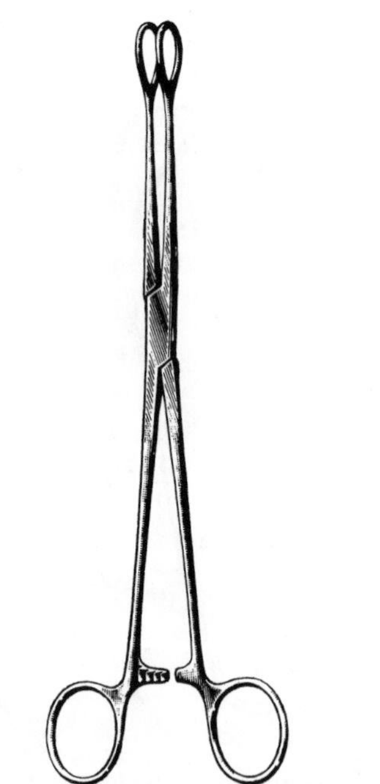

10. Name: ______________________
    Use: ______________________
    ____

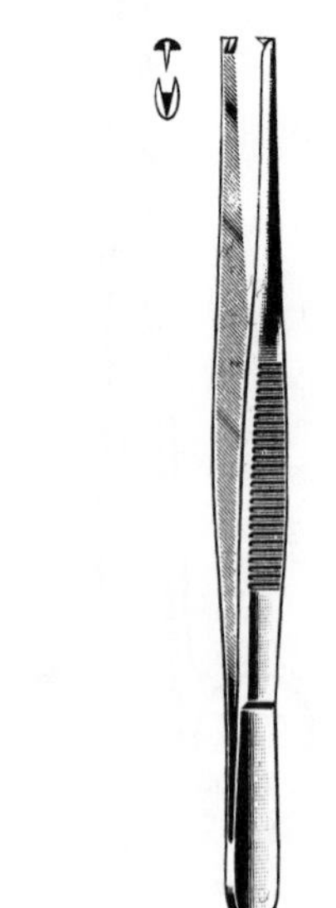

11. Name: ______________________
    Use: ______________________
    ____

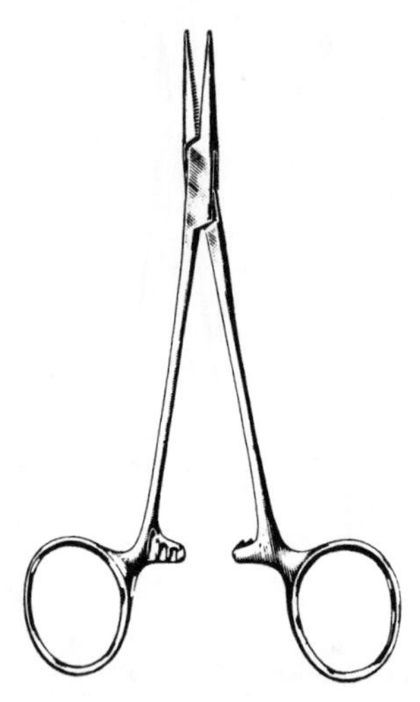

12. Name: ______________________
    Use: ______________________
    ____

(Courtesy of Elmed Incorporated, Addison, IL.)

Copyright © 2008, 2004, 2000, 1995, 1990 by Saunders, an imprint of Elsevier Inc. All rights reserved.

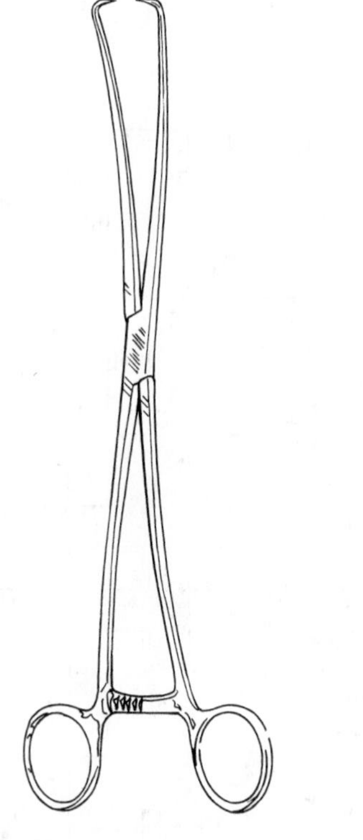

13. Name: ____________________

Use: ____________________

____

(Courtesy of Elmed Incorporated, Addison, IL.)

D. PIONEERS IN SURGICAL ASEPSIS

Using a reference source, in the space provided describe the contributions the following men made to medicine, especially regarding surgical asepsis:

1. Ignaz Semmelweis

____

____

____

2. Louis Pasteur

____

____

____

3. Joseph Lister

____

____

____

Copyright © 2008, 2004, 2000, 1995, 1990 by Saunders, an imprint of Elsevier Inc. All rights reserved.

E. CROSSWORD PUZZLE
Minor Office Surgery

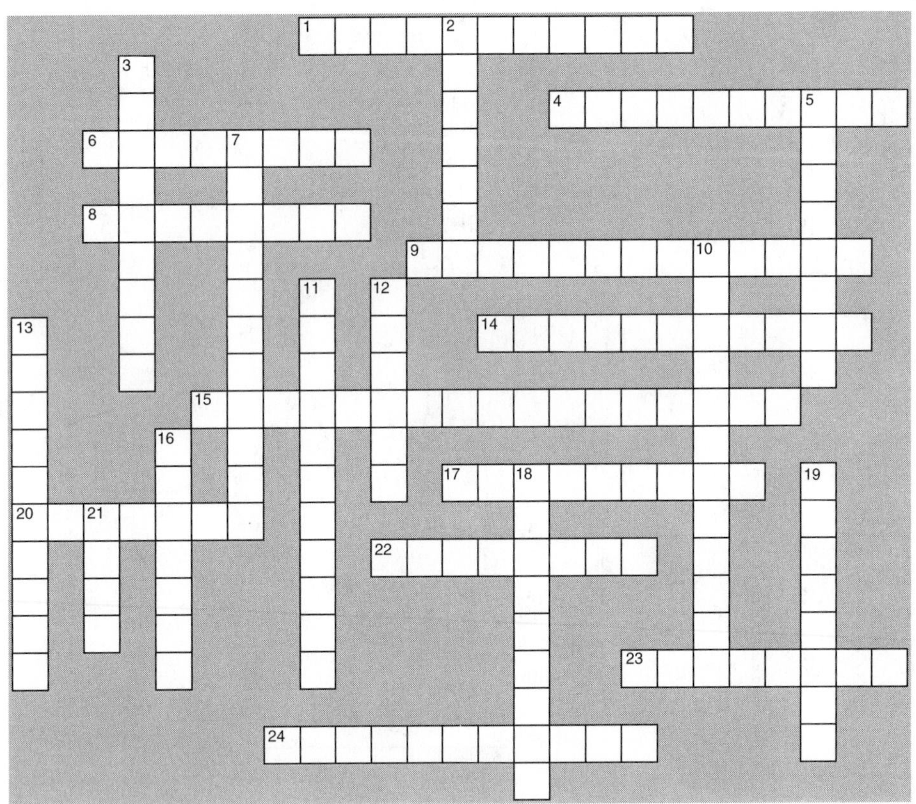

Directions: Complete the crossword puzzle using the clues presented below.

ACROSS

1 Drape with a hole
4 Produces collagen
6 Clean, smooth cut
8 Boil
9 Sac containing oil secretions
14 Pus formation
15 Clamps off blood vessels
17 Local anesthetic brand name
20 Pus in a cavity
22 Tetanus may grow here
23 A local sign of inflammation
24 Bring together

DOWN

2 Free of all MOs and spores
3 Bruise
5 Scrape
7 Exudate containing blood
10 Suture/needle combination
11 Tx for chronic cervicitis
12 Father of modern surgery
13 Ragged and irregular wound
16 Discovered penicillin
18 Position for colposcopy
19 Antiseptic brand name
21 Nonabsorbable suture material

Copyright © 2008, 2004, 2000, 1995, 1990 by Saunders, an imprint of Elsevier Inc. All rights reserved.

F. PATIENT INSTRUCTION SHEET

1. You are working for a surgeon and she would like you to develop a patient instruction sheet for minor surgery. Select one of the minor surgeries presented below. Using the following instruction sheet, develop a sheet that would be informative and visually appealing to a patient. Be as creative as possible in designing your sheet.
2. Select a partner. Have your partner play the role of a patient that is going to have the minor surgery performed and explain the information on the sheet. Ask the patient to sign the sheet and witness the patient's signature.

Minor Office Surgeries:

a. Sebaceous cyst removal

b. Needle biopsy

c. Ingrown toenail removal

d. Colposcopy and biopsy

e. Cervical cryosurgery

Copyright © 2008, 2004, 2000, 1995, 1990 by Saunders, an imprint of Elsevier Inc. All rights reserved.

Notes

Copyright © 2008, 2004, 2000, 1995, 1990 by Saunders, an imprint of Elsevier Inc. All rights reserved.

PATIENT INSTRUCTION SHEET

NAME OF THE PROCEDURE:

DESCRIPTION OF PROCEDURE:

PURPOSE OF THE PROCEDURE:

HOW TO PREPARE FOR THE PROCEDURE:

WHAT TO DO FOLLOWING THE PROCEDURE:

I have received and understand the above instructions:

Patient's Signature ______________________________

Witness: ______________________________ Date: ____________

Copyright © 2008, 2004, 2000, 1995, 1990 by Saunders, an imprint of Elsevier Inc. All rights reserved.

G. ROAD TO RECOVERY

Surgical Asepsis

Object: The object of the game is to lead your "patient" to recovery by correctly determining if an action violates sterile technique or does not violate sterile technique.

Needed: **Road to Recovery** game board (located at the end of this manual)
Game cards
A token for each player (such as a button or coin)
Dice (1)
Playing cards
Score card

Directions:

1. Get into a group of four students. Make a list of 16 actions that violate (**V**) surgical asepsis and 16 actions that do not violate (**NV**) surgical asepsis (for a total of 32). You can use the information in Critical Thinking Activity B for some of your actions that violate surgical asepsis. Each student should take four **V** actions and four **NV** actions and write them on his or her game cards (located on the following page), making sure to use the appropriate **V** or **NV** card.
2. Cut out the game cards and trade your group's set of 32 game cards with another group.
3. Place one complete set of cards on the game board with the action facing up (and the **V** or **NV** designation facing down).
4. Play **Road to Recovery** following the directions on the reverse side of the game board. A player should pick up a card, read the action, and respond by indicating whether the action violates sterile technique or does not violate sterile technique. Turn your card over to determine if you answered correctly. If you did, award yourself 5 points. If you answered incorrectly, you receive 0 points. If time permits, trade your set of cards with another group and continue playing. If a question arises as to the correct answer, consult your instructor for assistance.
5. Keep track of your points using the score card provided.

Copyright © 2008, 2004, 2000, 1995, 1990 by Saunders, an imprint of Elsevier Inc. All rights reserved.

ROAD TO RECOVERY
SCORE CARD

Name: ______________________________

Recording Points:
Using the Game Card Points box, cross off a number each time you answer a game card correctly (starting with 5 and continuing in sequence). Your total game card points will be equal to the last number you crossed off. Record this number in the space provided (1). Record any extra points you were awarded during the game (2), and any points that were deducted (3). To determine your total points, add (1) and (2) together and deduct (3). Record this number in the Total Points Earned space provided. Compare your score with the other players and determine where you placed. Place a check mark next to the level of recovery your patient attained.

Game Card Points:

5	75	145	215
10	80	150	220
15	85	155	225
20	90	160	230
25	95	165	235
30	100	170	240
35	105	175	245
40	110	180	250
45	115	185	255
50	120	190	260
55	125	195	265
60	130	200	270
65	135	205	275
70	140	210	280

Calculation of Points:

(1) Total Game Card Points: ________

(2) Additional Points Awarded: ________

(3) Deducted Points: ________

TOTAL POINTS EARNED: ________

LEVEL OF RECOVERY:

Patient's Name: ____________________

☐ First Place: **Fully Recovered**
☐ Second Place: **Almost Recovered**
☐ Third Place: **Still Recovering**
☐ Fourth Place: **Gasping for Air**

Copyright © 2008, 2004, 2000, 1995, 1990 by Saunders, an imprint of Elsevier Inc. All rights reserved.

Action:

Action:

Action:

Action:

Action:

Action:

Action:

Action:

V	V
V	V
NV	NV
NV	NV

PRACTICE FOR COMPETENCY

Sterile Technique

Procedure 10-1: Applying and Removing Sterile Gloves. Apply and remove sterile gloves.

Procedure 10-2: Sterile Package. Open a sterile package.

Commercially Prepared Sterile Packages. Add a sterile article to a sterile field using a peel-apart package. Practice each of the methods used to transfer articles to a sterile field as shown in Figure 10-3 of your textbook.

Procedure 10-3: Sterile Solution. Pour a sterile solution into a container on a sterile field.

Minor Surgical Procedures

Procedure 10-4: Sterile Dressing. Change a sterile dressing and record the procedure in the chart provided.

Procedure 10-5: Suture and Staple Removal. Practice the procedure for removing sutures and staples and record the procedure in the chart provided.

Procedure 10-6: Adhesive Skin Closures. Practice the procedure for applying and removing adhesive skin closures and record the procedure in the chart provided.

Procedure 10-7: Assisting with Minor Office Surgery. Obtain 8 index cards. For each of the following minor office surgeries, indicate (on one side of the card) the equipment and supplies required for the side table. On the other side of the card, indicate the equipment and supplies required for the sterile tray setup. Set up a surgical tray for the procedures listed below using your index cards, In the chart provided, record the instructions relayed to the patient following the surgery.

a. Suture insertion

b. Sebaceous cyst removal

c. Incision and drainage of a localized infection

d. Needle biopsy

e. Ingrown toenail removal

f. Colposcopy

g. Cervical punch biopsy

h. Cervical cryosurgery

Procedure 10-A: Bandage Turns

Practice the following bandage turns:

a. Circular turn

b. Spiral turn

c. Spiral-reverse turn

d. Figure-eight turn

e. Recurrent turn

Copyright © 2008, 2004, 2000, 1995, 1990 by Saunders, an imprint of Elsevier Inc. All rights reserved.

Procedure 10-8: Tubular Gauze Bandage. Practice the procedure for applying a tubular gauze bandage and record the procedure in the chart provided.

CHART	
Date	

Copyright © 2008, 2004, 2000, 1995, 1990 by Saunders, an imprint of Elsevier Inc. All rights reserved.

EVALUATION OF COMPETENCY

Procedure 10-1: Applying and Removing Sterile Gloves

Name: ______________________________ Date: ______________

Evaluated By: ______________________________ Score: ______________

Performance Objective

Outcome:	Apply and remove sterile gloves.
Conditions:	Given the appropriate sized sterile gloves.
	Using a clean flat surface.
Standards:	Time: 5 minutes. Student completed procedure in ____ minutes.
	Accuracy: Satisfactory score on the Performance Evaluation Checklist.

Performance Evaluation Checklist

Trial 1	*Trial 2*	*Point Value*	*Performance Standards*
			Application of Gloves
		•	Removed rings and washed hands with an antimicrobial soap.
		▷	Explained why the hands should be washed.
		•	Selected the appropriate sized gloves.
		•	Explained what might occur if the gloves are too small or too large.
		•	Placed the glove package on a clean flat surface.
		•	Opened the sterile glove package without touching the inside of the wrapper.
		•	Picked up the first glove on the inside of the cuff without contaminating.
		▷	Explained why the inside of the cuff can be touched with the bare hand.
		•	Did not touch the outside of the glove with the bare hand.
		•	Stepped back and pulled on glove and allowed the cuff to remain turned back on itself.
		•	Picked up the second glove by slipping sterile gloved fingers under its cuff and grasping the opposite side with the thumb..
		▷	Stated how the above step prevents contamination.
		•	Pulled the glove on and turned back the cuff.
		•	Turned back the cuff of the first glove without contaminating.
		•	Adjusted the gloves to a comfortable position.
		•	Inspected the gloves for tears.
		▷	Explained what should be done if a glove is torn.

Copyright © 2008, 2004, 2000, 1995, 1990 by Saunders, an imprint of Elsevier Inc. All rights reserved.

Trial 1	Trial 2	Point Value	Performance Standards
			Removal of Gloves
		•	Grasped the outside of the right glove 1 to 2 inches from the top with the gloved left hand.
		•	Slowly pulled right glove off the hand.
		•	Pulled the right glove free and scrunched it into a ball with the gloved left hand.
		•	Placed index and middle fingers of the right hand on the inside of left glove.
		•	Did not allow the clean hand to touch the outside of the glove.
		•	Pulled the glove off the left hand, enclosing the balled-up right glove.
		•	Discarded both gloves in an appropriate waste container.
		▷	Stated how to discard gloves if they are visibly contaminated with blood.
		•	Sanitized hands.
		✶	Completed the procedure within 5 minutes.
			TOTALS

Evaluation of Student Performance

EVALUATION CRITERIA			COMMENTS
Symbol	Category	Point Value	
✶	Critical Step	16 points	
•	Essential Step	6 points	
▷	Theory Question	2 points	
Score calculation: 100 points – ______ points missed ____ Score Satisfactory score: 85 or above			

AAMA/CAAHEP Competency Achieved:

☑ III. C. 3. b. (4) (f): Prepare patient for and assist with procedures, treatments, and minor office surgeries.

Copyright © 2008, 2004, 2000, 1995, 1990 by Saunders, an imprint of Elsevier Inc. All rights reserved.

EVALUATION OF COMPETENCY

Procedure 10-2: Opening a Sterile Package

Name: ______________________________ Date: ______________

Evaluated By: ______________________________ Score: ______________

Performance Objective

Outcome:	Open a sterile package.
Conditions:	Given a sterile package.
	Using a clean flat surface.
Standards:	Time: 5 minutes. Student completed procedure in ____ minutes.
	Accuracy: Satisfactory score on the Performance Evaluation Checklist.

Performance Evaluation Checklist

Trial 1	*Trial 2*	*Point Value*	*Performance Standards*
		•	Sanitized hands.
		•	Assembled equipment.
		•	Checked pack to make sure it is not wet, torn, or opened.
		•	Checked the autoclave tape on the pack.
		▷	Stated the purpose of autoclave tape.
		•	Positioned the pack on the table so that the top flap of wrapper will open away from the body.
		•	Removed the fastener on wrapped package and discarded it.
		•	Opened the first flap away from the body.
		•	Opened the left and right flaps without contaminating contents.
		•	Opened the flap closest to the body.
		•	In all cases, only touched the outside of the wrapper.
		•	In all cases, did not reach over the sterile contents of the package.
		▷	Stated why the medical assistant should not reach over the contents of the package.
		•	Adjusted the sterile wrapper by the corners as needed.
		•	Checked the sterilization indicator on the inside of the pack.
		*	Completed the procedure within 5 minutes.
			TOTALS

Copyright © 2008, 2004, 2000, 1995, 1990 by Saunders, an imprint of Elsevier Inc. All rights reserved.

Evaluation of Student Performance

EVALUATION CRITERIA			COMMENTS
Symbol	Category	Point Value	
*	Critical Step	16 points	
●	Essential Step	6 points	
▷	Theory Question	2 points	
Score calculation: 100 points – ______ points missed ____ Score Satisfactory score: 85 or above			

AAMA/CAAHEP Competency Achieved:

☑ III. C. 3. b. (4) (f): Prepare patient for and assist with procedures, treatments, and minor office surgeries.

Copyright © 2008, 2004, 2000, 1995, 1990 by Saunders, an imprint of Elsevier Inc. All rights reserved.

EVALUATION OF COMPETENCY

Using Commercially Prepared Sterile Packages

Name: ______________________________ Date: ______________

Evaluated By: ______________________________ Score: ______________

Performance Objective

Outcome:	Add a sterile article to a sterile field from a peel-apart package by ejecting its contents onto the field.
Conditions:	Given the following: peel-apart package and a sterile field.
Standards:	Time: 3 minutes. Student completed procedure in ____ minutes.
	Accuracy: Satisfactory score on the Performance Evaluation Checklist.

Performance Evaluation Checklist

Trial 1	Trial 2	Point Value	*Performance Standards*
		•	Sanitized hands.
		•	Grasped the two unsterile flaps of the peel-pack between thumbs.
		•	Pulled the package apart using a rolling-outward motion.
		▷	Stated what parts of the peel-pack must remain sterile.
		•	Stepped back slightly from the sterile field.
		▷	Explained the reason for stepping back.
		•	Gently ejected contents of the peel-pack onto the center of the sterile field.
		*	Completed the procedure within 3 minutes.
			TOTALS

Copyright © 2008, 2004, 2000, 1995, 1990 by Saunders, an imprint of Elsevier Inc. All rights reserved.

Evaluation of Student Performance

EVALUATION CRITERIA			COMMENTS
Symbol	**Category**	**Point Value**	
✶	Critical Step	16 points	
●	Essential Step	6 points	
▷	Theory Question	2 points	
Score calculation: 100 points – ______ points missed ____ Score Satisfactory score: 85 or above			

AAMA/CAAHEP Competency Achieved:

☑ III. C. 3. b. (4) (f): Prepare patient for and assist with procedures, treatments, and minor office surgeries.

Copyright © 2008, 2004, 2000, 1995, 1990 by Saunders, an imprint of Elsevier Inc. All rights reserved.

EVALUATION OF COMPETENCY

DVD Procedure 10-3: Pouring a Sterile Solution

Name: ______________________________ Date: ______________

Evaluated By: ______________________________ Score: ______________

Performance Objective

Outcome:	Pour a sterile solution.
Conditions:	Given the following: sterile solution, sterile container, and a sterile towel.
Standards:	Time: 5 minutes Student completed procedure in ____ minutes.
	Accuracy: Satisfactory score on the Performance Evaluation Checklist.

Performance Evaluation Checklist

Trial 1	*Trial 2*	*Point Value*	*Performance Standards*
		•	Checked the label of the solution.
		•	Checked expiration date on the solution.
		•	Checked solution label a second time.
		•	Palmed the label of the bottle.
		▷	Explained why the label should be palmed.
		•	Removed cap and placed it on a flat surface with the open end up.
		▷	Stated why cap should be placed with the open end up.
		•	Rinsed the lip of the bottle.
		▷	Explained why the lip of the bottle should be rinsed.
		•	Poured the proper amount of solution into a sterile container.
		•	Did not allow the neck of the bottle to come in contact with container.
		•	Did not allow any of the solution to splash onto the sterile field.
		▷	Explained why the sterile solution should not be allowed to splash onto the sterile field.
		•	Replaced cap on container without contaminating.
		•	Checked the label a third time.
		*	Completed the procedure within 5 minutes.
			TOTALS

Copyright © 2008, 2004, 2000, 1995, 1990 by Saunders, an imprint of Elsevier Inc. All rights reserved.

Evaluation of Student Performance

EVALUATION CRITERIA			COMMENTS
Symbol	Category	Point Value	
*	Critical Step	16 points	
●	Essential Step	6 points	
▷	Theory Question	2 points	
Score calculation: 100 points – ______ points missed ____ Score Satisfactory score: 85 or above			

AAMA/CAAHEP Competency Achieved:

☑ III. C. 3. b. (4) (f): Prepare patient for and assist with procedures, treatments, and minor office surgeries.

Copyright © 2008, 2004, 2000, 1995, 1990 by Saunders, an imprint of Elsevier Inc. All rights reserved.

EVALUATION OF COMPETENCY

Procedure 10-4: Changing a Sterile Dressing

Name: ______________________________ Date: ______________

Evaluated By: ______________________________ Score: ______________

Performance Objective

Outcome:	Change a sterile dressing.
Conditions:	Given the following: clean disposable gloves, antiseptic swabs, sterile gloves, plastic waste bag, adhesive tape and scissors, biohazard waste container, sterile dressing, and thumb forceps.
Standards:	Time: 10 minutes. Student completed procedure in ____ minutes.
	Accuracy: Satisfactory score on the Performance Evaluation Checklist.

Performance Evaluation Checklist

Trial 1	*Trial 2*	*Point Value*	*Performance Standards*
		•	Washed hands with an antimicrobial soap.
		•	Assembled equipment.
		•	Set up nonsterile items.
		•	Positioned the plastic waste bag in a convenient location.
		•	Greeted the patient and introduced yourself.
		•	Identified patient and explained the procedure.
		•	Instructed patient not to move during procedure.
		•	Adjusted the light.
		•	Applied clean gloves.
		•	Loosened the tape and carefully removed soiled dressing.
		•	Did not touch inside of dressing next to the wound.
		▷	Explained why the inside of the dressing should not be touched.
		▷	Described what should be done if the dressing is stuck to the wound.
		•	Placed soiled dressing in the waste bag without touching outside of bag.
		•	Inspected the wound.
		▷	Stated what type of inspection should be performed.
		•	Opened the antiseptic swabs and placed the pouch in a convenient location or held them.
		•	Applied the antiseptic to the wound.
		•	Used a new swab for each motion.
		•	Discarded each contaminated swab in the waste bag after use.

Copyright © 2008, 2004, 2000, 1995, 1990 by Saunders, an imprint of Elsevier Inc. All rights reserved.

Trial 1	Trial 2	Point Value	Performance Standards
		•	Removed gloves and discarded them without contaminating.
		•	Sanitized hands and prepared the sterile field.
		•	Opened sterile glove package and applied sterile gloves.
		•	Picked up sterile dressing from the tray using sterile gloves or sterile forceps.
		•	Placed sterile dressing over the wound by lightly dropping it in place.
		▷	Explained why the dressing should be dropped onto the wound.
		•	Did not move dressing after dropping it in place.
		▷	Stated why the dressing should not be moved.
		•	Discarded gloves (and forceps) in the waste bag.
		•	Applied hypoallergenic tape to hold sterile dressing in place.
		•	Instructed patient in wound care.
		▷	Described the wound care that should be relayed to the patient.
		•	Provided the patient with written instructions.
		•	Asked patient to sign instruction sheet.
		•	Witnessed the patient's signature.
		•	Gave a signed copy to the patient.
		•	Filed original in the patient's medical record.
		▷	Stated purpose of filing original in patient's chart.
		•	Returned equipment.
		•	Disposed of plastic bag in a biohazard waste container.
		•	Sanitized hands.
		•	Charted the procedure correctly.
		*	Completed the procedure within 10 minutes.
			TOTALS

CHART

Date	

Copyright © 2008, 2004, 2000, 1995, 1990 by Saunders, an imprint of Elsevier Inc. All rights reserved.

Evaluation of Student Performance

EVALUATION CRITERIA			COMMENTS
Symbol	Category	Point Value	
*	Critical Step	16 points	
•	Essential Step	6 points	
▷	Theory Question	2 points	
Score calculation: 100 points – ____ points missed ____ Score Satisfactory score: 85 or above			

AAMA/CAAHEP Competency Achieved:

☑ III. C. 3. b. (4) (f): Prepare patient for and assist with procedures, treatments, and minor office surgeries.
☑ III. C. 3. c. (3) (c): Provide instruction for health maintenance and disease prevention.

Copyright © 2008, 2004, 2000, 1995, 1990 by Saunders, an imprint of Elsevier Inc. All rights reserved.

Notes

Copyright © 2008, 2004, 2000, 1995, 1990 by Saunders, an imprint of Elsevier Inc. All rights reserved.

EVALUATION OF COMPETENCY

Procedure 10-5: Removing Sutures and Staples

Name: ______________________________ Date: ____________

Evaluated By: ______________________________ Score: ____________

Performance Objective

Outcome:	Remove sutures and staples.
Conditions:	Given the following: antiseptic swabs, clean disposable gloves, sterile 4 × 4 gauze, surgical tape, biohazard waste container, suture removal kid, and staple removal kit.
Standards:	Time: 10 minutes. Student completed procedure in ____ minutes.
	Accuracy: Satisfactory score on the Performance Evaluation Checklist.

Performance Evaluation Checklist

Trial 1	*Trial 2*	*Point Value*	*Performance Standards*
		•	Washed hands with an antimicrobial soap.
		•	Assembled equipment.
		•	Greeted the patient and introduced yourself.
		•	Identified patient and explained the procedure.
		•	Positioned the patient as required.
		•	Adjusted the light.
		•	Checked to make sure the sutures (or staples) were intact.
		•	Checked to make sure the incision line was approximated and free from infection.
		▷	Explained what to do if the incision line is not approximated.
		•	Opened the suture or staple removal kit.
		•	Applied clean gloves.
		•	Cleaned the incision line with antiseptic swabs using a new swab for each motion.
		•	Allowed the skin to dry.
			Removed Sutures as Follows:
		•	Informed the patient that he or she would feel a pulling sensation.
		•	Picked up the knot of suture with thumb forceps.
		•	Placed curved tip of suture scissors under the suture.
		•	Cut suture below the knot on the side of suture closest to the skin.
		•	Gently pulled suture out of the skin, using a smooth continuous motion.

Copyright © 2008, 2004, 2000, 1995, 1990 by Saunders, an imprint of Elsevier Inc. All rights reserved.

Trial 1	Trial 2	Point Value	*Performance Standards*
		•	Did not allow any portion of suture previously on the outside to be pulled through the tissue lying beneath the incision line.
		•	Placed the suture on the gauze.
		•	Repeated above sequence until all sutures were removed.
			Removed Staples as Follows:
		• •	Gently placed the jaws of the staple remover under the staple. Squeezed the staple handles until they were closed.
		• •	Lifted the staple remover upward to remove the staple. Placed staple on gauze.
		•	Continued until all the staples were removed.
		•	Counted number of sutures or staples and checked number with chart.
		•	Cleansed the site with an antiseptic swab.
		•	Applied adhesive skin closures if directed by physician.
		•	Applied DSD, if directed to do so by physician.
		•	Disposed of sutures or staples and gauze in biohazard waste container.
		•	Removed gloves and sanitized hands.
		•	Charted the procedure correctly.
		✶	Completed the procedure within 10 minutes.
			TOTALS

CHART	
Date	

Evaluation of Student Performance

EVALUATION CRITERIA			COMMENTS
Symbol	Category	Point Value	
✶	Critical Step	16 points	
•	Essential Step	6 points	
▷	Theory Question	2 points	
Score calculation: 100 points – ____ points missed ____ Score Satisfactory score: 85 or above			

AAMA/CAAHEP Competency Achieved:

☑ III. C. 3. b. (4) (f): Prepare patient for and assist with procedures, treatments, and minor office surgeries.
☑ III. C. 3. c. (3) (c): Provide instruction for health maintenance and disease prevention.

Copyright © 2008, 2004, 2000, 1995, 1990 by Saunders, an imprint of Elsevier Inc. All rights reserved.

EVALUATION OF COMPETENCY

Procedure 10-6: Applying and Removing Adhesive Skin Closures

Name: ______________________________ Date: ______________

Evaluated By: ______________________________ Score: ______________

Performance Objective

Outcome: Apply and remove adhesive skin closures.

Conditions: Given the following: clean disposable gloves, sterile gloves, antiseptic solution, surgical scrub brush, antiseptic swabs, tincture of benzoin, sterile cotton-tipped applicator, adhesive skin closure strips, sterile 4 × 4 gauze pads, surgical tape, and a biohazard waste container.

Standards: Time: 10 minutes. Student completed procedure in ____ minutes.

Accuracy: Satisfactory score on the Performance Evaluation Checklist.

Performance Evaluation Checklist

Trial 1	Trial 2	Point Value	*Performance Standards*
			Application of Adhesive Skin Closures
		•	Washed hands with an antimicrobial soap.
		•	Assembled equipment.
		•	Greeted patient and introduced yourself.
		•	Identified patient and explained the procedure.
		•	Positioned the patient as required.
		•	Adjusted the light.
		•	Applied clean gloves.
		•	Inspected the wound.
		•	Scrubbed the wound with an antiseptic solution.
		•	Allowed the skin to dry or patted dry.
		•	Applied antiseptic using a new swab for each motion.
		•	Allowed the skin to dry.
		•	Applied tincture of benzoin without letting it touch the wound.
		▷	Stated the purpose of tincture of benzoin.
		•	Allowed the skin to dry.
		•	Removed gloves and washed hands.
		•	Opened the package of adhesive strips and laid them on a flat surface.
		•	Applied sterile gloves and tear tab off card of strips.

Copyright © 2008, 2004, 2000, 1995, 1990 by Saunders, an imprint of Elsevier Inc. All rights reserved.

Trial 1	Trial 2	Point Value	*Performance Standards*
		•	Peeled a strip of tape off the card.
		•	Checked to make sure the skin surface was dry.
		•	Secured one end of the strip to the skin by pressing down firmly.
		•	Stretched the strip across the incision until the edges of the wound were approximated.
		•	Secured the strip to the skin on the other side of the wound.
		•	Applied the next strip on one side of center strip at an ⅛-inch interval.
		•	Applied a third strip at an ⅛-inch interval on the other side of the center strip.
		•	Continued applying the strips at ⅛-inch intervals until the edges of the wound were approximated.
		▷	Explained why the strips should be spaced at ⅛-inch intervals.
		•	Applied two closures approximately ½-inch from the ends of the strips.
		▷	Stated the purpose of applying a strip along each edge.
		•	Applied a sterile dressing over the strips if indicated by the physician.
		•	Removed gloves and sanitized hands.
		•	Instructed the patient in wound care and provided written instructions.
		•	Charted the procedure correctly.
			Removal of Adhesive Skin Closures
		•	Sanitized hands.
		•	Greeted patient and introduced yourself.
		•	Identified patient and explained the procedure.
		•	Positioned the patient as required.
		•	Checked to make sure the incision line was approximated and free from infection.
		•	Positioned a 4 × 4 gauze pad in a convenient location.
		•	Applied clean gloves.
		•	Peeled off each half of the strip from the outside toward the wound margin.
		•	Lifted the strip away from the wound and placed on the gauze.
		•	Continued until all closures were removed.
		•	Cleansed the site with an antiseptic swab.
		•	Applied a sterile dressing if indicated by the physician.
		•	Disposed of strips and gauze in a biohazard waste container.
		•	Removed gloves and sanitized hands.
		•	Charted the procedure correctly.
		*	Completed the procedure within 10 minutes.
			TOTALS

Copyright © 2008, 2004, 2000, 1995, 1990 by Saunders, an imprint of Elsevier Inc. All rights reserved.

CHART	
Date	

Evaluation of Student Performance

EVALUATION CRITERIA			COMMENTS
Symbol	Category	Point Value	
✶	Critical Step	16 points	
●	Essential Step	6 points	
▷	Theory Question	2 points	
Score calculation: 100 points			
− ______ points missed			
____ Score			
Satisfactory score: 85 or above			

AAMA/CAAHEP Competency Achieved:

☑ III. C. 3. b. (4) (f): Prepare patient for and assist with procedures, treatments, and minor office surgeries.
☑ III. C. 3. c. (3) (c): Provide instruction for health maintenance and disease prevention.

Copyright © 2008, 2004, 2000, 1995, 1990 by Saunders, an imprint of Elsevier Inc. All rights reserved.

Notes

Copyright © 2008, 2004, 2000, 1995, 1990 by Saunders, an imprint of Elsevier Inc. All rights reserved.

EVALUATION OF COMPETENCY

Procedure 10-7: Assisting with Minor Office Surgery

Name: ______________________________ Date: ______________

Evaluated By: ______________________________ Score: ______________

Performance Objective

Outcome: Set up the surgical tray and assist with minor office surgery.

Conditions: Given the instruments and supplies required for a specific minor office surgery as designed by the instructor.

Standards: Time: 15 minutes. Student completed procedure in ____ minutes.

Accuracy: Satisfactory score on the Performance Evaluation Checklist.

Performance Evaluation Checklist

Trial 1	Trial 2	Point Value	*Performance Standards*
		•	Determined the type of minor office surgery to be performed.
		•	Prepared examining room.
		•	Sanitized hands.
		•	Set up articles required that are not sterile on a side table or counter.
		•	Labeled the specimen container (if included).
		•	Washed hands with an antimicrobial soap.
		•	Set up the minor office surgery tray on a clean, dry, flat surface, using the principles of surgical asepsis.
			Prepackaged Sterile Set-Up
		•	Selected the appropriate package from supply shelf and placed it on a flat surface.
		•	Opened the setup using the inside of wrapper as the sterile field.
		•	Checked the sterilization indicator on inside of pack.
		•	Added any additional articles required for the surgery and covered tray setup with a sterile towel.
			Transferring Articles to a Sterile Field
		•	Placed sterile towel on a flat surface by two corner ends, making sure not to contaminate it.
		•	Transferred sterile articles to the field, using peel-apart packages.
		•	Applied sterile glove.
		•	Arranged articles neatly on the sterile field with sterile glove.
		•	Checked to make sure all articles were available on the sterile field.

Copyright © 2008, 2004, 2000, 1995, 1990 by Saunders, an imprint of Elsevier Inc. All rights reserved.

Trial 1	Trial 2	Point Value	*Performance Standards*
		•	Covered the tray setup with a sterile towel without allowing arms to pass over the sterile field.
			Prepared the Patient
		•	Greeted the patient and introduced yourself.
		•	Identified patient, explained the procedure, and reassured the patient.
		•	Asked patient if he or she needs to void before the surgery.
		•	Instructed patient on clothing removal.
		•	Instructed patient not to move during procedure or to talk, laugh, sneeze, or cough over the sterile field.
		•	Positioned patient as required for the type of surgery to be performed.
		•	Adjusted the light so that it was focused on the operative site.
			Prepared the Patient's Skin
		•	Applied clean disposable gloves.
		•	Shaved skin (if required).
		•	Cleansed skin with an antiseptic solution.
		•	Rinsed and dried the area.
		•	Applied antiseptic using antiseptic swabs.
		•	Allowed the skin to dry.
		•	Removed gloves and sanitized hands.
		•	Checked to make sure that everything was ready and informed physician.
			Assisted the Physician
		•	Uncovered the tray set-up.
		•	Opened the outer glove wrapper for physician.
		•	Held the vial while physician withdrew the local anesthetic.
		•	Adjusted the light as required.
		•	Restrained patient.
		•	Relaxed and reassured patient.
		•	Handed instruments and supplies to physician. (Sterile gloves required.)
		•	Kept the sterile field neat and orderly. (Sterile gloves required.)
		•	Held basin for physician to deposit soiled instruments and supplies. (Clean gloves required.)
		•	Retracted tissue. (Sterile gloves required.)
		•	Sponged blood from operative site. (Sterile gloves required.)
		•	Added instruments and supplies as necessary to the sterile field.
		•	Held specimen container to accept specimen. (Clean gloves required.)
		•	Cut ends of suture material after insertion by physician. (Sterile gloves required.)
			Following the Surgery
		•	Applied sterile dressing to the surgical wound if ordered by physician.

Copyright © 2008, 2004, 2000, 1995, 1990 by Saunders, an imprint of Elsevier Inc. All rights reserved.

Trial 1	Trial 2	Point Value	Performance Standards
		•	Stayed with patient as a safety precaution.
		•	Assisted and instructed patient as required.
		•	Verified that patient understood postoperative instructions.
		•	Provided patient with verbal and written wound care instructions.
		▷	Stated the patient instructions that should be relayed for wound and suture care.
		•	Relayed information regarding the return visit
		•	Assisted patient off table.
		•	Instructed patient to get dressed.
		•	Transferred any specimens collected to the laboratory with a completed biopsy request.
		•	Charted correctly.
		•	Cleaned examining room.
		•	Discarded disposable contaminated articles in a biohazard waste container.
		•	Sanitized and sterilized instruments.
		*	Completed the procedure within 15 minutes.
			TOTALS

CHART	
Date	

Evaluation of Student Performance

EVALUATION CRITERIA			COMMENTS
Symbol	Category	Point Value	
*	Critical Step	16 points	
•	Essential Step	6 points	
▷	Theory Question	2 points	
Score calculation: 100 points – ______ points missed ____ Score Satisfactory score: 85 or above			

AAMA/CAAHEP Competency Achieved:

☑ III. C. 3. b. (4) (f): Prepare patient for and assist with procedures, treatments, and minor office surgeries.
☑ III. C. 3. c. (2) (a): Identify and respond to issues of confidentiality.
☑ III. C. 3. c. (3) (b): Perform within legal and ethical boundaries.
☑ III. C. 3. c. (3) (c): Provide instruction for health maintenance and disease prevention.

Copyright © 2008, 2004, 2000, 1995, 1990 by Saunders, an imprint of Elsevier Inc. All rights reserved.

Notes

Copyright © 2008, 2004, 2000, 1995, 1990 by Saunders, an imprint of Elsevier Inc. All rights reserved.

EVALUATION OF COMPETENCY

Procedure 10-A: Bandage Turns

Name: ______________________________ Date: ____________

Evaluated By: ______________________________ Score: ____________

Performance Objective

Outcome:	Apply the following bandage turns: circular, spiral, spiral-reverse, figure-eight, and recurrent.
Conditions:	Given the following: a roller bandage and an elastic bandage.
Standards:	Time: 15 minutes. Student completed procedure in ____ minutes.
	Accuracy: Satisfactory score on the Performance Evaluation Checklist.

Performance Evaluation Checklist

Trial 1	*Trial 2*	*Point Value*	*Performance Standards*
			Circular Turn
		•	Placed the end of a bandage on a slant.
		•	Encircled the body part while allowing the corner of the bandage to extend.
		•	Turned down corner of bandage.
		•	Made another circular turn around the body part.
		▷	Stated a use of the circular turn.
			Spiral Turn
		•	Anchored bandage using a circular turn.
		•	Encircled the body part while keeping bandage at a slant.
		•	Carried each spiral turn upward at a slight angle.
		•	Overlapped each previous turn by one half to two thirds the width of bandage.
		▷	Stated a use of the spiral turn.
			Spiral-Reverse Turn
		•	Anchored bandage using a circular turn.
		•	Encircled the body part while keeping bandage at a slant.
		•	Reversed the spiral turn using the thumb or index finger.
		•	Directed bandage downward and folded it on itself.
		•	Kept bandage parallel to the lower edge of the previous turn.
		•	Overlapped each previous turn by two thirds the width of the bandage.
		▷	Stated a use of the spiral-reverse turn.

Copyright © 2008, 2004, 2000, 1995, 1990 by Saunders, an imprint of Elsevier Inc. All rights reserved.

Trial 1	Trial 2	Point Value	Performance Standards
			Figure-Eight Turn
		•	Anchored bandage using a circular turn.
		•	Slanted bandage turns to alternately ascend and descend around the body part.
		•	Crossed the turns over one another in the middle to resemble a figure eight
		•	Overlapped each previous turn by two thirds the width of bandage.
		▷	Stated a use of the figure-eight turn.
			Recurrent Turn
		•	Anchored bandage using two circular turns.
		•	Passed bandage back and forth over the tip of the body part being bandaged.
		•	Overlapped each previous turn by two thirds of the width of the bandage.
		▷	Stated a use of the recurrent turn.
		*	Completed the procedure within 15 minutes.
			TOTALS

CHART	
Date	

Evaluation of Student Performance

EVALUATION CRITERIA			COMMENTS
Symbol	Category	Point Value	
*	Critical Step	16 points	
•	Essential Step	6 points	
▷	Theory Question	2 points	
Score calculation: 100 points –______ points missed ____ Score Satisfactory score: 85 or above			

AAMA/CAAHEP Competency Achieved:

☑ III. C. 3. b. (4) (f): Prepare patient for and assist with procedures, treatments, and minor office surgeries.

Copyright © 2008, 2004, 2000, 1995, 1990 by Saunders, an imprint of Elsevier Inc. All rights reserved.

EVALUATION OF COMPETENCY

Procedure 10-8: Applying a Tubular Gauze Bandage

Name: ______________________________ Date: ______________

Evaluated By: ______________________________ Score: ______________

Performance Objective

Outcome:	Apply a tubular gauze bandage.
Conditions:	Given the following: applicator, tubular gauze, adhesive tape, bandage scissors.
Standards:	Time: 5 minutes. Student completed procedure in ____ minutes.
	Accuracy: Satisfactory score on the Performance Evaluation Checklist.

Performance Evaluation Checklist

Trial 1	*Trial 2*	*Point Value*	*Performance Standards*
		•	Sanitized hands.
		•	Greeted the patient and introduced yourself.
		•	Identified patient and explained the procedure.
		•	Assembled equipment.
		•	Selected the proper applicator.
		•	Pulled a sufficient length of gauze from dispensing box roll.
		•	Spread apart the open end of gauze.
		•	Slid gauze over one end of applicator.
		•	Continuing loading applicator by gathering enough gauze on it to complete the bandage.
		•	Cut roll of gauze near the opening of box.
		•	Placed applicator over the proximal end of patient's finger.
		•	Moved applicator from the proximal to the distal end of patient's finger.
		•	Held bandage in place with the fingers.
		▷	Explained why bandage should be held in place.
		•	Pulled applicator 1 to 2 inches past the end of patient's finger.
		•	Rotated applicator one full turn to anchor bandage.
		•	Moved applicator forward toward the proximal end of patient's finger.
		•	Moved applicator forward approximately 1 inch past the original starting point of bandage.
		•	Rotated the applicator one full turn.
		▷	Stated the reason for rotating the applicator.

Copyright © 2008, 2004, 2000, 1995, 1990 by Saunders, an imprint of Elsevier Inc. All rights reserved.

Trial 1	Trial 2	Point Value	*Performance Standards*
		•	Repeated procedure for the number of layers desired.
		•	Finished the last layer at the proximal end.
		•	Cut gauze from applicator.
		•	Removed applicator.
		•	Applied adhesive tape at the base of patient's finger.
		•	Sanitized hands.
		•	Charted the procedure correctly.
		*	Completed the procedure within 5 minutes.
			TOTALS

CHART	
Date	

Evaluation of Student Performance

EVALUATION CRITERIA			COMMENTS
Symbol	Category	Point Value	
*	Critical Step	16 points	
•	Essential Step	6 points	
▷	Theory Question	2 points	
Score calculation: 100 points – ______ points missed ____ Score Satisfactory score: 85 or above			

AAMA/CAAHEP Competency Achieved:

☑ III. C. 3. b. (4) (f): Prepare patient for and assist with procedures, treatments, and minor office surgeries.

Copyright © 2008, 2004, 2000, 1995, 1990 by Saunders, an imprint of Elsevier Inc. All rights reserved.

11

Administration of Medication and Intravenous Therapy

CHAPTER ASSIGNMENTS

√ After Completing	Date Due	Textbook Page(s)	TEXTBOOK ASSIGNMENTS	Possible Points	Points You Earned
		417-492	Read Chapter 11: Administration of Medication and Intravenous Therapy		
		420 487	Read Case Study 1 Case Study 1 questions	5	
		448 487	Read Case Study 2 Case Study 2 questions	5	
		471 487	Read Case Study 3 Case Study 3 questions	5	
		488	Apply Your Knowledge questions	10	
			TOTAL POINTS		
√ After Completing	**Date Due**	**Study Guide Page(s)**	**STUDY GUIDE ASSIGNMENTS (CTA: Critical Thinking Activity)**	**Possible Points**	**Points You Earned**
		465	Pretest	10	
		466	Key Term Assessment	30	
		467-473	Evaluation of Learning questions	80	
		473-476	CTA A: Using the PDR	34	
		476-477	CTA B: Locating Information in a Drug Insert	12	
		477	CTA C: Drug Classifications (3 points each)	30	
		478	CTA D: Seven Rights of Medication Administration	35	
			CD Activity: Chapter 11 Script It! (Record points earned)		
		479	CTA E: Liquid Measurement	11	
		479	CTA F: Parts of a Needle and Syringe	11	

Copyright © 2008, 2004, 2000, 1995, 1990 by Saunders, an imprint of Elsevier Inc. All rights reserved.

√ After Completing	Date Due	Study Guide Page(s)	STUDY GUIDE ASSIGNMENTS (CTA: Critical Thinking Activity)	Possible Points	Points You Earned
			CD Activity: Chapter 11 Take the Plunge (Record points earned)		
		479	CTA G: Hypodermic Syringe Calibrations	20	
			CD Activity: Chapter 11 Which Needle? (Record points earned)		
		480	CTA H: Insulin Syringe Calibrations	20	
		480	CTA I: Tuberculin Syringe Calibrations	30	
			Activity: Chapter 11 Draw It Up! (Record points earned)		
		481	CTA J: Syringe and Needle Labels (3 points each)	12	
		481	CTA K: Angle of Insertion for Injections	3	
		481-482	CTA L: Preparing and Administering Parenteral Medication	18	
		482-483	CTA M: Anaphylactic Reaction	20	
		484-485	CTA N: Mantoux Test Results	30	
		485-495	CTA O: Researching Drugs (5 points/drug researched)	200	
		496	CTA P: Crossword Puzzle	40	
		497	CTA Q: Road to Recovery: Drug Categories (Team Players) (Record points earned)		
			CD Activity: Chapter 11 Road to Recovery: Drug Categories (Individual Player) (Record points earned)		
			CD Activity: Chapter 11 Animations	20	
		465	Posttest	10	
			ADDITIONAL ASSIGNMENTS		
			TOTAL POINTS		

Copyright © 2008, 2004, 2000, 1995, 1990 by Saunders, an imprint of Elsevier Inc. All rights reserved.

√ After Completing	Date Due	Study Guide Page(s)	STUDY GUIDE ASSIGNMENTS DRUG DOSAGE CALCULATION: SUPPLEMENTAL EDUCATION FOR CHAPTER 11	Possible Points	Points You Earned
		527	**Unit 1: The Metric System** A. Units of Measurement	10	
		528	**Unit 1: The Metric System** B. Metric Abbreviations	7	
		528	**Unit 1: The Metric System** C. Metric Notation	20	
		529	**Unit 2: The Apothecary System** A. Units of Measurement	14	
		529	**Unit 2: The Apothecary System** B. Apothecary Abbreviations	10	
		530	**Unit 2: The Apothecary System** C. Apothecary Notation	20	
		530	**Unit 3: The Household System** Practice Problems for Units of Measurement	4	
		531	**Unit 4: Medication Orders** A. Medical Abbreviations	30	
		532-533	**Unit 4: Medication Orders** B. Interpreting Medication Orders (3 points each)	30	
		533-534	**Unit 5: Converting Units of Measurement** A. Using Conversion Tables (2 points each)	50	
		534-536	**Unit 5: Converting Units of Measurement** B. Converting Units Within the Metric System (2 points each)	40	
		536-538	**Unit 5: Converting Units of Measurement** C. Converting Units Within the Apothecary System (2 points each)	50	
		538-540	**Unit 5: Converting Units of Measurement** D. Converting Units Within the Household System (2 points each)	20	
		540-542	**Unit 6: Ratio and Proportion** A. Ratio and Proportion Guidelines (6 points each)	48	
		542-544	**Unit 6: Ratio and Proportion** B. Converting Units Using Ratio and Proportion (2 points each)	40	
		544-550	**Unit 7: Determining Drug Dosage** A. Oral Administration Oral Solid Medications (2 points each)	20	

Copyright © 2008, 2004, 2000, 1995, 1990 by Saunders, an imprint of Elsevier Inc. All rights reserved.

√ After Completing	Date Due	Study Guide Page(s)	STUDY GUIDE ASSIGNMENTS DRUG DOSAGE CALCULATION: SUPPLEMENTAL EDUCATION FOR CHAPTER 11	Possible Points	Points You Earned
		544-550	**Unit 7: Determining Drug Dosage** A. Oral Administration Oral Liquid Medications (2 points each)	10	
		550-555	**Unit 7: Determining Drug Dosage** B. Parenteral Administration (2 points each)	20	
			ADDITIONAL ASSIGNMENTS		
			TOTAL POINTS		

Copyright © 2008, 2004, 2000, 1995, 1990 by Saunders, an imprint of Elsevier Inc. All rights reserved.

√ When Assigned By Your Instructor	Study Guide Page(s)	Practices Required	LABORATORY ASSIGNMENTS (Procedure Number and Name)	*Score
	507-508	5	**Practice for Competency** 11-1: Administering Oral Medication Textbook reference: pp. 451-452	
	509-510		**Evaluation of Competency** 11-1: Administering Oral Medication	*
	507-508	Vial: 5 Ampule: 5	DVD **Practice for Competency** 11-2: Preparing an Injection Textbook reference: pp. 462-465	
	511-513		**Evaluation of Competency** 11-2: Preparing an Injection	*
	507-508	3	DVD **Practice for Competency** 11-3: Reconstituting Powdered Drugs Textbook reference: pp. 465-466	
	515-516		**Evaluation of Competency** 11-3: Reconstituting Powdered Drugs	*
	507-508	5	DVD **Practice for Competency** 11-4: Administering a Subcutaneous Injection Textbook reference: pp. 466-468	
	517-518		**Evaluation of Competency** 11-4: Administering a Subcutaneous Injection	*
	507-508	5	DVD **Practice for Competency** 11-5: Administering an Intramuscular Injection Textbook reference: pp. 468-470	
	519-520		**Evaluation of Competency** 11-5: Administering an Intramuscular Injection	*
	507-508	5	DVD **Practice for Competency** 11-6: Z-Tract Intramuscular Injection Technique Textbook reference: p. 471	
	521-523	5	**Evaluation of Competency** 11-6: Z-Tract Intramuscular Injection Technique	*
	507-508	5	DVD **Practice for Competency** 11-7: Administering an Intradermal Injection Textbook reference: pp. 479-481	

Copyright © 2008, 2004, 2000, 1995, 1990 by Saunders, an imprint of Elsevier Inc. All rights reserved.

√ When Assigned By Your Instructor	Study Guide Page(s)	Practices Required	LABORATORY ASSIGNMENTS (Procedure Number and Name)	*Score
	523-525		**Evaluation of Competency** 11-7: Administering an Intradermal Injection	*
			ADDITIONAL ASSIGNMENTS	

Copyright © 2008, 2004, 2000, 1995, 1990 by Saunders, an imprint of Elsevier Inc. All rights reserved.

Name ______________________________ Date ______________

PRETEST

True or False

_____ 1. A drug is a chemical that is used for treatment, prevention, or diagnosis of disease.

_____ 2. The generic name of a drug is assigned by the pharmaceutical manufacturer who develops the drug.

_____ 3. The Rx symbol comes from the Latin word *recipe* and means "take."

_____ 4. An anaphylactic reaction can be life threatening.

_____ 5. The dorsogluteal site is the most common site for administering injections in infants.

_____ 6. A subcutaneous injection is given into muscle tissue.

_____ 7. The purpose of aspirating when administering an injection is to make sure the needle is not in a blood vessel.

_____ 8. The Mantoux tuberculin test is administered through a subcutaneous injection.

_____ 9. The peripheral veins of the arm and hand are used most often for administering IV therapy.

_____ 10. Chemotherapy is the use of chemicals to treat disease.

POSTTEST

True or False

_____ 1. OSHA is responsible for determining if drugs are safe before release for human use.

_____ 2. An enteric-coated tablet does not dissolve until it reaches the intestines.

_____ 3. The apothecary system is most often used to administer medication in the medical office.

_____ 4. The parenteral route of administering medications is used when the patient is allergic to the oral form of the drug.

_____ 5. Hypodermic syringes are calibrated in cubic centimeters.

_____ 6. The maximum amount of medication that can be administered through the subcutaneous route is 2 cc.

_____ 7. A patient with latent tuberculosis infection has a negative reaction to a TB test.

_____ 8. A tuberculin skin test result should be read 15 to 20 minutes after administering.

_____ 9. Intermittent IV administration involves the administration of IV medication over a specific amount of time at specified intervals.

_____ 10. Immune globulin consists of pooled human plasma that contains clotting factors.

Copyright © 2008, 2004, 2000, 1995, 1990 by Saunders, an imprint of Elsevier Inc. All rights reserved.

KEY TERM ASSESSMENT

Directions: Match each medical term with its definition.

_____ 1. Adverse reaction
_____ 2. Allergen
_____ 3. Allergy
_____ 4. Ampule
_____ 5. Anaphylactic reaction
_____ 6. Autoimmune disease
_____ 7. Chemotherapy
_____ 8. Controlled drug
_____ 9. Dose
_____ 10. Drug
_____ 11. Enteral nutrition
_____ 12. Gauge
_____ 13. Hemophilia
_____ 14. Immune globulins
_____ 15. Induration
_____ 16. Infusion
_____ 17. Inhalation administration
_____ 18. Intradermal injection
_____ 19. Intramuscular injection
_____ 20. Intravenous therapy
_____ 21. Oral administration
_____ 22. Parenteral
_____ 23. Pharmacology
_____ 24. Prescription
_____ 25. Subcutaneous injection
_____ 26. Sublingual administration
_____ 27. Topical administration
_____ 28. Transfusion
_____ 29. Vial
_____ 30. Wheal

A. Application of a drug to a particular spot, usually for a local action
B. Introduction of medication into the dermal layer of the skin
C. A small sealed glass container that holds a single dose of medication
D. A physician's order authorizing the dispensing of drugs by a pharmacist
E. An unintended and undesirable effect produced by a drug
F. An abnormal hypersensitivity of the body to substances that are ordinarily harmless
G. The administration of a liquid agent directly into a patient's vein where it is distributed throughout the body by way of the circulatory system
H. A small raised area of the skin
I. Introduction of medication beneath the skin, into the subcutaneous or fatty layer of the body
J. An area of hardened tissue
K. A closed glass container with a rubber stopper that holds medication
L. The administration of medication by way of air or other vapor being drawn into the lungs
M. A serious allergic reaction that requires immediate treatment
N. Administration of medication by mouth
O. A drug that has restrictions placed on it by the federal government because of its potential for abuse
P. Introduction of medication into the muscular layer of the body
Q. Administration of medication by placing it under the tongue
R. The quantity of a drug to be administered at one time
S. A substance that is capable of causing an allergic reaction
T. A chemical used for the treatment, prevention, or diagnosis of disease
U. The diameter of the lumen of a needle used to administer medication
V. Administration of medication by injection
W. The study of drugs
X. A condition in which the body's immune system produces antibodies that attack the body's own cells
Y. The use of chemicals to treat disease; most often used to refer to the treatment of cancer using antineoplastic medications
Z. The delivery of nutrients through a tube inserted into the GI tract
AA. An inherited bleeding disorder caused by a deficiency of a clotting factor needed for proper coagulation of the blood
BB. A blood product consisting of pooled human plasma containing antibodies
CC. The administration of fluids, medications or nutrients into a vein
DD. The administration of whole blood or blood products through the intravenous route

Copyright © 2008, 2004, 2000, 1995, 1990 by Saunders, an imprint of Elsevier Inc. All rights reserved.

EVALUATION OF LEARNING

Directions: Fill in each blank with the correct answer.

1. What is the difference between administering, prescribing, and dispensing medication at the medical office?

2. What is the difference between the generic name and the brand name of a drug?

3. What is a liniment?

4. What is a spray?

5. What is a syrup?

6. What is a tablet?

7. What is the purpose of scoring a tablet?

8. List two drugs that come in the form of chewable tablets.

9. List two reasons for enterically coating a tablet.

10. What is a capsule?

11. Why must a suppository have a cylindrical or conical shape?

Copyright © 2008, 2004, 2000, 1995, 1990 by Saunders, an imprint of Elsevier Inc. All rights reserved.

12. What is a transdermal patch?

____

____

13. Why is the metric system used most often to administer medication?

____

____

14. Define the term volume.

____

15. Describe the use of the household system of measurement.

____

____

16. When is conversion required?

____

____

17. What is a controlled drug?

____

18. In what forms can a prescription be authorized?

____

____

____

19. What requirements must be followed when writing a prescription for a Schedule II drug?

____

____

____

20. List five brand names of Schedule II analgesics.

____

____

21. What requirements must be followed when writing a prescription for a Schedule III drug?

____

____

____

22. What is a Schedule IV drug?

____

____

Copyright © 2008, 2004, 2000, 1995, 1990 by Saunders, an imprint of Elsevier Inc. All rights reserved.

23. List three brand names of Schedule IV analgesics.

24. List four brand names of Schedule IV antianxiety agents.

25. What is included in each of the following parts of a prescription?
    a. Superscription
    b. Inscription
    c. Subscription
    d. Signatura

26. Why is it important for the patient's age to be indicated on a prescription?

27. What types of medications should be recorded on a medication record form?

28. List and describe three factors that affect the action of drugs in the body.

29. What are the symptoms and treatment of an anaphylactic reaction?

30. What are the advantages and disadvantages of using the parenteral route of administration?

31. How do safety-engineered syringes reduce the risk of a needlestick injury?

32. What is the purpose of using a filter needle when withdrawing medication from an ampule?

33. What sites are used most frequently to administer a subcutaneous injection?

Copyright © 2008, 2004, 2000, 1995, 1990 by Saunders, an imprint of Elsevier Inc. All rights reserved.

34. List three medications commonly administered through a subcutaneous injection.

35. Why is medication absorbed faster through the intramuscular route than through the subcutaneous route?

36. List the four intramuscular (IM) injection sites and explain why these sites must be used to administer an IM injection.

37. What types of medication are given using the Z-track technique?

38. What sites are used most frequently to administer an intradermal injection?

39. What is the most frequent use of an intradermal injection?

40. What are the symptoms of active pulmonary tuberculosis?

41. What is latent tuberculosis infection?

42. Who should have a tuberculin test?

43. What is induration and what causes it?

44. What procedures are performed if a patient has a positive reaction to a tuberculin skin test?

45. What are 10 examples of common allergens?

46. What is the general treatment for allergies?

Copyright © 2008, 2004, 2000, 1995, 1990 by Saunders, an imprint of Elsevier Inc. All rights reserved.

47. What is the purpose of patch testing?

48. How long does it take for a reaction to occur with a skin-prick test?

49. Explain what is meant by each of the following intradermal skin test reactions.
   a. ±1
   b. +2
   c. +3

50. What are the advantages of RAST testing over direct skin testing?

Intravenous Therapy

1. What is intravenous therapy?

2. Which veins are most often used for IV therapy?

3. What type of liquid agents are administered through IV therapy?

4. List examples of outpatient sites in which IV therapy may be administered.

5. What are the advantages of outpatient IV therapy?

6. What requirements must be met before an entry-level medical assistant can perform IV therapy at a medical office?

7. What must be determined by the physician before prescribing IV therapy?

8. What are the responsibilities of the physician in prescribing IV therapy?

Copyright © 2008, 2004, 2000, 1995, 1990 by Saunders, an imprint of Elsevier Inc. All rights reserved.

9. What instructions should the medical assistant relay to a patient scheduled for outpatient IV therapy?

____

____

10. List six reasons for using the IV route to administer medication.

____

____

____

11. How is medication administered using the direct IV injection method?

____

____

12. How is medication administered using the intermittent IV administration method?

____

____

13. What is continuous IV medication administration?

____

____

14. List five conditions for which a physician may prescribe IV antibiotic therapy in an outpatient setting.

____

____

15. How do antineoplastic drugs work to treat cancer?

____

16. Why must the IV route be used to administer chemotherapy?

____

17. What criteria are used to determine the frequency and length of a chemotherapy treatment?

____

____

18. How does Remicade (infliximab) work to treat inflammatory diseases?

____

____

19. IV Remicade therapy may be prescribed for what conditions?

____

____

20. Outpatient IV analgesic therapy may be prescribed for what conditions?

____

____

Copyright © 2008, 2004, 2000, 1995, 1990 by Saunders, an imprint of Elsevier Inc. All rights reserved.

21. What is a PCA pump?

22. List four conditions that may cause a depletion of fluids and electrolytes in the body.

23. List three examples of IV fluids.

24. List five conditions for which outpatient IV nutritional supplements might be prescribed.

25. List three examples of autoimmune diseases.

26. How are immune globulins obtained?

27. What is hemophilia?

28. What is the treatment for hemophilia?

29. What may occur if hemophilia treatment is delayed?

30. What medical office emergency situations might benefit from establishing IV access?

CRITICAL THINKING ACTIVITIES

A. USING THE PDR

The following is an activity to assist you in learning how to use the PDR. Refer to Figure 11-1 in your textbook to answer the following questions.

Manufacturer's Index

1. What information is included in the Manufacturer's Index?

2. What company manufactures the drugs listed in this section of the Manufacturer's Index?

3. What number would you call if you had an emergency on the weekend regarding one of these drugs?

Copyright © 2008, 2004, 2000, 1995, 1990 by Saunders, an imprint of Elsevier Inc. All rights reserved.

4. What page would you turn to in the PDR for product information on Nitrostat tablets?

5. Is a photograph included in the PDR for Loestrin 21 tablets?

6. What page would you turn to in the PDR to find a color photograph of Nardil tablets?

Brand and Generic Name Index

1. To what page in this PDR edition would you turn to find product information on Lipitor tablets manufactured by Parke-Davis?

2. What is the generic name of Prinivil tablets?

3. What company manufactures Prinivil tablets?

4. What page would you turn to in the PDR to find product information on Prinivil tablets?

5. What page would you turn to in the PDR to find product identification information on Prinivil tablets?

6. Who manufactures Zestril tablets?

7. Does the PDR contain full product information on Zestril tablets?

Product Category Index

1. What is the drug category for Flexeril tablets?

2. Who manufactures Soma tablets?

3. What page would you turn to in this PDR edition to find product information on Skelaxin tablets?

4. Who manufactures Valium tablets?

Product Identification Guide

1. What is included in the Product Identification Guide?

Copyright © 2008, 2004, 2000, 1995, 1990 by Saunders, an imprint of Elsevier Inc. All rights reserved.

2. How can this section assist the user?

____

____

Product Information

Under which heading would you look in this section to find information on:

1. Conditions the drug is approved by the FDA to treat

____

____

2. Information to relay to the patient to ensure safe and effective use of the drug

____

____

3. Route of administration

____

4. Symptoms associated with an overdose of the drug

____

____

____

5. Situations that require special consideration when the drug is used

____

____

6. Generic name of the drug

____

7. How the drug functions in the body to produce its therapeutic effect

____

____

8. Situations in which the drug should not be used

____

____

9. Recommended adult dosage and duration of treatment

____

10. How to pronounce the brand name of the drug

____

11. Handling and storage conditions

____

____

____

Copyright © 2008, 2004, 2000, 1995, 1990 by Saunders, an imprint of Elsevier Inc. All rights reserved.

12. Serious adverse reactions that may occur with the drug

13. Symptoms associated with an overdose of the drug

14. Unintended and undesirable effects that may occur with the use of the drug

15. Modification of dosage needed for children

B. LOCATING INFORMATION IN A DRUG INSERT

Obtain a drug insert for a prescription drug and answer the following questions.

1. What is the brand name of the drug?

2. What is the generic name of the drug?

3. What is the drug category of this medication?

4. What are the dosage forms for this drug?

5. What is the route of administration of this medication?

6. What are the indications and usage for this medication?

7. What are the contraindications for this medication?

Copyright © 2008, 2004, 2000, 1995, 1990 by Saunders, an imprint of Elsevier Inc. All rights reserved.

8. List the warnings for this drug.

____

____

____

9. What are the general precautions for this medication?

____

____

____

10. What information should be relayed to patients regarding this medication?

____

____

____

11. What are the adverse reactions for this medication?

____

____

____

12. What is the dosage and administration for this medication?

____

____

C. DRUG CLASSIFICATIONS

Inspect the package labels of 10 drugs (or use other means) to assess the classification of each drug based on preparation and action. List the name of each drug along with its appropriate category in the spaces provided. Compare results. Example: Drug: Tylenol elixir. Classification based on preparation: elixir. Classification based on action: analgesic, antipyretic.

		Classification Based On:	
	Drug	**Preparation**	**Action**
1.			
2.			
3.			
4.			
5.			
6.			
7.			
8.			
9.			
10.			

Copyright © 2008, 2004, 2000, 1995, 1990 by Saunders, an imprint of Elsevier Inc. All rights reserved.

D. SEVEN RIGHTS OF MEDICATION ADMINISTRATION

You are the office manager at a large clinic. Six new medical assistants were just hired. Your physician asks you to design an illustrated poster portraying the seven rights of medication administration to remind the new employees of the importance of following these guidelines. Use the diagram below to design your poster.

Follow the Seven "Rights"	
Right Drug	Right Dose
Right Time	Right Patient
Right Route	Right Technique
Right Documentation	

Copyright © 2008, 2004, 2000, 1995, 1990 by Saunders, an imprint of Elsevier Inc. All rights reserved.

E. LIQUID MEASUREMENT

Obtain a medicine cup that is graduated into the metric (milliliters), apothecary (drams and ounces), and household (teaspoons and tablespoons) systems. Complete the following:

1. What is its capacity? ______________________ ounce(s)
   ______________________ milliliter(s)
   ______________________ tablespoon(s)
   ______________________ dram(s)
2. Practice pouring oral liquid medication by pouring the following amounts of water into the medicine cup. Place a check mark by each amount after it has been properly poured.
   20 ml ______________________
   4 drams ______________________
   1 ounce ______________________
   10 ml ______________________
   ½ ounce ______________________
   1 tablespoon ______________________
   2 drams ______________________

F. PARTS OF A NEEDLE AND SYRINGE

Obtain a needle and syringe. Locate the following parts of each and explain their function.

Needle **Function**

1. hub ____
2. shaft ____
3. lumen ____
4. point ____
5. bevel ____
6. What is the gauge of the needle? ______________________
7. What is the length of the needle? ______________________

Syringe **Function**

8. barrel ____
9. flange ____
10. plunger ____
11. What is the capacity of the syringe? ______________________

G. HYPODERMIC SYRINGE CALIBRATIONS

1. Obtain a 3-cc syringe that is divided into tenths of a cubic centimeter. Locate the following calibrations on the syringe. Place a check mark in the blank next to each calibration after it has been correctly located.

   Calibration (cc)
   0.5 _______
   1.0 _______
   1.2 _______
   2.5 _______
   2.7 _______
2. Locate each calibration (listed above) on the illustration of the hypodermic syringe by placing an arrow on the correct calibration line and labeling it with the calibration.

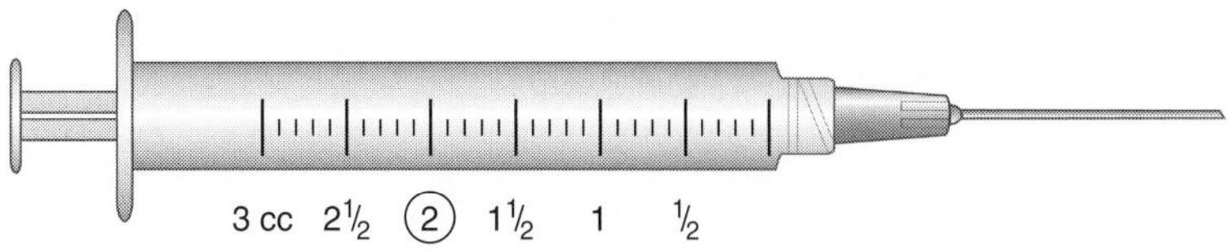

Copyright © 2008, 2004, 2000, 1995, 1990 by Saunders, an imprint of Elsevier Inc. All rights reserved.

H. INSULIN SYRINGE CALIBRATIONS

1. Obtain a U-100 insulin syringe. Locate the following calibrations on the syringe. Place a check mark in the blank next to each calibration after it has been correctly located.
   Calibration (units)
   10 _______
   16 _______
   20 _______
   44 _______
   60 _______
   68 _______
   70 _______
   86 _______
   90 _______
   100 _______
2. Locate each calibration (listed on p. 409) on the illustration of the insulin syringe by placing an arrow on the correct calibration line and labeling it with the calibration.

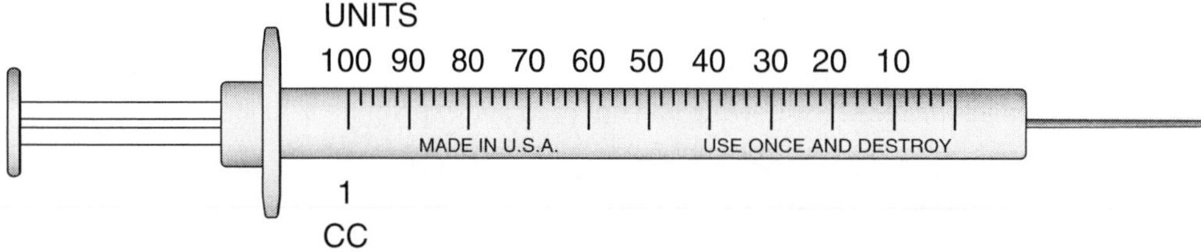

I. TUBERCULIN SYRINGE CALIBRATIONS

1. Obtain a 1-cc tuberculin syringe that is divided into tenths and hundredths of a cubic centimeter. Locate the following calibrations on the syringe. Place a check mark in the blank next to each calibration after it has been correctly located.
   Calibration (cc)
   0.05 _______
   0.10 _______
   0.15 _______
   0.34 _______
   0.52 _______
   0.75 _______
   0.92 _______
2. Locate each calibration (listed above) on the illustration of the tuberculin syringe by placing an arrow on the correct calibration line and labeling it with the calibration.

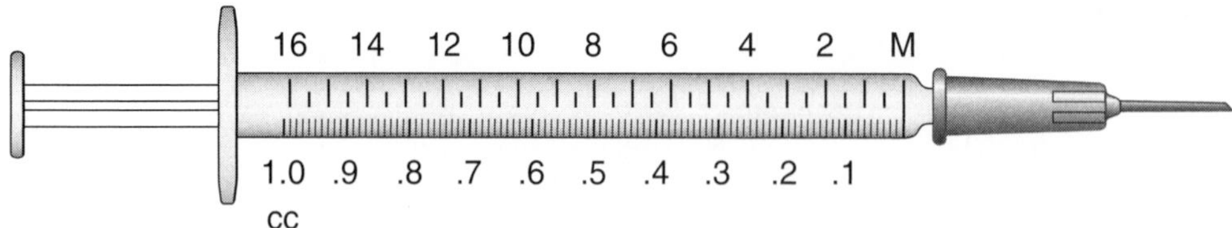

Copyright © 2008, 2004, 2000, 1995, 1990 by Saunders, an imprint of Elsevier Inc. All rights reserved.

J. SYRINGE AND NEEDLE LABELS

Refer to Figure 11-5 in your textbook and indicate the following information for each syringe and needle: the syringe capacity and the gauge and length of the needle.

____

____

____

____

____

K. ANGLE OF INSERTION FOR INJECTIONS

In the diagram that follows, draw three lines indicating the angle of insertion into the correct body tissue for an intradermal, a subcutaneous, and an intramuscular injection. Label the lines.

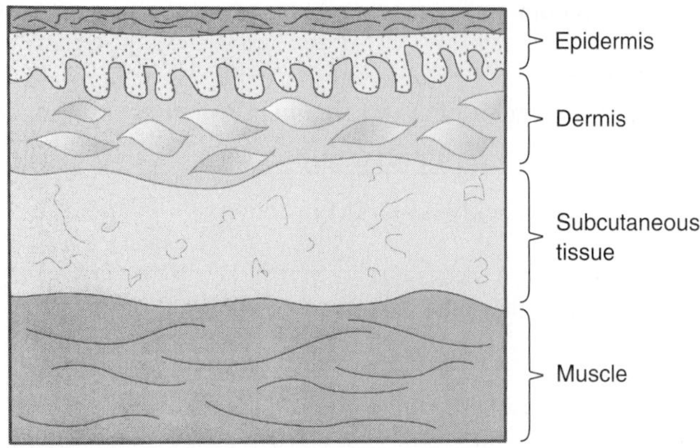

L. PREPARING AND ADMINISTERING PARENTERAL MEDICATION

For each of the following situations involving the preparation and administration of medication, write **C** if the technique is correct and **I** if it is incorrect. If the technique is correct, state the principle underlying the technique. If the technique is incorrect, explain what might happen if it were performed.

_______ 1. The expiration date of the medication is checked before administering the medication.

____

_______ 2. The medical assistant is unfamiliar with the drug to be administered, so he or she looks it up in a drug reference.

____

_______ 3. The medical assistant compares the medication label with the physician's instructions three times: as it is taken from the shelf, before preparing the medication, and after preparing the medication.

____

_______ 4. The rubber stopper of the multidose vial is cleansed with an antiseptic wipe before withdrawing the medication.

____

Copyright © 2008, 2004, 2000, 1995, 1990 by Saunders, an imprint of Elsevier Inc. All rights reserved.

_______ 5. Air is not injected into the multidose vial before withdrawing the medication.

____

_______ 6. Air bubbles are present in the medication in the syringe that has been withdrawn from an ampule.

____

_______ 7. The injection sites are not rotated when repeated injections are given.

____

_______ 8. The antiseptic is not allowed to dry before administering an injection.

____

_______ 9. The skin is stretched taut before an intramuscular injection is given.

____

_______ 10. The needle is inserted slowly and steadily for an IM injection.

____

_______ 11. An IM injection is given in the deltoid site to a patient who has a tight sleeve.

____

_______ 12. An IM injection is given into the dorsogluteal site when the site is not fully exposed.

____

_______ 13. The medical assistant does not aspirate when giving an intramuscular injection.

____

_______ 14. The medication is injected quickly for an IM injection.

____

_______ 15. The needle is withdrawn at the same angle as for insertion.

____

_______ 16. The intradermal needle is inserted with the bevel facing downward.

____

_______ 17. The medical assistant does not aspirate when giving an intradermal injection.

____

_______ 18. The injection site is gently massaged after an intramuscular injection is given.

____

M. ANAPHYLACTIC REACTION

Create a profile of an individual who is experiencing an anaphylactic reaction following these guidelines:

1. Using colored pencils, crayons, or markers, draw a figure of an individual exhibiting the symptoms of an anaphylactic reaction. Be as creative as possible.
2. Do not use any text on your drawing, other than to label items you have drawn in your picture. (A picture is worth a thousand words!)
3. Try to include as many of the symptoms of an anaphylactic reaction as possible.
4. In the classroom, find a partner and trade drawings. Identify the symptoms in your partner's drawing. With your partner, discuss what causes an anaphylactic reaction and how to prevent it. Also discuss the method of treatment for an anaphylactic reaction.

Copyright © 2008, 2004, 2000, 1995, 1990 by Saunders, an imprint of Elsevier Inc. All rights reserved.

ANAPHYLACTIC REACTION

Copyright © 2008, 2004, 2000, 1995, 1990 by Saunders, an imprint of Elsevier Inc. All rights reserved.

N. MANTOUX TEST RESULTS

1. In the space provided, indicate whether the following Mantoux test results are positive, doubtful, or negative:
   a. 12 mm of induration ______________________________
   b. 7 mm of induration ______________________________
   c. 5 mm induration (the patient is infected with HIV) ______________________________
   d. 2 mm of induration ______________________________
   e. Erythema: 6 mm wide (no induration) ______________________________
2. Complete a tuberculosis test record card for each of the above results. (Use patient names of your choice. The brand name of the Mantoux test is Tubersol 5 TU.)

TUBERCULOSIS TEST RECORD			
Name	Date Admin:		
	Date Read:		
MANTOUX TEST	RESULT		
	Negative	Doubtful	Positive
	____ mm	____ mm	____ mm
Logan Family Practice 401 St. George St. St. Augustine, FL 32084 (555) 824-3933			
Performed by ______________________________			

TUBERCULOSIS TEST RECORD			
Name	Date Admin:		
	Date Read:		
MANTOUX TEST	RESULT		
	Negative	Doubtful	Positive
	____ mm	____ mm	____ mm
Logan Family Practice 401 St. George St. St. Augustine, FL 32084 (555) 824-3933			
Performed by ______________________________			

Copyright © 2008, 2004, 2000, 1995, 1990 by Saunders, an imprint of Elsevier Inc. All rights reserved.

TUBERCULOSIS TEST RECORD

Name		Date Admin:	
		Date Read:	
MANTOUX TEST	RESULT		
	Negative	Doubtful	Positive
	___ mm	___ mm	___ mm

Logan Family Practice
401 St. George St.
St. Augustine, FL 32084
(555) 824-3933

Performed by ______________________________

TUBERCULOSIS TEST RECORD

Name		Date Admin:	
		Date Read:	
MANTOUX TEST	RESULT		
	Negative	Doubtful	Positive
	___ mm	___ mm	___ mm

Logan Family Practice
401 St. George St.
St. Augustine, FL 32084
(555) 824-3933

Performed by ______________________________

TUBERCULOSIS TEST RECORD

Name		Date Admin:	
		Date Read:	
MANTOUX TEST	RESULT		
	Negative	Doubtful	Positive
	___ mm	___ mm	___ mm

Logan Family Practice
401 St. George St.
St. Augustine, FL 32084
(555) 824-3933

Performed by ______________________________

O. RESEARCHING DRUGS

Obtain a drug reference book and look up the following information for each of the drugs listed on the Pharmacology Drug Sheets: generic name and drug classification, indications, patient teaching. Record this information in the appropriate space on the Pharmacology Drug Sheets.

Copyright © 2008, 2004, 2000, 1995, 1990 by Saunders, an imprint of Elsevier Inc. All rights reserved.

Pharmacology Drug Sheet

Name: ______________________________

Generic Name and Drug Classification	Indications	Patient Teaching
Accupril		
Adderall		
Adrenalin		
Ambien		

Copyright © 2008, 2004, 2000, 1995, 1990 by Saunders, an imprint of Elsevier Inc. All rights reserved.

Pharmacology Drug Sheet

Name: ____________________

Generic Name and Drug Classification	Indications	Patient Teaching
Amoxil		
Bentyl		
Cardizem		
Catapres		

Copyright © 2008, 2004, 2000, 1995, 1990 by Saunders, an imprint of Elsevier Inc. All rights reserved.

Pharmacology Drug Sheet

Name: ______________________________

Generic Name and Drug Classification	Indications	Patient Teaching
Celebrex		
Cipro		
Coumadin		
Cozaar		

Copyright © 2008, 2004, 2000, 1995, 1990 by Saunders, an imprint of Elsevier Inc. All rights reserved.

Pharmacology Drug Sheet

Name: ____________________

Generic Name and Drug Classification	Indications	Patient Teaching
Depo-Medrol		
Diflucan		
Dilantin		
Flagyl		

Copyright © 2008, 2004, 2000, 1995, 1990 by Saunders, an imprint of Elsevier Inc. All rights reserved.

Pharmacology Drug Sheet

Name: ______________________________

Generic Name and Drug Classification	Indications	Patient Teaching
Flexeril		
Fosamax		
Glucotrol XL		
Inderal		

Copyright © 2008, 2004, 2000, 1995, 1990 by Saunders, an imprint of Elsevier Inc. All rights reserved.

Pharmacology Drug Sheet

Name: ______________________________

Generic Name and Drug Classification	Indications	Patient Teaching
InFeD		
Lanoxin		
Lasix		
Levoxyl		

Copyright © 2008, 2004, 2000, 1995, 1990 by Saunders, an imprint of Elsevier Inc. All rights reserved.

Pharmacology Drug Sheet

Name: ____________________

Generic Name and Drug Classification	Indications	Patient Teaching
Lipitor		
Lomotil		
Meridia		
Nitro-Bid		

Copyright © 2008, 2004, 2000, 1995, 1990 by Saunders, an imprint of Elsevier Inc. All rights reserved.

Pharmacology Drug Sheet

Name: ______________________________

Generic Name and Drug Classification	Indications	Patient Teaching
Phenergan		
Plavix		
Prevacid		
Prozac		

Copyright © 2008, 2004, 2000, 1995, 1990 by Saunders, an imprint of Elsevier Inc. All rights reserved.

Pharmacology Drug Sheet

Name: ______________________________

Generic Name and Drug Classification	Indications	Patient Teaching
Singulair		
Tessalon		
Viagra		
Vicodin		

Copyright © 2008, 2004, 2000, 1995, 1990 by Saunders, an imprint of Elsevier Inc. All rights reserved.

Pharmacology Drug Sheet

Name: ______________________________

Generic Name and Drug Classification	Indications	Patient Teaching
Xanax		
Zithromax		
Zyloprim		
Zyrtec		

Copyright © 2008, 2004, 2000, 1995, 1990 by Saunders, an imprint of Elsevier Inc. All rights reserved.

P. CROSSWORD PUZZLE
Administration of Medication

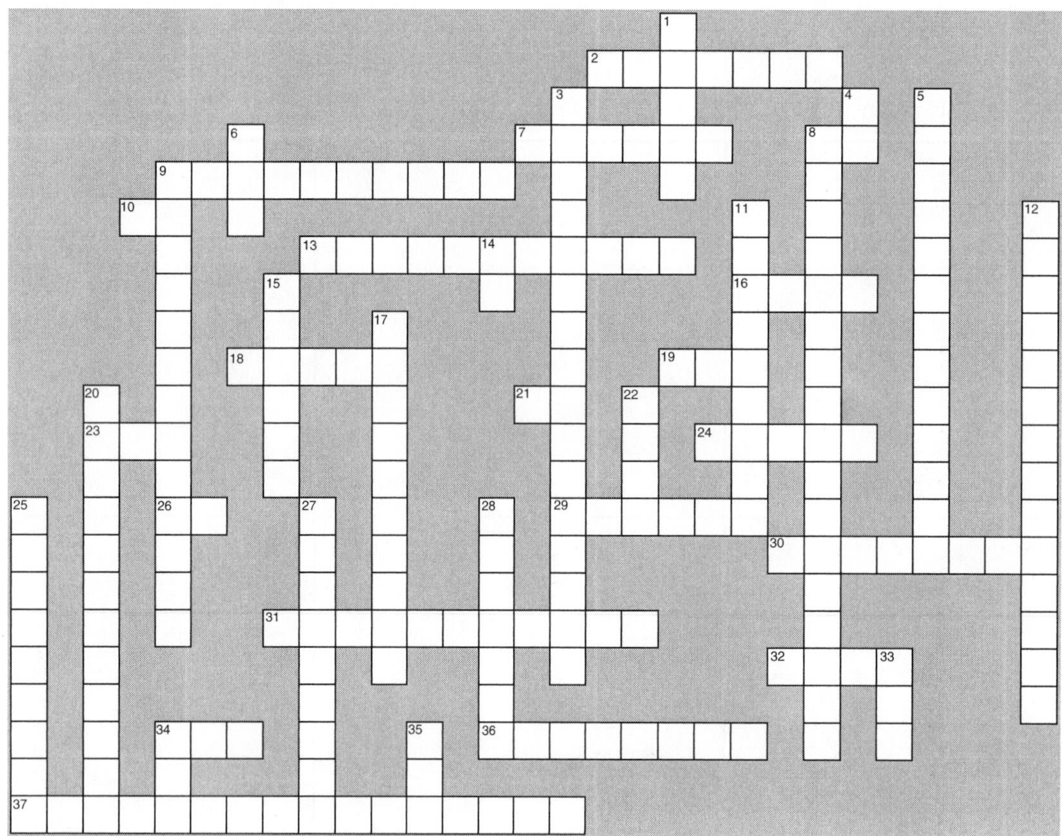

Directions: Complete the crossword puzzle using the clues presented below.

ACROSS

2 Discovered penicillin
7 Most aggressive Hymenoptera
8 1 ml = 1 _______
9 Present with a + Mantoux
10 Right ear
13 Used to tx anaphylactic R
16 Metric weight unit
18 Ranges between 18 and 27
19 Aspirin
21 Every day
23 Available w/o a Rx
24 Needle opening
26 Before meals
29 Sym: wheezing and dyspnea
30 Allergy to molds and pollen
31 Conditions a drug is approved to tx
32 Immediately!
34 Tuberculin is made of this
36 Causes house dust allergy
37 Runny and inflamed allergic nose

DOWN

1 Slant of the needle
3 Do not use this drug!
4 Route of admin for allergy inj
5 Drug to d/c before allergy testing
6 Approves drugs
8 Poison ivy causes this
9 Abnormal or peculiar reaction
11 Means "label" in Latin
12 Calibrated in units
14 By mouth
15 Prevents syringe from rolling
17 This drug may cause an allergic R
20 Site for deep IM injection
22 Blood test for allergies
25 Hives
27 Rx requirement for controlled drug
28 Max of 1 cc at this site
33 Three times a day
34 Drug reference (ex)
35 As needed

Copyright © 2008, 2004, 2000, 1995, 1990 by Saunders, an imprint of Elsevier Inc. All rights reserved.

Q. ROAD TO RECOVERY

Drug Categories

Object: The object of the game is to lead your "patient" to recovery by correctly defining drug categories based on action.

Needed: **Road to Recovery** game board (located at the end of this manual)
Game cards
A token for each player (such as a button or coin)
Dice (1)
Score card

Directions:

1. Cut out the pharmacology game cards on the following pages.
2. Study the drug categories/definitions of drugs based on action in preparation for the game.
3. Place one complete set of game cards on the game board with the definitions facing up (and the drug category facing down).
4. Play **Road to Recovery** following the directions on the reverse side of the game board.
5. Keep track of your points using the score card provided.
6. If time permits, place the set of cards on the game board again with the drug category face-up and the definitions face-down, and continue playing the game until all the cards have been used.

ROAD TO RECOVERY
SCORE CARD

Name: ______________________________

Recording Points:
Using the Game Card Points box, cross off a number each time you answer a game card correctly (starting with 5 and continuing in sequence). Your total game card points will be equal to the last number you crossed off. Record this number in the space provided (1). Record any extra points you were awarded during the game (2), and any points that were deducted (3). To determine your total points, add (1) and (2) together and deduct (3). Record this number in the Total Points Earned space provided. Compare your score with the other players and determine where you placed. Place a check mark next to the level of recovery your patient attained.

Game Card Points:			
5	75	145	215
10	80	150	220
15	85	155	225
20	90	160	230
25	95	165	235
30	100	170	240
35	105	175	245
40	110	180	250
45	115	185	255
50	120	190	260
55	125	195	265
60	130	200	270
65	135	205	275
70	140	210	280

Calculation of Points:

(1) Total Game Card Points: ________

(2) Additional Points Awarded: ________

(3) Deducted Points: ________

TOTAL POINTS EARNED: ________

LEVEL OF RECOVERY:

Patient's Name: ______________________

☐ First Place: **Fully Recovered**
☐ Second Place: **Almost Recovered**
☐ Third Place: **Still Recovering**
☐ Fourth Place: **Gasping for Air**

Copyright © 2008, 2004, 2000, 1995, 1990 by Saunders, an imprint of Elsevier Inc. All rights reserved.

Notes

Copyright © 2008, 2004, 2000, 1995, 1990 by Saunders, an imprint of Elsevier Inc. All rights reserved.

Analgesic (opioid)	Analgesic/Antipyretic	Local Anesthetic	Antacid
Antianemic	Antianginal	Antianxiety	Anticholinergic
Anticoagulant	Anticonvulsant	Antidepressant	Antidiabetic
Antidiarrheal	Antidysrhythmic	Antiemetic	Antiflatulent

Neutralizes gastric acid to relieve gastric pain and irritation	Produces a loss of feeling to a part of the body	Used to manage mild to moderate pain and to reduce fever	Used to manage moderate to severe pain
Used preoperatively to decrease oral and respiratory secretions	Used to treat anxiety	Relieves or prevents angina attacks	Prevents or cures anemia
Used to manage diabetes	Prevents, cures, or alleviates depression	Prevents or relieves seizures	Delays or prevents blood coagulation
Relieves gas and bloating in the GI tract	Prevents or relieves nausea and vomiting	Controls or prevents cardiac dysrhythmias	Works by inhibiting peristalsis and reducing fecal volume

Antifungal

Antigout

Anthelmintics

Antihistamine

Antihypertensive

Antiimpotence Agent

Antiinfective

Antiinflammatory

Antimanic

Antimigraine

Antineoplastic

Antiparkinson

Antiprotozoal

Antipsychotic

Antiretroviral

Antispasmodic

Relieves the symptoms associated with allergies	Used to treat worm infections	Inhibits the production of uric acid	Kills or inhibits the growth of fungi
Relieves symptoms of osteoarthritis and rheumatoid arthritis	Kills or inhibits the growth of bacteria	Used to treat erectile dysfunction	Used to manage high blood pressure
Used to treat symptoms of Parkinson's disease	Used to treat tumors	Causes vasocontriction in large intracranial arteries	Used to treat bipolar affective disorder
Controls hypermotility in irritable bowel syndrome	Used to manage HIV infections	Used to treat psychotic disorders	Destroys protozoa

Antitubercular	Antitussive	Antiulcer	Antiviral
Bone Resorption Inhibitor	Bronchodilator	Cardiac Glycoside	Contraceptive
Corticosteroid	Decongestant	Diuretic	Electrolyte Replacement
Emetic	Expectorant	Hormone Replacement	Immunization

Used to manage herpes infections	Prevents the accumulation of acid in the stomach	Used to prevent or relieve coughs	Kills or inhibits the growth of mycobacteria
Inhibits ovulation	Increases the strength and force of myocardial contractions and slows the heart rate	Relaxes the smooth muscle in the respiratory tract	Used to treat and prevent osteoporosis
Treats or prevents electrolyte depletion	Removes excess fluid from the body by increasing urine output	Produces vasoconstriction in respiratory tract mucosa	Suppresses inflammation and modifies the normal immune response
Stimulates the body to produce antibodies	Used to treat vasomotor symptoms of menopause	Promotes clearance of mucus from the respiratory tract	Induces vomiting

Immunosuppressant	Laxative	Lipid-Lowering	Muscle Relaxant
Ophthalmic Antiinfective	Otic Preparation	Platelet Inhibitor	Sedative and Hypnotic
Smoking Deterrent	Thrombolytic	Thyroid Hormones	Vasopressor
Weight Control			

Used to treat acute, painful musculoskeletal conditions	Used to lower cholesterol	Used to relieve constipation	Used to treat, prevent, and treat rejection of transplanted organs
Promotes sleep by CNS depression	Interferes with the ability of platelets to adhere to each other	Used to treat ear conditions	Used to treat eye infections
Used to treat severe allergic reactions	Increases basal metabolism rate	Dissolves existing clots	Used to manage nicotine withdrawal
			Used to manage obesity

PRACTICE FOR COMPETENCY

Prerequisite. Complete the Drug Dosage Calculation: Supplemental Education for Chapter 11 (pages 527-555 in this manual).

Procedure 11-1: Oral Medication. Administer oral solid and liquid medication and record the procedure in the chart provided.

Procedure 11-2: Preparing the Injection. Prepare an injection from an ampule and a vial.

Procedure 11-3: Reconstituting Powdered Drugs. Reconstitute a powdered drug for parenteral administration.

Procedure 11-4: Subcutaneous Injection. Administer a subcutaneous injection and record the procedure in the chart provided.

Procedure 11-5: Intramuscular Injection. Administer an intramuscular injection and record the procedure in the chart provided.

Procedure 11-6: Z-track method. Administer an intramuscular injection using the Z-track method. Record the procedure in the chart provided.

Procedure 11-7: Intradermal Injection. Administer an intradermal injection and record the procedure in the chart provided. Read and interpret the test results and record them in the chart.

CHART	
Date	

Copyright © 2008, 2004, 2000, 1995, 1990 by Saunders, an imprint of Elsevier Inc. All rights reserved.

CHART

Date	

Copyright © 2008, 2004, 2000, 1995, 1990 by Saunders, an imprint of Elsevier Inc. All rights reserved.

EVALUATION OF COMPETENCY

Procedure 11-1: Administering Oral Medication

Name: ______________________________ Date: ______________

Evaluated By: ______________________________ Score: ______________

Performance Objective

Outcome:	Administer oral solid and liquid medication.
Conditions:	Given the following: appropriate medication, medicine cup, and a medication tray.
Standards:	Time: 10 minutes. Student completed procedure in ____ minutes.
	Accuracy: Satisfactory score on the Performance Evaluation Checklist.

Performance Evaluation Checklist

Trial 1	*Trial 2*	*Point Value*	*Performance Standards*
		•	Sanitized hands.
		•	Assembled equipment.
		•	Worked in a quiet, well-lit atmosphere.
		*	Selected the correct medication from the shelf.
		•	Compared the medication with the physician's instructions.
		•	Checked the drug label.
		•	Checked the expiration date.
		*	Calculated the correct dose to be given, if needed.
		•	Removed the bottle cap.
		•	Checked the drug label and poured the medication.
			Solid Medication
		*	Poured the correct number of capsules or tablets into the bottle cap.
		▷	Explained why the medication is poured into the bottle cap.
		•	Transferred the medication to a medicine cup.
			Liquid Medication
		•	Placed lid of bottle on a flat surface with the open end facing up.
		•	Palmed the surface of the drug label.
		▷	Explained why the surface of the drug label should be palmed.
		•	Placed thumbnail at the proper calibration on medicine cup.
		•	Held medicine cup at eye level.

Copyright © 2008, 2004, 2000, 1995, 1990 by Saunders, an imprint of Elsevier Inc. All rights reserved.

Trial 1	Trial 2	Point Value	Performance Standards
		✶	Poured the correct amount of medication and read the dose at the lowest level of the meniscus.
		●	Replaced the bottle cap.
		●	Checked the drug label and returned the medication to its storage location.
		●	Greeted the patient and introduced yourself.
		●	Identified the patient and explained the procedure.
		●	Handed the medicine cup to the patient.
		●	Offered water to patient.
		▷	Stated one instance when water should not be offered.
		●	Remained with patient until the medication was swallowed.
		●	Sanitized hands.
		●	Charted the procedure correctly.
		✶	Completed the procedure within 10 minutes.
			TOTALS

CHART	
Date	

Evaluation of Student Performance

EVALUATION CRITERIA			COMMENTS
Symbol	Category	Point Value	
✶	Critical Step	16 points	
●	Essential Step	6 points	
▷	Theory Question	2 points	
Score calculation: 100 points – ____ points missed ____ Score Satisfactory score: 85 or above			

AAMA/CAAHEP Competency Achieved:

☑ III. C. 3. b. (4) (g): Apply pharmacology principles to prepare and administer oral and parenteral medication.

Copyright © 2008, 2004, 2000, 1995, 1990 by Saunders, an imprint of Elsevier Inc. All rights reserved.

EVALUATION OF COMPETENCY

Procedure 11-2: Preparing an Injection

Name: ______________________________ Date: ______________

Evaluated By: ______________________________ Score: ______________

Performance Objective

Outcome:	Prepare an injection from an ampule and a vial.
Conditions:	Given the following: medication ordered by the physician, needle and syringe, antiseptic wipe, and medication tray.
Standards:	Time: 10 minutes. Student completed procedure in ____ minutes.
	Accuracy: Satisfactory score on the Performance Evaluation Checklist.

Performance Evaluation Checklist

Trial 1	*Trial 2*	*Point Value*	*Performance Standards*
		•	Sanitized hands.
		•	Assembled equipment.
		•	Worked in a quiet, well-lit atmosphere.
		*	Selected the proper medication from its storage location.
		•	Checked the drug label.
		•	Compared the medication with the physician's instructions.
		•	Checked the expiration date.
		*	Calculated the correct dose to be given, if needed.
		•	Opened syringe and needle package(s).
		•	Assembled needle and syringe if necessary.
		•	Checked to make sure that needle is attached firmly to syringe and moved the plunger back and forth.
		•	Checked the drug label a second time.
		•	If required, mixed the medication.
			Withdrew Medication from a Vial
		•	Removed metal or plastic cap if vial is new.
		•	Cleansed the rubber stopper of the vial with an antiseptic wipe.
		•	Placed vial in an upright position on a flat surface.
		•	Removed the needle guard.
		•	Drew air into syringe equal to the amount of medication to be withdrawn.
		•	Inserted needle through rubber stopper until it reached the empty space between stopper and the fluid level.

Copyright © 2008, 2004, 2000, 1995, 1990 by Saunders, an imprint of Elsevier Inc. All rights reserved.

Trial 1	Trial 2	Point Value	*Performance Standards*
		•	Pushed down on plunger to inject air into the vial.
		•	Kept needle above the fluid level.
		▷	Explained why air must be injected into the vial.
		•	Inverted the vial while holding onto syringe and plunger.
		✶	Held syringe at eye level and withdrew the proper amount of medication.
		•	Kept the needle opening below the fluid level.
		▷	Explained why the needle opening must be kept below the fluid level.
		•	Removed any air bubbles in syringe by tapping barrel with the finger tips.
		▷	Explained why air bubbles should be removed from the syringe.
		•	Removed any air remaining at the top of syringe by pushing the plunger forward.
		•	Removed the needle from rubber stopper and replaced the needle guard.
		•	Checked the drug label for a third time and returned the medication to its storage location.
			Withdrew Medication from an Ampule
		•	Removed regular needle from syringe and attached a filter needle.
		▷	Stated the purpose of a filter needle.
		•	Cleansed the neck of the vial with an antiseptic wipe.
		•	Tapped the stem of ampule lightly to remove any medication in the neck of ampule.
		•	Checked the medication label a second time.
		•	Placed piece of gauze around the neck of ampule.
		•	Broke off the stem by snapping it quickly and firmly away from the body.
		•	Discarded stem and gauze in a biohazard sharps container.
		•	Placed ampule on a flat surface.
		•	Removed needle guard.
		•	Inserted needle opening below the fluid level.
		✶	Withdrew the proper amount of medication.
		•	Kept needle opening below the fluid level.
		▷	Explained why needle opening must be kept below the fluid level.
		•	Removed needle from ampule and replaced needle guard.
		•	Checked drug label for a third time.
		•	Discarded the ampule in a biohazard sharps container.
		•	Removed the filter needle and reapplied the regular needle (and guard) to the syringe.
		•	Tapped syringe to remove air bubbles in syringe.
		•	Removed needle guard and expelled air remaining at the top of syringe.
		•	Replaced the needle guard.
		✶	Completed the procedure within 10 minutes.
			TOTALS

Copyright © 2008, 2004, 2000, 1995, 1990 by Saunders, an imprint of Elsevier Inc. All rights reserved.

Evaluation of Student Performance

EVALUATION CRITERIA			COMMENTS
Symbol	Category	Point Value	
✶	Critical Step	16 points	
●	Essential Step	6 points	
▷	Theory Question	2 points	
Score calculation: 100 points –_____ points missed ____ Score Satisfactory score: 85 or above			

AAMA/CAAHEP Competency Achieved:

☑ III. C. 3. b. (4) (g): Apply pharmacology principles to prepare and administer oral and parenteral medication.

Copyright © 2008, 2004, 2000, 1995, 1990 by Saunders, an imprint of Elsevier Inc. All rights reserved.

Notes

Copyright © 2008, 2004, 2000, 1995, 1990 by Saunders, an imprint of Elsevier Inc. All rights reserved.

EVALUATION OF COMPETENCY

Procedure 11-3: Reconstituting Powdered Drugs

Name: ____ Date: ______________

Evaluated By: ____ Score: ______________

Performance Objective

Outcome:	Reconstitute a powdered drug for parenteral administration.
Conditions:	Given the following: vial containing the powdered drug, reconstituting liquid, and a needle and syringe.
Standards:	Time: 5 minutes. Student completed procedure in ____ minutes.
	Accuracy: Satisfactory score on the Performance Evaluation Checklist.

Performance Evaluation Checklist

Trial 1	Trial 2	Point Value	*Performance Standards*
		•	Withdrew an amount of air equal to the amount of liquid to be injected into the vial from the vial containing the powdered drug.
		•	Injected the air into the vial of diluent.
		*	Inverted the diluent vial and withdrew the proper amount of liquid into the syringe.
		•	Removed air bubbles from the syringe and removed the needle from the vial.
		•	Inserted the needle into the powdered drug vial.
		•	Injected the diluent into the vial.
		•	Removed the needle from the vial and discarded the syringe and needle in a biohazard sharps container.
		•	Rolled the vial between hands to mix it.
		•	Labeled multiple-dose vials with the date of preparation and your initials.
		•	Administer the medication.
		•	Stored multiple-dose vials as indicated in the manufacturer's instructions.
		▷	Explained the importance of checking the date of preparation of a reconstituted multiple-dose vial before administering it.
		*	Completed the procedure within 5 minutes.
			TOTALS

Copyright © 2008, 2004, 2000, 1995, 1990 by Saunders, an imprint of Elsevier Inc. All rights reserved.

Evaluation of Student Performance

EVALUATION CRITERIA			COMMENTS
Symbol	**Category**	**Point Value**	
*	Critical Step	16 points	
•	Essential Step	6 points	
▷	Theory Question	2 points	
Score calculation: 100 points – ____ points missed ____ Score Satisfactory score: 85 or above			

AAMA/CAAHEP Competency Achieved:

☑ III. C. 3. b. (4) (g): Apply pharmacology principles to prepare and administer oral and parenteral medication.

Copyright © 2008, 2004, 2000, 1995, 1990 by Saunders, an imprint of Elsevier Inc. All rights reserved.

EVALUATION OF COMPETENCY

Procedure 11-4: Administering a Subcutaneous Injection

Name: ______________________________ Date: ______________

Evaluated By: ______________________________ Score: ______________

Performance Objective

Outcome:	Administer a subcutaneous injection.
Conditions:	Given the following: appropriate medication, appropriate needle and syringe, antiseptic wipe, 2 × 2 gauze pad, disposable gloves, and a biohazard sharps container.
Standards:	Time: 5 minutes. Student completed procedure in ____ minutes.
	Accuracy: Satisfactory score on the Performance Evaluation Checklist.

Performance Evaluation Checklist

Trial 1	*Trial 2*	*Point Value*	*Performance Standards*
		•	Sanitized hands.
		•	Prepared the injection.
		•	Greeted the patient and introduced yourself.
		•	Identified the patient and explained the procedure and purpose of the injection.
		•	Selected an appropriate subcutaneous injection site.
		▷	Stated what tissue layer of the body the medication will be injected into.
		•	Cleansed area with an antiseptic wipe and allowed it to dry completely.
		▷	Explained why the site should be allowed to dry.
		•	Applied gloves.
		•	Removed needle guard.
		•	Properly positioned the hand on area surrounding the injection site.
		▷	Explained when the area should be grasped and when it should be held taut.
		•	Inserted needle to the hub at a 45-degree or 90-degree angle (depending on the length of the needle) with a quick, smooth motion.
		•	Removed the hand from the skin.
		▷	Explained why the hand should be removed from the skin.
		*	Aspirated to make sure that the needle was not in a blood vessel.
		▷	Explained what should be done if needle is in a blood vessel.
		•	Injected the medication slowly and steadily.
		▷	Described what would happen if the medication were injected rapidly.

Copyright © 2008, 2004, 2000, 1995, 1990 by Saunders, an imprint of Elsevier Inc. All rights reserved.

Trial 1	Trial 2	Point Value	*Performance Standards*
		•	Placed an antiseptic wipe or gauze pad gently over the injection site and removed needle quickly at the same angle as insertion.
		▷	Explained why the needle should be removed at the angle of insertion.
		•	Applied gentle pressure to the injection site.
		▷	Stated why the site should not be vigorously massaged.
		•	Activated the safety shield on the needle.
		•	Properly disposed of needle and syringe.
		•	Removed gloves and sanitized hands.
		•	Charted the procedure correctly.
		•	Remained with patient to make sure there were no unusual reactions.
		▷	Stated the steps to follow if the patient has been given an allergy injection.
		✶	Completed the procedure within 5 minutes.
			TOTALS

CHART	
Date	

Evaluation of Student Performance

EVALUATION CRITERIA			COMMENTS
Symbol	Category	Point Value	
✶	Critical Step	16 points	
•	Essential Step	6 points	
▷	Theory Question	2 points	
Score calculation: 100 points – ____ points missed ____ Score Satisfactory score: 85 or above			

AAMA/CAAHEP Competency Achieved:

☑ III. C. 3. b. (4) (g): Apply pharmacology principles to prepare and administer aral and parenteral medication.
☑ III. C. 3. c. (2) (d): Document appropriately.

Copyright © 2008, 2004, 2000, 1995, 1990 by Saunders, an imprint of Elsevier Inc. All rights reserved.

EVALUATION OF COMPETENCY

Procedure 11-5: Administering an Intramuscular Injection

Name: ______________________ Date: __________

Evaluated By: ______________________ Score: __________

Performance Objective

Outcome: Administer an intramuscular injection.

Conditions: Given the following: appropriate medication, appropriate needle and syringe, antiseptic wipe, 2 x 2 gauze pad, disposable gloves, and a biohazard sharps container.

Standards: Time: 5 minutes. Student completed procedure in ____ minutes.

Accuracy: Satisfactory score on the Performance Evaluation Checklist.

Performance Evaluation Checklist

Trial 1	Trial 2	Point Value	*Performance Standards*
		•	Sanitized hands.
		•	Prepared the injection.
		•	Greeted the patient and introduced yourself.
		•	Identified the patient and explained the procedure and purpose of the injection.
			Located the Intramuscular Injection Sites
		*	Dorsogluteal
		*	Deltoid
		*	Vastus lateralis
		*	Ventrogluteal
		▷	Stated what tissue layer of the body the medication will be injected into.
		•	Cleansed area with an antiseptic wipe and allowed it to dry completely.
		•	Applied gloves.
		•	Removed needle guard.
		•	Stretched the skin taut over the injection site.
		▷	Explained why the skin should be stretched taut.
		•	Held the barrel of syringe like a dart and inserted needle quickly at a 90-degree angle to the patient's skin with a firm motion.
		•	Inserted the needle to the hub.
		▷	Explained why the needle should be inserted quickly and smoothly.
		*	Aspirated to make sure that the needle was not in a blood vessel.
		▷	Described what would happen if the medication was injected into a blood vessel.

Copyright © 2008, 2004, 2000, 1995, 1990 by Saunders, an imprint of Elsevier Inc. All rights reserved.

Trial 1	Trial 2	Point Value	*Performance Standards*
		•	Injected the medication slowly and steadily.
		•	Placed an antiseptic wipe or gauze pad gently over the injection site and removed needle quickly at the same angle as insertion.
		•	Applied gentle pressure to the injection site.
		▷	Stated the reason for applying pressure to the injection site.
		•	Activated the safety shield on the needle.
		•	Properly disposed of needle and syringe.
		•	Removed gloves and sanitized hands.
		•	Charted the procedure correctly.
		▷	Stated the purpose of the lot number on the medication vial.
		•	Remained with patient to make sure there were no unusual reactions.
		*	Completed the procedure within 5 minutes.
			TOTALS

CHART	
Date	

Evaluation of Student Performance

EVALUATION CRITERIA			COMMENTS
Symbol	Category	Point Value	
*	Critical Step	16 points	
•	Essential Step	6 points	
▷	Theory Question	2 points	
Score calculation: 100 points – ____ points missed ____ Score Satisfactory score: 85 or above			

AAMA/CAAHEP Competency Achieved:

☑ III. C. 3. b. (4) (g): Apply pharmacology principles to prepare and administer oral and parenteral medication.
☑ III. C. 3. c. (2) (d): Document appropriately.

Copyright © 2008, 2004, 2000, 1995, 1990 by Saunders, an imprint of Elsevier Inc. All rights reserved.

EVALUATION OF COMPETENCY

Procedure 11-6: Z-Track Intramuscular Injection Technique

Name: ______________________________ Date: ____________

Evaluated By: ______________________________ Score: ____________

Performance Objective

Outcome: Administer an intramuscular injection using the Z-track method.

Conditions: Given the following: appropriate medication, appropriate needle and syringe, antiseptic wipe, disposable gloves, and a biohazard sharps container.

Standards: Time: 5 minutes. Student completed procedure in ____ minutes.

Accuracy: Satisfactory score on the Performance Evaluation Checklist.

Performance Evaluation Checklist

Trial 1	*Trial 2*	*Point Value*	*Performance Standards*
		•	Sanitized hands.
		•	Prepared the injection.
		•	Greeted the patient and introduced yourself.
		•	Identified the patient and explained the procedure and purpose of the injection.
		•	Selected and properly located the intramuscular injection site.
		•	Cleansed area with an antiseptic wipe and allowed it to dry completely.
		•	Applied gloves.
		•	Removed needle guard.
		•	Pulled the skin away laterally from the injection site with the nondominant hand.
		•	Inserted needle quickly and smoothly at a 90-degree angle.
		*	Aspirated to make sure that the needle was not in a blood vessel.
		•	Injected the medication slowly and steadily.
		•	Waited 10 seconds before withdrawing the needle.
		▷	Explained why there should be a 10-second waiting period.
		•	Withdrew needle quickly at the same angle as that of insertion.
		•	Released the traction on the skin.
		▷	Described what occurs when the skin traction is released.
		•	Did not apply pressure to the injection site.
		•	Activated the safety shield on the needle.
		•	Properly disposed of needle and syringe.

Copyright © 2008, 2004, 2000, 1995, 1990 by Saunders, an imprint of Elsevier Inc. All rights reserved.

Trial 1	Trial 2	Point Value	Performance Standards
		▷	Stated why pressure should not be applied.
		•	Removed gloves and sanitized hands.
		•	Charted the procedure correctly.
		•	Remained with patient to make sure there were no unusual reactions.
		✶	Completed the procedure within 5 minutes.
			TOTALS

CHART	
Date	

Evaluation of Student Performance

EVALUATION CRITERIA			COMMENTS
Symbol	Category	Point Value	
✶	Critical Step	16 points	
•	Essential Step	6 points	
▷	Theory Question	2 points	

Score calculation: 100 points
– ______ points missed
____ Score

Satisfactory score: 85 or above

AAMA/CAAHEP Competency Achieved:

☑ III. C. 3. b. (4) (g): Apply pharmacology principles to prepare and administer oral and parenteral medication.
☑ III. C. 3. c. (2) (d): Document appropriately.

Copyright © 2008, 2004, 2000, 1995, 1990 by Saunders, an imprint of Elsevier Inc. All rights reserved.

EVALUATION OF COMPETENCY

Procedure 11-7: Administering an Intradermal Injection

Name: ______________________ Date: ____________

Evaluated By: ______________________ Score: ____________

Performance Objective

Outcome: Administer an intradermal injection and read the test results.

Conditions: Given the following: appropriate medication, appropriate needle and syringe, antiseptic wipe, 2 x 2 gauze pad, disposable gloves, millimeter ruler, TB test record card, and a biohazard sharps container.

Standards: Time: 10 minutes. Student completed procedure in ____ minutes.

Accuracy: Satisfactory score on the Performance Evaluation Checklist.

Performance Evaluation Checklist

Trial 1	*Trial 2*	*Point Value*	*Performance Standards*
		•	Sanitized hands.
		•	Prepared the injection.
		•	Greeted the patient and introduced yourself.
		•	Identified the patient and explained the procedure and purpose of the injection.
		•	Selected an appropriate intradermal injection site.
		▷	Stated what tissue layer of the body the medication will be injected into.
		•	Cleansed area with an antiseptic wipe and allowed it to dry completely.
		•	Applied gloves.
		•	Removed needle guard.
		•	Stretched the skin taut at the site of administration.
		▷	Explained why the skin is held taut.
		•	Inserted needle at an angle of 10 to 15 degrees, with the bevel upward.
		•	The bevel of the needle just penetrated the skin.
		▷	Stated why the bevel should face upward.
		•	Injected the medication slowly and steadily, ensuring that a wheal formed.
		▷	Explained what to do if a wheal does not form.
		•	Placed an antiseptic wipe or gauze pad gently over the injection site and removed the needle quickly at the same angle as that of insertion.
		•	Did not apply pressure to the injection site.
		▷	Explained why pressure should not be applied to the site.
		•	Activated the safety shield on the needle.

Copyright © 2008, 2004, 2000, 1995, 1990 by Saunders, an imprint of Elsevier Inc. All rights reserved.

Trial 1	Trial 2	Point Value	Performance Standards
		•	Properly disposed of needle and syringe.
		•	Removed gloves and sanitized hands.
		•	Remained with patient to make sure that there were no unusual reactions.
			Allergy Skin Tests
		•	Read the test results within 20 to 30 minutes.
		•	Inspected and palpated the site of the skin tests.
		•	Interpreted the skin test results.
		•	Charted the procedure correctly.
			Mantoux Tuberculin Test
		•	Instructed the patient in the care of the test site.
		▷	Stated the instructions that must be relayed to the patient.
		•	Informed the patient to return in 48 to 72 hours to have the results read.
		•	Charted the procedure correctly.
			READING MANTOUX TEST RESULTS
		•	Greeted and introduced yourself.
		•	Identified the patient and explained the procedure.
		•	Worked in a quiet, well-lit atmosphere.
		•	Checked the patient's chart to determine the site of administration of the test.
		•	Sanitized hands and applied gloves.
		•	Asked the patient to flex the arm at the elbow.
		•	Located the application site.
		•	Gently rubbed finger over the test site.
		•	If induration is present, rubbed the area lightly, going from the area of normal skin to the indurated area.
		•	Measured the diameter of the induration with a millimeter ruler.
		*	The measurement was identical to the evaluator's measurement.
		•	Interpreted the test results.
		▷	Explained how the test results are interpreted.
		•	Removed gloves and sanitized hands.
		•	Charted the results correctly.
		•	Completed a TB test record card and gave it to the patient.
		*	Completed the procedure within 10 minutes.
			TOTALS

CHART	
Date	

Copyright © 2008, 2004, 2000, 1995, 1990 by Saunders, an imprint of Elsevier Inc. All rights reserved.

TUBERCULOSIS TEST RECORD			
Name	Date Admin:		
	Date Read:		
MANTOUX TEST	RESULT		
	Negative	Doubtful	Positive
	____ mm	____ mm	____ mm
Logan Family Practice 401 St. George St. St. Augustine, FL 32084 (555) 824-3933 Performed by ____________________			

Evaluation of Student Performance

EVALUATION CRITERIA			COMMENTS
Symbol	Category	Point Value	
✶	Critical Step	16 points	
●	Essential Step	6 points	
▷	Theory Question	2 points	
Score calculation: 100 points – ______ points missed ____ Score Satisfactory score: 85 or above			

AAMA/CAAHEP Competency Achieved:

☑ III. C. 3. b. (4) (g): Apply pharmacology principles to prepare and administer oral and parenteral medication.
☑ III. C. 3. c. (2) (d): Document appropriately.

Copyright © 2008, 2004, 2000, 1995, 1990 by Saunders, an imprint of Elsevier Inc. All rights reserved.

Notes

Copyright © 2008, 2004, 2000, 1995, 1990 by Saunders, an imprint of Elsevier Inc. All rights reserved.

DRUG DOSAGE CALCULATION: SUPPLEMENTAL EDUCATION FOR CHAPTER 11

This section is designed as supplemental education for Chapter 11 (Administration of Medication) in your textbook. Completion of the exercises in this section will enable you to calculate drug dosage effectively and accurately, which is essential for administering the proper amount of medication to patients and preventing medication errors. This section is organized so that each unit builds on the next one; therefore, it is important that you are completely familiar with each step before proceeding to the next.

Learning Objectives

After completing this chapter, you should be able to:

1. Identify metric abbreviations.
2. Indicate dose quantity using metric notation guidelines.
3. Identify apothecary abbreviations.
4. Indicate dose quantity using apothecary notations.
5. Identify common medical abbreviations used in writing medication orders.
6. Interpret medication orders.
7. Convert units of measurement within the following systems: metric, apothecary, and household.
8. Convert units of measurement using ratio and proportion.
9. Convert units of measurement between the metric, apothecary, and household systems.
10. Determine oral drug dosage.
11. Determine parenteral drug dosage.

UNIT 1: THE METRIC SYSTEM

A. Units of Measurement

The basic units of measurement in the metric system are the gram, liter, and meter. The gram is a unit of weight used to measure solids; the liter is a unit of measure used to measure liquids; and the meter is a unit of linear measure used to measure length or distance.

Practice Problems: Units of Measurement
Directions: In the space provided below, indicate whether each of the following metric units of measurement is a unit of weight (W), volume (V), or length (L).

_______ 1. milligram

_______ 2. cubic centimeter

_______ 3. meter

_______ 4. kilogram

_______ 5. liter

_______ 6. milliliter

_______ 7. kiloliter

_______ 8. millimeter

_______ 9. microgram

_______ 10. gram

Copyright © 2008, 2004, 2000, 1995, 1990 by Saunders, an imprint of Elsevier Inc. All rights reserved.

B. Metric Abbreviations

Practice Problems: Metric Abbreviations

Review the metric abbreviations in your textbook before completing these problems.

Directions: In the space provided, indicate the correct abbreviation for each of the metric units of measurement listed below.

_______ 1. milligram

_______ 2. gram

_______ 3. kilogram

_______ 4. liter

_______ 5. cubic centimeter

_______ 6. microgram

_______ 7. milliliter

C. Metric Notation

Practice Problems: Metric Notations

In order to read prescriptions and medication orders, to record medication administration, and to avoid medication errors, the medical assistant must be familiar with and be able to use metric notation guidelines. Review the Metric Notation Guidelines on page 439 of your textbook before completing the following practice problems.

Directions: In the space provided, use metric notation guidelines to indicate the following dose quantities.

_______ 1. 25 milligrams

_______ 2. 5 grams

_______ 3. 1 ½ liters

_______ 4. 1 cubic centimeter

_______ 5. 10 milliliters

_______ 6. ½ gram

_______ 7. 50 milligrams

_______ 8. ½ cubic centimeter

_______ 9. 4 milliliters

_______ 10. 2 kilograms

_______ 11. 120 milliliters

_______ 12. 3 cubic centimeters

_______ 13. ¼ gram

_______ 14. 250 milligrams

_______ 15. ½ liter

_______ 16. 500 milliliters

_______ 17. 1 cubic centimeter

_______ 18. 5 kilograms

_______ 19. 2 ½ grams

_______ 20. 10 milligrams

Copyright © 2008, 2004, 2000, 1995, 1990 by Saunders, an imprint of Elsevier Inc. All rights reserved.

UNIT 2: THE APOTHECARY SYSTEMS

A. Units of Measurement

The basic units of measurement in the apothecary system are the grain, minim, and inch. The grain is a unit of weight used to measure solids; the minim is a unit of measure used to measure liquids; and the inch is a unit of linear measure used to measure length or distance.

Practice Problems: Units of Measurement

Directions: In the space provided, indicate whether each of the following units of measurement is a unit of weight (W), volume (V), or length (L).

_______ 1. grain

_______ 2. inch

_______ 3. minim

_______ 4. fluid dram

_______ 5. foot

_______ 6. quart

_______ 7. ounce

_______ 8. gallon

_______ 9. yard

_______ 10. fluid ounce

_______ 11. pound

_______ 12. pint

_______ 13. dram

_______ 14. mile

B. Apothecary Abbreviations

Practice Problems: Apothecary Abbreviations

Review the apothecary abbreviations in your textbook before completing these problems.

Directions: In the space provided, indicate the correct abbreviation or symbol for each of the apothecary units of measurement listed below.

_______ 1. grain

_______ 2. dram

_______ 3. ounce

_______ 4. minim

_______ 5. fluid dram

_______ 6. fluid ounce

_______ 7. pint

_______ 8. quart

_______ 9. gallon

_______ 10. inch

Copyright © 2008, 2004, 2000, 1995, 1990 by Saunders, an imprint of Elsevier Inc. All rights reserved.

C. Apothecary Notation

Practice Problems: Apothecary Notation

Although the apothecary system is used less frequently than the metric system, the medical assistant must still be familiar with and be able to use apothecary notation guidelines. Review the Apothecary Notation Guidelines on page 440 of your textbook before completing the following practice problems.

Directions: In the space provided, use apothecary notations to indicate the following dose quantities.

_______ 1. 4 ounces

_______ 2. 10 grains

_______ 3. 5 drams

_______ 4. ½ ounce

_______ 5. 6 fluid drams

_______ 6. 7 ½ grains

_______ 7. 3 ½ ounces

_______ 8. 10 minims

_______ 9. 3 fluid ounces

_______ 10. 2 drams

_______ 11. ¼ grain

_______ 12. 16 ounces

_______ 13. 12 minims

_______ 14. 1 dram

_______ 15. 9 fluid drams

_______ 16. 4 grains

_______ 17. 8 drams

_______ 18. 32 fluid ounces

_______ 19. 30 minims

_______ 20. 8 ounces

UNIT 3: THE HOUSEHOLD SYSTEM

The household system is more complicated and less accurate for administering medication than the metric and apothecary systems. However, most individuals are familiar with this system because of its frequent use in the United States. Thus, this unit of measurement may be the only one the patient can fully relate to and therefore may safely use to administer liquid medication at home.

A. Units of Measurement

Volume is the only household unit of measurement used to administer medication. The basic unit of liquid volume is the drop. The remaining units, in order of increasing volume, are the teaspoon, tablespoon, ounce, cup, and glass.

Practice Problems: Units of Measurement

Directions: In the space provided, indicate the correct abbreviation for each of the household units of measurement listed below.

_______ 1. drop

_______ 2. teaspoon

_______ 3. tablespoon

_______ 4. ounce

Copyright © 2008, 2004, 2000, 1995, 1990 by Saunders, an imprint of Elsevier Inc. All rights reserved.

UNIT 4: MEDICATION ORDERS

To safely administer medication, the medical assistant should be completely familiar with common medical abbreviations. Review Table 11-5 in your textbook before completing the following practice problems.

A. Medical Abbreviations

Practice Problems: Medical Abbreviations

Directions: In the space provided, write the meaning of the following medical abbreviations.

_______ 1. NPO

_______ 2. prn

_______ 3. AS

_______ 4. hs

_______ 5. tab

_______ 6. OD

_______ 7. ac

_______ 8. pc

_______ 9. qid

_______ 10. c̄

_______ 11. OU

_______ 12. s̄

_______ 13. bid

_______ 14. tid

_______ 15. qh

_______ 16. gtts

_______ 17. qd

_______ 18. q4h

_______ 19. AU

_______ 20. qs

_______ 21. IM

_______ 22. caps

_______ 23. qod

_______ 24. po

_______ 25. OS

_______ 26. ad lib

_______ 27. āā

_______ 28. DAW

_______ 29. INH

_______ 30. OTC

Copyright © 2008, 2004, 2000, 1995, 1990 by Saunders, an imprint of Elsevier Inc. All rights reserved.

B. Interpreting Medication Orders

Practice Problems: Interpreting Medication Orders

To safely administer medication and instruct patients on administering medication at home, the medical assistant should be able to interpret medication orders.

Directions: Interpret the following medication orders. Using a drug reference, indicate the drug category based on action and a brand name for each medication.

1. tetracycline 250 mg po qid × 10 days

   ____

   Drug category: ______________________________

   Brand name: ______________________________

2. lansoprazole 30 mg po qd ac

   ____

   Drug category: ______________________________

   Brand name: ______________________________

3. alprazolam 0.25 mg po tid

   ____

   Drug category: ______________________________

   Brand name: ______________________________

4. diltiazem 50 mg po q4h

   ____

   Drug category: ______________________________

   Brand name: ______________________________

5. ciprofloxacin 500 mg q12h

   ____

   Drug category: ______________________________

   Brand name: ______________________________

6. hydrocodone/acetaminophen 5 mg q4h prn

   ____

   Drug category: ______________________________

   Brand name: ______________________________

7. furosemide 40 mg po q AM

   ____

   Drug category: ______________________________

   Brand name: ______________________________

8. paroxetine 20 mg po qd in AM

   ____

   Drug category: ______________________________

   Brand name: ______________________________

Copyright © 2008, 2004, 2000, 1995, 1990 by Saunders, an imprint of Elsevier Inc. All rights reserved.

9. cetirizine 5 mg po qd

___

Drug category: ___

Brand name: ___

10. cyclobenzaprine 10 mg po tid × 1 wk

___

Drug category: ___

Brand name: ___

UNIT 5: CONVERTING UNITS OF MEASUREMENT

A. Using Conversion Tables

Changing from one unit of measurement to another is known as conversion. Conversion is required when medication is ordered in one unit of measurement and the medication label expresses the drug strength in a different unit. The dose quantity must be mathematically translated or converted to the unit of measurement of the medication on hand. For example, if the physician orders 5 grams of an oral solid medication and the medication label expresses the drug strength in milligrams, the medical assistant will need to convert the grams into milligrams to know how much medication to administer.

Converting units of measurement can be classified into the following categories:

1. Conversion of units within a measurement system.
2. Conversion of units from one measurement system to another.

Converting units within a measurement system allows a quantity to be expressed in a different but equal unit of measurement within the same system. An example of converting between units of weight within the metric system is as follows: 1 gram is equal to 1000 milligrams.

Converting from one measurement system to another allows a quantity to be expressed in a unit of measurement of another system. An example of a conversion between the apothecary and metric systems is as follows: 1 grain (apothecary system) is equivalent to 60 milligrams (metric system). Methods used to convert units of measurement are presented in this unit and in Unit 6.

Conversion requires the use of a conversion table to indicate the equivalent values between units of measurement. The practice problems that follow will assist you in attaining competency in conversion table utilization.

Practice Problems: Conversion Tables

Refer to the conversion tables at the end of this chapter. Locate and record the equivalent value for each of the units of measurement listed on the following page. In the space provided, indicate the conversion table you used to locate the equivalent value (e.g., metric, apothecary, metric to apothecary, etc.).

		ANSWER	CONVERSION TABLE
1. 1 g	=	___ mg	___
2. 1 ounce	=	___ drams	___
3. 1 tablespoon	=	___ teaspoons	___
4. 1 grain	=	___ mg	___
5. 1 liter	=	___ ml	___
6. 1 dram	=	___ grains	___
7. 1 pint	=	___ fluid ounces	___
8. 1 teaspoon	=	___ drops	___
9. 1 ml	=	___ cc	___
10. 1 ml	=	___ minims	___
11. 1 fluid ounce	=	___ ml	___

Copyright © 2008, 2004, 2000, 1995, 1990 by Saunders, an imprint of Elsevier Inc. All rights reserved.

12. 1 kg = ______ g ______
13. 1 fluid dram = ______ minims ______
14. 1 gallon = ______ quarts ______
15. 1 ounce = ______ tablespoons ______
16. 1 quart = ______ pints ______
17. 1 fluid dram = ______ ml ______
18. 1 g = ______ grains ______
19. 1 quart = ______ ml ______
20. 1 drop = ______ minims ______
21. 1 fluid ounce = ______ tablespoons ______
22. 1 fluid dram = ______ teaspoons ______
23. 1 tablespoon = ______ fluid drams ______
24. 1 kg = ______ pounds ______
25. 1 glass = ______ ml ______

B. Converting Units within the Metric System

Drug administration often requires conversion within the metric system to prepare the correct dosage. Metric conversion involves either converting a larger unit to a smaller unit (e.g., grams to milligrams) or converting a smaller unit to a larger unit (e.g., milliliters to liters).

Methods used to convert one metric unit to another are described as follows.

Converting a Larger Unit to a Smaller Unit

Converting a larger unit to a smaller unit within the metric system can be accomplished using one of three methods of conversion, outlined below. The method you use is based on your personal preference as well as the level of difficulty of the conversion problem; for example, more difficult problems will require the use of ratio and proportion as the method of conversion.

Examples of converting a larger unit to a smaller unit are as follows:

1. grams to milligrams
2. liters to milliliters
3. kilograms to grams

METHOD OF CONVERSION: To convert a larger unit to a smaller unit within the metric system:

Method 1: Multiply the unit to be changed by 1000.
Method 2: Move the decimal point of the unit to be changed three places to the right.
Method 3: Ratio and proportion (see Unit 6).

GUIDELINE: If you are converting a larger unit to a smaller unit, you should expect the quantity to become larger. Use this guideline as a reference to assist in making accurate conversions. Refer to the example problems below as an illustration of this guideline.

Examples

PROBLEM 2 L = ______ ml

Method 1: Multiply the unit to be changed by 1000.
$2 \times 1000 = 2000$ ml

Method 2: Move the decimal point of the unit to be changed three places to the right.
2.0 0 0. = 2000 ml

Answer 2 L = 2000 ml

Copyright © 2008, 2004, 2000, 1995, 1990 by Saunders, an imprint of Elsevier Inc. All rights reserved.

PROBLEM 4 g = _______ mg

Method 1: Multiply the unit to be changed by 1000.
4 × 1000 = 4000 mg

Method 2: Move the decimal point of the unit to be changed three places to the right.
4.0 0 0. = 4000 mg

Answer	4 g = 4000 mg

Converting a Smaller Unit to a Larger Unit

Converting a smaller unit to a larger unit within the metric system can be accomplished using one of three methods of conversion as outlined below.

Examples of converting a smaller unit to a larger unit are as follows:

1. milligrams to grams
2. milliliters to liters
3. grams to kilograms

METHOD OF CONVERSION: To convert a smaller unit to a larger unit within the metric system:

Method 1: Divide the unit to be changed by 1000.
Method 2: Move the decimal point of the unit to be changed three places to the left.
Method 3: Ratio and proportion (see Unit 6).

GUIDELINE: If you are converting a smaller unit to a larger unit, you should expect the quantity to become smaller. Refer to the problems below as an illustration of this guideline.

Examples

PROBLEM 250 mg = _______ g

Method 1: Divide the unit to be changed by 1000.
250 ÷ 1000 = 0.25 g

Method 2: Move the decimal point of the unit to be changed three places to the left.
.2 5 0. = 0.25 g

Answer	250 mg = 0.25 g

PROBLEM 1500 ml = _______ L

Method 1: Divide the unit to be changed by 1000.
1500 ÷ 1000 = 1.5 L

Method 2: Move the decimal point of the unit to be changed three places to the left.
1.5 0 0. = 1.5 L

Answer	1500 ml = 1.5 L

Practice Problems: Converting Units within the Metric System

Directions: Convert the following metric units of measurement using either Method 1 or Method 2. In the space provided, indicate if the conversion is going from a larger to smaller unit (L→S) or smaller to larger unit (S→L).

		ANSWER	CONVERSION TABLE
1. 1 g	=	_______ mg	____________________
2. 750 mg	=	_______ g	____________________
3. 2 kg	=	_______ g	____________________
4. 1000 g	=	_______ kg	____________________
5. 1.5 L	=	_______ ml	____________________

Copyright © 2008, 2004, 2000, 1995, 1990 by Saunders, an imprint of Elsevier Inc. All rights reserved.

6. 250 ml = ______ L ____________________
7. 5 g = ______ mg ____________________
8. 0.25 kg = ______ g ____________________
9. 1000 mg = ______ g ____________________
10. 2.5 g = ______ mg ____________________
11. 475 ml = ______ L ____________________
12. 0.05 g = ______ mg ____________________
13. 0.5 L = ______ ml ____________________
14. 1000 ml = ______ L ____________________
15. 500 g = ______ kg ____________________
16. 50 mg = ______ g ____________________
17. 1 L = ______ ml ____________________
18. 40 g = ______ mg ____________________
19. 50 ml = ______ L ____________________
20. 1 kg = ______ g ____________________

C. Converting Units within the Apothecary System

Drug administration may sometimes require conversion within the apothecary system to prepare the correct dosage. Apothecary conversion involves converting a larger unit to a smaller unit (e.g., drams to grains) or converting a smaller unit to a larger unit (e.g., ounces to pounds). Methods used to convert one apothecary unit to another are described below.

Converting a Larger Unit to a Smaller Unit

Converting a larger unit to a smaller unit within the apothecary system is accomplished through either the equivalent value method or the ratio and proportion method. Examples of converting a larger unit to a smaller unit are as follows:

Weight:
drams to grains
ounces to drams
pounds to ounces

Volume:
fluid drams to minims
fluid ounces to fluid drams
pints to fluid ounces
quarts to pints
gallons to quarts

METHOD OF CONVERSION: To convert a larger unit to a smaller unit within the apothecary system:

Method 1:
a. Look at the Apothecary Conversion Table at the end of this chapter to determine the equivalent value between the two units of measurement.
b. Multiply the equivalent value by the number next to the larger unit of measurement.
Method 2: Ratio and proportion (see Unit 6).

Examples
PROBLEM 4 drams = ______ grains
Method 1:
a. Look at the conversion table to determine the equivalent value:
1 dram = 60 grains
60 = the equivalent value

Copyright © 2008, 2004, 2000, 1995, 1990 by Saunders, an imprint of Elsevier Inc. All rights reserved.

b. Multiply the equivalent value by the number next to the larger unit of measurement:
 4 × 60 = 240 grains

Answer 4 drams = 240 grams

PROBLEM 1 ½ pints = _______ fluid ounces

Method 1:

a. Look at the conversion table to determine the equivalent value:
 1 pint = 16 fluid ounces
 16 = the equivalent value
b. Multiply the equivalent value by the number next to the larger unit of measurement:
 1.5 × 16 = 24 fluid ounces

Answer 1 ½ pints = 24 fluid ounces

Converting a Smaller Unit to a Larger Unit

Converting a smaller unit to a larger unit within the apothecary system can also be accomplished using either the equivalent value method or the ratio and proportion method. Examples of converting from a smaller unit to a larger unit are as follows:

Weight:	*Volume:*
grains to drams	minims to fluid drams
drams to ounces	fluid drams to fluid ounces
ounces to pounds	fluid ounces to pints
	pints to quarts
	quarts to gallons

METHOD OF CONVERSION: To convert a smaller unit to a larger unit within the apothecary system:

Method 1:

a. Look at the Apothecary Conversion Table at the end of this chapter to determine the equivalent value between the two units of measurement.
b. Divide the equivalent value into the number next to the smaller unit of measurement.

Method 2: Ratio and proportion (see Unit 6).

Examples

PROBLEM 30 grains = _______ drams

Method 1:

a. Look at the conversion table to determine the equivalent value:
 60 grains = 1 dram
 60 = the equivalent value
b. Divide the equivalent value into the number next to the smaller unit of measurement:
 30 ÷ 60 = ½ dram

Answer 30 grains = ½ dram

PROBLEM 16 fluid drams = _______ fluid ounces

Method 1:

a. Look at the conversion table to determine the equivalent value:
 8 fluid drams = 1 fluid ounce
 8 = the equivalent value
b. Divide the equivalent value into the number next to the smaller unit of measurement:
 16 ÷ 8 = 2 fluid ounces

Answer 16 fluid drams = 2 fluid ounces

Copyright © 2008, 2004, 2000, 1995, 1990 by Saunders, an imprint of Elsevier Inc. All rights reserved.

Practice Problems: Converting Units within the Apothecary

Convert the following apothecary units of measurement using the equivalent value method of conversion. In the space provided, indicate the equivalent value for each problem.

		ANSWER	EQUIVALENT VALUE
1. 2 quarts	=	_______ pints	______________
2. 4 drams	=	_______ grains	______________
3. ½ ounce	=	_______ drams	______________
4. 300 grains	=	_______ drams	______________
5. 2 fluid drams	=	_______ minims	______________
6. 8 pints	=	_______ quarts	______________
7. 16 drams	=	_______ ounces	______________
8. 24 fluid drams	=	_______ fluid ounces	______________
9. 18 ounces	=	_______ pounds	______________
10. 32 fluid ounces	=	_______ pints	______________
11. ½ quart	=	_______ pints	______________
12. ½ dram	=	_______ grains	______________
13. 3 ounces	=	_______ drams	______________
14. 210 grains	=	_______ drams	______________
15. 4 ½ fluid drams	=	_______ minims	______________
16. 3 pints	=	_______ quarts	______________
17. 4 drams	=	_______ ounces	______________
18. 24 ounces	=	_______ pounds	______________
19. 8 fluid ounces	=	_______ pints	______________
20. 2 quarts	=	_______ gallons	______________
21. 120 minims	=	_______ fluid drams	______________
22. 2 fluid ounces	=	_______ fluid drams	______________
23. ½ pound	=	_______ ounces	______________
24. 4 pints	=	_______ fluid ounces	______________
25. 2 gallons	=	_______ quarts	______________

D. Converting Units within the Household System

Household system conversion involves converting a larger unit to a smaller unit (e.g., tablespoons to teaspoons) or converting a smaller unit to a larger unit (e.g., tablespoons to ounces). Methods used to convert one unit to another are described below.

Converting a Larger Unit to a Smaller Unit

Converting a larger unit to a smaller unit within the household system is accomplished using either the equivalent value method or the ratio and proportion method. The method you use is based upon your personal preference as well as the level of difficulty of the conversion problem. Examples of converting a larger unit to a smaller unit are as follows:

Volume:
teaspoons to drops
tablespoons to teaspoons
ounces to teaspoons
ounces to tablespoons
teacup to ounces
glass to ounces

Copyright © 2008, 2004, 2000, 1995, 1990 by Saunders, an imprint of Elsevier Inc. All rights reserved.

METHOD OF CONVERSION: To convert a larger unit to a smaller unit within the household system:

Method 1:

a. Look at the Household Conversion Table at the end of this chapter to determine the equivalent value between the two units of measurement.
b. Multiply the equivalent value by the number next to the larger unit of measurement.

Method 2: Ratio and proportion (see Unit 6).

Examples

PROBLEM 2 tablespoons = _______ teaspoons

Method 1:

a. Look at the conversion table to determine the equivalent value:
   1 tablespoon = 3 teaspoons
   3 = the equivalent value
b. Multiply the equivalent value by the number next to the larger unit of measurement:
   $2 \times 3 = 6$ teaspoons

Answer 2 tablespoons = 6 teaspoons

PROBLEM ½ teaspoon = _______ drops

Method 1:

a. Look at the conversion table to determine the equivalent value:
   1 teaspoon = 60 drops
   60 = the equivalent value
b. Multiply the equivalent value by the number next to the larger unit of measurement:
   $\frac{1}{2} \times 60 = 30$ drops

Answer ½ teaspoon = 30 drops

Converting a Smaller Unit to a Larger Unit

Converting a smaller unit to a larger unit within the household system is accomplished using either the equivalent value method or the ratio and proportion method. Examples of converting from a smaller unit to a larger unit are as follows:

Volume:
drops to teaspoons
teaspoons to tablespoons
teaspoons to ounces
tablespoons to ounces
ounces to teacups
ounces to glasses

METHOD OF CONVERSION: To convert a smaller unit to a larger unit within the household system:

Method 1:

a. Look at the Household Conversion Table at the end of this chapter to determine the equivalent value between the two units of measurement.
b. Divide the equivalent value into the number next to the smaller unit of measurement.

Method 2: Ratio and proportion (see Unit 6).

Examples

PROBLEM 4 tablespoons = _______ ounces

Method 1:

a. Look at the conversion table to determine the equivalent value:
   1 ounce = 2 tablespoons
   2 = the equivalent value

Copyright © 2008, 2004, 2000, 1995, 1990 by Saunders, an imprint of Elsevier Inc. All rights reserved.

b. Divide the equivalent value into the number next to the smaller unit of measurement:
4 ÷ 2 = 2 ounces

> ***Answer*** 4 tablespoons = 2 ounces

PROBLEM 24 ounces = _______ glasses

Method 1:

a. Look at the conversion table to determine the equivalent value:
1 glass = 8 ounces
8 = the equivalent value

b. Divide the equivalent value into the number next to the smaller unit of measurement:
24 ÷ 8 = 3 glasses

> ***Answer*** 24 ounces = 3 glasses

Practice Problems: Converting Units within the Household System

Directions: Convert the following household units of measurement using the equivalent value method of conversion. In the space provided, indicate the equivalent value for each problem.

		ANSWER	EQUIVALENT VALUE
1. 12 teaspoons	=	_______ ounces	____________________
2. 4 ounces	=	_______ glasses	____________________
3. 90 drops	=	_______ teaspoons	____________________
4. ½ ounce	=	_______ tablespoons	____________________
5. 6 teaspoons	=	_______ tablespoons	____________________
6. 3 tablespoons	=	_______ ounces	____________________
7. 18 ounces	=	_______ teacups	____________________
8. ½ ounce	=	_______ teaspoons	____________________
9. 3 tablespoons	=	_______ teaspoons	____________________
10. ½ teaspoon	=	_______ drops	____________________

UNIT 6: RATIO AND PROPORTION

Ratio and proportion are also used to convert units of measurement.This method of conversion has the advantage of clarifying the mathematical rationale for the methods of conversion previously presented. It is also useful in converting units of measurement that are more difficult to calculate, such as converting between systems, for example, when converting an apothecary unit of measurement to a metric unit of measurement.

A. Ratio and Proportion Guidelines

Some basic guidelines must be followed when using ratio and proportion. These guidelines are described below.

1. A **ratio** is composed of two related numbers separated by a colon. It indicates the relationship between two quantities or numbers. The ratio example below shows a relationship between milligrams and grams, i.e., 1000 mg = 1 g.

   EXAMPLE 1000 mg : 1 g

2. A **proportion** shows the relationship between two equal ratios. The proportion consists of two ratios separated by an equal sign (=) which indicates that the two ratios are equal. This proportion example shows the relationship between two equal ratios of milligrams and grams.

   EXAMPLE 1000 mg : 1 g = 2000 mg : 2 g

3. The units of measurement in the two ratios of a proportion must be expressed in the same sequence. The correct sequencing in the proportion example below is mg : g = mg : g, *not* mg : g = g : mg.

Copyright © 2008, 2004, 2000, 1995, 1990 by Saunders, an imprint of Elsevier Inc. All rights reserved.

EXAMPLE *Correct:* 1000 mg : 1 g = 2000 mg : 2 g
Incorrect: 1000 mg : 1 g = 2 g: 2000 mg

4. The numbers on the ends of a proportion are called the **extremes** while the numbers in the middle of the proportion are known as the **means**. In this example, the means consist of 1 g and 2000 mg, and the extremes are 1000 mg and 2 g.

EXAMPLE 1000 mg : 1 g = 2000 mg : 2g
(1 g and 2000 mg: means; 1000 mg and 2g: extremes)

5. The product of the means equals the product of the extremes. The calculation of the product of the means in the example is as follows: 1 × 2000 = 2000. The calculation of the product of the extremes is as follows: 1000 · 2 = 2000. Hence, the product of the means equals the product of the extremes or 2000 = 2000.

EXAMPLE 1000 mg: 1 g = 2000 mg : 2 g
1 × 2000 = 1000 × 2
2000 = 2000

6. In setting up a proportion, one side of the equation consists of the known quantities, and the other side of the equation consists of the unknown quantity. The letter **x** is commonly used to express the unknown quantity. To be consistent, the known quantities are indicated on the left side of the equation and the unknown quantity is indicated on the right side of the equation. Using the above proportion, but inserting an unknown quantity, or **x**, the equation is set up as follows:

EXAMPLE 1000 mg : 1 g = x mg : 2 g
(known quantities) (unknown quantity)

Practice Problems: Ratio and Proportion

Answer the following questions:

1. What is a ratio? ______________________________

____

2. In the space provided, place a check mark next to each correct example of a ratio.

_______ a. 15 drops : 15 minims : 1 ml

_______ b. 1000 ml = 1 L

_______ c. 1 ounce : 8 drams

_______ d. 60 minims/1 fluid dram

_______ e. 1 dram : 60 grains

_______ f. 1 ml : 1 cc

3. What is a proportion?

____

____

____

4. In the space provided, place a check mark next to each correct example of a proportion.

_______ a. 1 ml : 1 cc

_______ b. 1 grain : 60 mg = 4 grains : 240 mg

_______ c. 2x = 60 mg

_______ d. 1000 ml : 1 L = 500 ml : 0.5 L

_______ e. 1000 mg : 1 grain = 1000 ml : 1 L

Copyright © 2008, 2004, 2000, 1995, 1990 by Saunders, an imprint of Elsevier Inc. All rights reserved.

5. In the space provided, place a check mark next to each proportion that has correct sequencing for the units of measurement.

    _______ a. 1000 g : 1 kg = 1500 g : 1.5 kg

    _______ b. 60 grains : 1 dram = 2 drams : 120 grains

    _______ c. 1000 mg : 1 g = 2000 mg : x g

6. Circle the means and underline the extremes in each of the following proportions:

    a. 1000 mg : 1 g = 500 mg : 0.5 g

    b. 2 pints : 1 quart = 4 pints : 2 quarts

    c. 1 ml : 1 cc = 2 ml : 2cc

7. In each of the following proportions, what is the product of the means and the product of the extremes?

    a. 1000 g : 1 kg = 1500 g : 1.5 kg

    _______ product of the means

    _______ product of the extremes

    b. 60 minims : 1 fluid dram = 120 minims : 2 fluid drams

    _______ product of the means

    _______ product of the extremes

    c. 60 mg : 1 grain = 300 mg : 5 grains

    _______ product of the means

    _______ product of the extremes

8. In each of the following proportions, circle the known quantities and underline the unknown quantity.

    a. 1000 mg : 1 g = 500 mg : x g

    b. 1 g : 15 grains = 2 g : x grains

    c. 8 drams : 1 ounce = x drams : 4 ounces

B. Converting Units Using Ratio and Proportion

The method to follow to convert units using ratio and proportion is outlined below.

METHOD OF CONVERSION: To convert a unit of measurement using ratio and proportion:

a. Look at the appropriate conversion table at the end of this chapter to determine what is known about the two units of measurement (equivalent value).
b. State the known quantities as a ratio.
c. Determine the unknown quantity.
d. State the unknown quantity as a ratio.
e. Set up the proportion with the known quantities on the left side and the unknown quantity on the right side of the equation.
f. Solve the equation as follows: Multiply the product of the means and the product of the extremes. Divide the equation by the number(s) before the x.
g. Include the unit of measure corresponding to x in the original equation with the answer.

Copyright © 2008, 2004, 2000, 1995, 1990 by Saunders, an imprint of Elsevier Inc. All rights reserved.

Examples

PROBLEM 2 g = _______ mg

a. Look at the metric conversion table to determine what is known about the two units of measurement:

1000 mg = 1 g

b. State the known quantities as a ratio:

1000 mg = 1 g

c. Determine the unknown quantity:

2 g = x mg

d. State the unknown quantity as a ratio using the correct unit of measurement sequencing:

x mg : 2 g

e. Set up the proportion with the known quantities on the left side and the unknown quantity on the right side of the equation:

1000 mg : 1 g = x mg : 2 g

f. Solve the equation by multiplying the product of the means and the product of the extremes and dividing the equation by the number before the x:

1000 mg : 1 g = x mg : 2 g
$1 \times x = 1000 \times 2$
1x = 2000
x = 2000

g. Include the unit of measure corresponding to x in the original equation with the answer:

x = 2000 mg

Answer 2 g = 2000 mg

PROBLEM
300 mg = _______ grains
The steps outlined above are followed here also. However, they are combined as they would be in working an actual conversion problem.

60 mg : 1 grain = 300 mg: x grains
$1 \times 300 = 60 \times x$
300 = 60x
$300 \div 60 = 60x \div 60$
x = 5 grains

Answer 300 mg = 5 grains

Practice Problems: Converting Units Using Ratio and Proportion

Directions: Use ratio and proportion to convert between the apothecary, metric, and household systems by completing the problems below. In the space at the right, indicate what is known regarding the two units of measurement.

		ANSWER	KNOWN QUANTITIES
1. 30 minims	=	_______ ml	_______________
2. 4 kg	=	_______ pounds	_______________
3. 90 ml	=	_______ fluid ounces	_______________
4. 30 mg	=	_______ grains	_______________
5. 60 mg	=	_______ ounces	_______________
6. 250 ml	=	_______ pints	_______________

Copyright © 2008, 2004, 2000, 1995, 1990 by Saunders, an imprint of Elsevier Inc. All rights reserved.

7. 6 g = _______ drams _______________
8. 1 ½ quarts = _______ ml _______________
9. 3 g = _______ grains _______________
10. 5 fluid drams = _______ ml _______________
11. 80 pounds = _______ kg _______________
12. 500 ml = _______ quarts _______________
13. 8 ml = _______ teaspoons _______________
14. 4 grains = _______ mg _______________
15. 32 ml = _______ fluid drams _______________
16. 120 mg = _______ grains _______________
17. 30 ml = _______ tablespoons _______________
18. 60 drops = _______ ml _______________
19. 1 ½ fluid ounces = _______ tablespoons _______________
20. ½ fluid ounce = _______ ml _______________

UNIT 7: DETERMINING DRUG DOSAGE

A. Oral Administration

Dosage refers to the amount of medication to be administered to the patient. Each medication has a certain dosage range or range of quantities that produce therapeutic effects. It is important to administer the exact drug dosage. If the dose is too small, it will not produce a therapeutic effect, whereas too large a dose could be harmful or even fatal to the patient.

The steps to follow in determining drug dosage depend on the unit of measurement in which the drug is ordered and the unit of measurement of the drug you have available, or the dose on-hand. A general discussion of the method for determining drug dosage is as follows:

1. If the dose on-hand is the same as that which has been ordered, no calculation is required. In this example, both the dose ordered and the dose on-hand are in the same unit of measurement, and one tablet is administered to the patient.

EXAMPLE The physician orders 50 mg of a medication po.
The drug label reads 50 mg/tablet.

2. If the dosage ordered is in the same unit of measurement as that indicated on the medication label, only one calculation step is required. In this example, both the dose ordered and the dose on-hand are in the same unit of measurement, or grains. The calculation step performed will be to determine the number of tablets to administer to the patient.

EXAMPLE The physician orders gr $\bar{\text{v}}$ of a medication po.
The drug label reads gr $\bar{\text{x}}$ tablet.

3. If the dosage ordered is in a different unit of measurement than indicated on the drug label, two calculation steps are required to determine the amount of medication to administer to the patient. In this example, the dose ordered and the dose on-hand are stated in different units of measurement, or in grams and milligrams. The first step requires conversion of the dose ordered to the unit of measurement of the dose on-hand; in this example, grams must be converted to milligrams. The second step is to determine the number of tablets to administer to the patient.

EXAMPLE The physician orders 1 g of a medication po.
The drug label reads 500 mg/tablet.

A detailed discussion of determining drug dosage for administration of oral medication follows. The method used to calculate drug dosage when the units of measurement are the same is presented first, followed by the method used when the units of measurement are different.

Copyright © 2008, 2004, 2000, 1995, 1990 by Saunders, an imprint of Elsevier Inc. All rights reserved.

Determining Drug Dosage with the Same Units of Measurement

Determining the correct drug dosage to be administered when the units of measurement are the same requires the use of a formula that is explained below.

DRUG DOSAGE FORMULA

$$\frac{\text{D } (\textit{dose ordered})}{\text{H } (\textit{on hand})} \times \text{V } (\textit{vehicle}) = \text{x (Amount of medication to be administered)}$$

D (*dose ordered*): This is the amount of medication ordered by the physician.

H (*drug strength on-hand*): This is the dosage strength available as indicated on the medication label or the dose on-hand.

V (*vehicle*): The vehicle refers to the type of preparation containing the dose on-hand (e.g., tablet, capsule, liquid).

x: The letter x is used to express the unknown quantity or the amount of medication to be administered.

GUIDELINES

1. The units of measurement must be included when setting up the problem.
2. The values for D and H must be in the same unit of measurement.
3. The value of x is expressed in the same unit as V.
4. When determining the drug dosage for oral liquid medication, the vehicle must also include the amount of liquid in which the available drug is contained. For example, if the medication label reads 250 mg/5 ml, the value of V is 5 ml.

The method to follow to determine drug dosage using this formula is outlined below. The first example illustrates determining dosage for oral solid medication.

Examples

PROBLEM *Oral Solid Medication*:
The physician orders 50 mg of a medication po.
The medication label reads 25 mg/tablet.
How much medication should be administered to the patient?

Drug Dosage Formula:

$$\frac{D}{H} \times V = x$$

a. Identify the dose ordered.
D = 50 mg

b. Identify the strength of the drug on-hand.
H = 25 mg

c. Determine the vehicle containing the dose on-hand.
V = 1 tablet

d. Calculate the amount of medication to administer to the patient. The units of measurement must be included when setting up the problem, and the values for D and H must be in the same unit of measurement. The value of x is expressed in the same unit as V; in this problem V = 1 tablet.

$$\frac{50 \text{ mg}}{25 \text{ mg}} \times 1 \text{ tablet} = x$$

$$(50 \div 25 = 2) \times 1 \text{ tablet} = x$$

$$2 \times 1 \text{ tablet} = x$$

$$x = 2 \text{ tablets}$$

Answer 2 tablets are administered to the patient.

Copyright © 2008, 2004, 2000, 1995, 1990 by Saunders, an imprint of Elsevier Inc. All rights reserved.

The next problem illustrates the determination of drug dosage for oral liquid medication.The steps outlined above are followed; however, they are combined as should be done when working out drug dosage problems. Remember, with oral liquid medication, the vehicle must also include the amount of liquid in which the available drug is contained; in the problem below, V = 5 ml.

PROBLEM *Oral Liquid Medication:*
The physician orders 500 mg of a medication.
The medication label reads 250 mg/5 ml.
How much medication should be administered to the patient?

$\frac{D}{H} \times V = x$

$\frac{500 \text{ mg}}{250 \text{ mg}} \times 1 \text{ tablet} = x$

$(500 \div 250 = 2) \times 5 \text{ ml} = x$

$2 \times 5 \text{ ml} = x$

$x = 10 \text{ ml}$

Answer 10 ml of medication is administered to the patient.

Determining Drug Dosage with Different Units of Measurement

At times the medication ordered is in a different unit of measurement than indicated on the drug label. In this case, the desired dose quantity must be converted to the unit of measurement of the dose on-hand before the drug dosage is determined.The method you use to convert a unit of measurement is based on your personal preference. Refer to Units 5 and 6 to review methods of conversion before completing this section.

The following steps are required to determine drug dosage when the units of measurement are different:

Step 1: Convert the dose quantities to the same unit of measurement. For consistency, it is best to convert to the unit of measurement of the drug on-hand.

Step 2: Determine the amount of medication to administer to the patient, using the drug dosage formula.

Examples

PROBLEM *Oral Solid Medication:*
The physician orders gr $\bar{x}$ of medication po.
The medication label reads 300 mg/tablet.
How much medication should be administered to the patient?

*Step 1:*The dosage ordered must be converted to the unit of measurement of the medication on-hand. In this problem, 10 grains must be converted to milligrams. The ratio and proportion method of conversion is used to make the conversion.

gr $\bar{x}$ = _______ mg

1 grain : 60 mg = 10 grains: x mg

600 = 1x

x = 600 mg

Answer gr $\bar{x}$ = 600 mg

The medication ordered is now in the same unit of measurement as the medication on-hand.

Step 2: Determine the amount of medication to administer to the patient using the drug dosage formula.

$\frac{D}{H} \times V = x$

600 mg × 1 tablet = x
300 mg

$(600 \div 300 = 2) \times 1 \text{ tablet} = x$

Copyright © 2008, 2004, 2000, 1995, 1990 by Saunders, an imprint of Elsevier Inc. All rights reserved.

2 × 1 tablet = x
x = 2 tablets

Answer 2 tablets are administered to the patient.

PROBLEM *Oral Liquid Medication:*
The physician order gr xv of a medication po.
The medication label reads 300 mg/fluid dram.
How much medication should be administered to the patient?

Step 1: Convert 15 grains to milligrams using ratio and proportion:
gr $\overline{xv}$= _______ mg
60 mg : 1 grain = x mg : 15 grains
1x = 900 mg
x = 900 mg

Answer gr $\overline{xv}$ = 900 mg

Step 2: Determine the amount of medication to administer to the patient using the drug dosage formula.

$\frac{D}{H} \times V = x$

900 mg × 1 fluid dram = x
300 mg
(900 ÷ 300 = 3) ×1 fluid dram = x
3 × 1 fluid dram = x
x = 3 fluid drams

Answer 3 fluid drams of medication are administered to the patient.

Practice Problems: Oral Administration

Directions: Determine the drug dosage to be administered for each of the following oral medication orders and record your answer below. In the space provided, indicate the drug category based on action for each medication using a drug reference.

Oral Solid Medications:

1. The physician orders Inderal 160 mg po.
Medication label:

Inderal propranolol 80 mg/capsule

How much medication should be administered? ______________________________

Drug category: ______________________________

2. The physician orders Tagamet gr $\overline{v}$ po.
Medication label:

Tagament cimetidine 300 mg/tablet

Copyright © 2008, 2004, 2000, 1995, 1990 by Saunders, an imprint of Elsevier Inc. All rights reserved.

How much medication should be administered? ____________________

Drug category: ____________________

3. The physician orders Amoxil 0.5 g po.
   Medication label:

   Amoxil
   amoxicillin
   250 mg/capsule

How much medication should be administered? ____________________

Drug category: ____________________

4. The physician orders Lasix 80 mg po.
   Medication label:

   Lasix
   furosemide
   40 mg/tablet

How much medication should be administered? ____________________

Drug category: ____________________

5. The physician orders Lomotil 5 mg po.
   Medication label:

   Lomotil
   diphenoxylate/atropine
   2.5 mg/tablet

How much medication should be administered? ____________________

Drug category: ____________________

6. The physician orders Zithromax 0.5 g po.
   Medication label:

   Zithromax
   azithromycin
   250 mg/tablet

How much medication should be administered? ____________________

Drug category: ____________________

7. The physician orders Calan gr ii po. ED: A bar needs to go between the lines and periods of ii
   Medication label:

   Calan
   verapamil
   40 mg/tablet

Copyright © 2008, 2004, 2000, 1995, 1990 by Saunders, an imprint of Elsevier Inc. All rights reserved.

How much medication should be administered? ____________________

Drug category: ____________________

8. The physician orders Xanax 0.5 mg po.
   Medication label:

Xanax alprazolam 0.25 mg/tablet

How much medication should be administered? ____________________

Drug category: ____________________

9. The physician orders Phenergan 25 mg po.
   Medication label:

Phenergan promethazine 12.5 mg/tablet

How much medication should be administered? ____________________

Drug category: ____________________

10. The physician orders Procardia XL gr $\overline{ss}$ po.
    Medication label:

Procardia nifedipine 10 mg/tablet

How much medication should be administered? ____________________

Drug category: ____________________

Oral Solid Medications:

1. The physician orders Sumycin Suspension 250 mg po.
   Medication label:

Sumycin Suspension tetracycline 125 mg/5 ml

How much medication should be administered? ____________________

Drug category: ____________________

2. The physician orders Tagamet liquid 300 mg po.
   Medication label:

Tagamet Cimetidine liquid 300 mg/5 ml

Copyright © 2008, 2004, 2000, 1995, 1990 by Saunders, an imprint of Elsevier Inc. All rights reserved.

How much medication should be administered? ______________________________

Drug category: ______________________________

3. The physician orders Tylenol Elixir grt po.
Medication label:

Tylenol Elixir acetaminophen 120 mg/5 ml

How much medication should be administered? ______________________________

Drug category: ______________________________

4. The physician orders Amoxil Suspension 0.5 g po.
Medication label:

Amoxil Suspension amoxicillin 125 mg/5 ml

How much medication should be administered? ______________________________

Drug category: ______________________________

5. The physician orders Gantanol Suspension 1 g po.
Medication label:

Gantanol Suspension sulfamethoxazole 500 mg/5 ml

How much medication should be administered? ______________________________

Drug category: ______________________________

B. Parenteral Administration

Medications for parenteral administration must be suspended in solution. The medication label indicates the amount of the drug contained in each milliliter of solution. For example, if a medication label reads 10 mg/ml, this means that there are 10 mg of medication for each ml of liquid volume. Some medications, such as penicillin, insulin, and heparin, are ordered and measured in terms of units (e.g., 300,000 units/ml). This refers to their biological activity in animal tests or the amount of the drug which is required to produce a particular response.

Parenteral medication is available in a number of dispensing forms which include ampules, single-dose vials, and multiple-dose vials. Once the proper drug dosage has been determined, the medication is drawn into a syringe from the dispensing unit. Since most syringes are calibrated in cubic centimeters (cc), it is important to remember the equivalent value between ml and cc, or 1 ml is equal to 1 cc.

Determining drug dosage for parenteral administration is calculated in a similar manner as that for oral liquid medication as explained below. The first problem illustrates the determination of drug dosage when the medication is ordered in a different unit of measurement from the dose on-hand, requiring two calculation steps.

Examples

PROBLEM The physician orders 0.5 g of a medication IM.
The medication label reads 250 mg/2 ml.
How much medication should be administered?

Copyright © 2008, 2004, 2000, 1995, 1990 by Saunders, an imprint of Elsevier Inc. All rights reserved.

Step 1: Convert 0.5 gram to milligrams.
0.5 g = _______ mg
1000 mg : 1 g = x mg : 0.5 g
1x = 500
x = 500 mg

> ***Answer*** 0.5 mg = 500 mg

Step 2: Determine the amount of medication to administer to the patient:

$$\frac{D}{H} \times V = x$$

$$\frac{500 \text{ mg}}{250 \text{ mg}} \times 2 \text{ ml} = x$$

(500 250 = 2) × 2 ml = x
2 × 2 ml = x
x = 4 ml (cc)

> ***Answer*** 4 cc of medication are administrated to the patient.

The next problem illustrates the determination of drug dosage with a medication ordered in units. Note that both the dose ordered and the dose on-hand are in the same unit of measurement; therefore, conversion of units of measurement is not necessary.

PROBLEM The physician orders 600,000 units of a medication IM.
The medication label reads 300,000 units/ml.
How much medication should be administered?

$$\frac{D}{H} \times V = x$$

$$\frac{600{,}000 \text{ units}}{300{,}000 \text{ units}} \times 1 \text{ ml} = x$$

(600,000 300,000 = 2) × 1 ml = x
x = 2 ml (cc)

> ***Answer*** 2 cc of medication are administrated to the patient.

Practice Problems: Parenteral Administration

Determine the drug dosage to be administered for each of the following parenteral medication orders and record your answer below. In the space provided, indicate the drug category based on action using a drug reference.

1. The physician orders Vistaril 75 mg IM.
   Medication label:

> Vistaril
> hydroxyzine injection
>
> 50 mg/ml

How much medication should be administered? ________________________________

Drug category: ________________________________

Copyright © 2008, 2004, 2000, 1995, 1990 by Saunders, an imprint of Elsevier Inc. All rights reserved.

2. The physician orders Cobex (Vitamin B_{12}) 200 mcg IM.
   Medication label:

Cobex cyanocobalamin injection 100 mcg/ml

How much medication should be administered? ___________________________________

Drug category: ___________________________________

3. The physician orders Depo-Medrol 40 mg IM.
   Medication label:

Depo-Medrol Methylprednisolone injection 80 mg/ml

How much medication should be administered? ___________________________________

Drug category: ___________________________________

4. The physician orders Wycillin 600,000 units IM.
   Medication label:

Wycillin procine penicillin G injection 300, 000 units/ml

How much medication should be administered? ___________________________________

Drug category: ___________________________________

5. The physician orders Rocephin 100 mg IM.
   Medication label:

Rocephin ceftriaxone injection 1 g/ml

How much medication should be administered? ___________________________________

Drug category: ___________________________________

6. The physician orders InFed 100 mg IM.
   Medication label:

Infed iron dextran injection 50 mg/ml

How much medication should be administered? ___________________________________

Drug category: ___________________________________

Copyright © 2008, 2004, 2000, 1995, 1990 by Saunders, an imprint of Elsevier Inc. All rights reserved.

7. The physician orders Bicillin 1.2 million units IM.
Medication label:

Bicillin benzathine penicillin G injection 600,000 units/ml

How much medication should be administered? ____________________

Drug category: ____________________

8. The physician orders Depo-Provera 150 mg IM.
Medication label:

Depo-Provera medroxyprogesterone 150 mg/ml

How much medication should be administered? ____________________

Drug category: ____________________

9. The physician orders Pronestyl 0.25 g IM.
Medication label:

Pronestyl procainamide injection 500 mg/ml

How much medication should be administered? ____________________

Drug category: ____________________

10. The physician orders Compazine 7 mg IM.
Medication label:

Compazine prochlorperazine injection 5 mg/ml

How much medication should be administered? ____________________

Drug category: ____________________

Copyright © 2008, 2004, 2000, 1995, 1990 by Saunders, an imprint of Elsevier Inc. All rights reserved.

Table 11-1. Metric System Conversion of Equivalent Values
WEIGHT
1000 micrograms = 1 milligram
1000 milligrams = 1 gram
1000 grams = 1 kilogram
VOLUME
1000 milliliters = 1 liter
1000 liters = 1 kiloliter
1 milliliter = 1 cubic centimeter

Table 11-2. Apothecary System: Conversion of Equivalent Values
WEIGHT
60 grains = 1 dram
8 drams = 1 ounce
12 ounces = 1 pound
VOLUME
60 minims = 1 fluid dram
8 fluid drams = 1 fluid ounce
16 fluid ounces = 1 pint
2 pints = 1 quart
4 quarts = 1 gallon

Table 11-3. Household System: Conversion of Equivalent Values
ABBREVIATIONS
drop: gtt
teaspoon: tsp
tablespoon: tbsp
ounce: oz
cup: c
VOLUME
60 drops = 1 teaspoon
3 teaspoons = 1 tablespoon
6 teaspoons = 1 ounce
2 tablespoons = 1 ounce
6 ounces = 1 teacup
8 ounces = 1 glass
8 ounces = 1 cup

Copyright © 2008, 2004, 2000, 1995, 1990 by Saunders, an imprint of Elsevier Inc. All rights reserved.

Table 11-4. Conversion Chart for Metric and Apothecary Systems (Commonly Used Approximate Equivalents)

METRIC SYSTEM TO APOTHECARY SYSTEM	APOTHECARY SYSTEM TO METRIC SYSTEM
WEIGHT	**WEIGHT**
60 mg = 1 grain	15 grains = 1000 mg (1 g)
1 g = 15 grains	10 grains = 600 mg
4 g = 1 dram	7.5 grains = 500 mg
30 mg = 1 ounce	5 grains = 300 mg
1 kg = 2.2 pounds	3 grains = 200 mg
	1.5 grains = 100 mg
VOLUME	1 grain = 60 mg
0.06 ml = 1 minim	$\frac{3}{4}$ grain = 50 mg
1 ml(cc) = 15 minims	$\frac{1}{2}$ grain = 30 mg
4 ml = 1 fluid dram	$\frac{1}{4}$ grain = 15 mg
30 ml = 1 fluid ounce	$\frac{1}{6}$ grain = 10 mg
500 ml = 1 pint	$\frac{1}{8}$ grain = 8 mg
1000 ml (1 L) = 1 quart	$\frac{1}{12}$ grain = 5 mg
	$\frac{1}{15}$ grain = 4 mg
	$\frac{1}{20}$ grain = 3 mg
	$\frac{1}{30}$ grain = 2 mg
	$\frac{1}{40}$ grain = 1.5 mg
	$\frac{1}{50}$ grain = 1.2 mg
	$\frac{1}{60}$ grain = 1 mg
	$\frac{1}{100}$ grain = 0.6 mg
	$\frac{1}{120}$ grain = 0.5 mg
	$\frac{1}{150}$ grain = 0.4 mg
	$\frac{1}{200}$ grain = 0.3 mg
	$\frac{1}{300}$ grain = 0.2 mg
	$\frac{1}{600}$ grain = 0.1 mg

Table 11-5. Conversion Chart for Apothecary and Metric Equivalents of Household Measures (Volume)

Household	Apothecary	Metric
1 drop	= 1 minim	= 0.06 ml
15 drops	= 15 minims	= 1 ml (cc)
1 teaspoon	= 1 fluid dram	= 5 (4) ml
1 tablespoon	= 4 fluid drams	= 15 ml
2 tablespoons	= 1 fluid ounce	= 30 ml
1 ounce	= 1 fluid ounce	= 30 ml
1 teacup	= 6 fluid ounces	= 180 ml
1 glass	= 8 fluid ounces	= 240 ml

Copyright © 2008, 2004, 2000, 1995, 1990 by Saunders, an imprint of Elsevier Inc. All rights reserved.

Notes

Copyright © 2008, 2004, 2000, 1995, 1990 by Saunders, an imprint of Elsevier Inc. All rights reserved.

12

Cardiopulmonary Procedures

CHAPTER ASSIGNMENTS

√ After Completing	Date Due	Textbook Page(s)	TEXTBOOK ASSIGNMENTS	Possible Points	Points You Earned
		493-525	Read Chapter 12: Cardiopulmonary Procedures		
		499 521	Read Case Study 1 Case Study 1 questions	 5	
		516 521	Read Case Study 2 Case Study 2 questions	 5	
		518 521	Read Case Study 3 Case Study 3 questions	 5	
		522-523	Apply Your Knowledge questions	12	
			TOTAL POINTS		
√ After Completing	**Date Due**	**Study Guide Page(s)**	**STUDY GUIDE ASSIGNMENTS (CTA: Critical Thinking Activity)**	**Possible Points**	**Points You Earned**
		561	Pretest	10	
		562	Key Term Assessment	15	
		564-568	Evaluation of Learning questions	30	
		568	CTA A: Chest Leads	5	
			CD Activity: Chapter 12 Find That Lead (Record points earned)		
		569	CTA B: ECG Cycle	10	
		570	CTA C: GO TO! Game (Team Players) (Record points earned)		
			CD Activity: Chapter 12 It's a Cycle (Individual Player) (Record points earned)		

Copyright © 2008, 2004, 2000, 1995, 1990 by Saunders, an imprint of Elsevier Inc. All rights reserved.

√ After Completing	Date Due	Study Guide Page(s)	STUDY GUIDE ASSIGNMENTS (CTA: Critical Thinking Activity)	Possible Points	Points You Earned
			CD Activity: Chapter 12 It's an Artifact (Record points earned)		
		577	CTA D: ECG Artifacts (10 points each)	30	
		577	CTA E: Myocardial Infarction	20	
		581	CTA F: Crossword Puzzle	27	
		582	CTA G: Road to Recovery Game (Record points earned)		
			CD Activity: Chapter 12 Animations	20	
		561	Posttest	10	
			ADDITIONAL ASSIGNMENTS		
			TOTAL POINTS		

Copyright © 2008, 2004, 2000, 1995, 1990 by Saunders, an imprint of Elsevier Inc. All rights reserved.

√ When Assigned By Your Instructor	Study Guide Page(s)	Practices Required	LABORATORY ASSIGNMENTS (Procedure Number and Name)	*Score
	585	3	DVD **Practice for Competency** 12-1: Running a 12-Lead, Three-Channel Electrocardiogram Textbook reference: pp. 505-507	
	587-589		**Evaluation of Competency** 12-1: Running a 12-Lead, Three-Channel Electrocardiogram	*
	585	3	**Practice for Competency** 12-2: Applying a Holter Monitor Textbook reference: pp. 510-511	
	591-593		**Evaluation of Competency** 12-2: Applying a Holter Monitor	*
	585	3	DVD **Practice for Competency** 12-3: Spirometry Testing Textbook reference: pp. 519-520	
	595-597		**Evaluation of Competency** 12-3: Spirometry Testing	*
			ADDITIONAL ASSIGNMENTS	

Copyright © 2008, 2004, 2000, 1995, 1990 by Saunders, an imprint of Elsevier Inc. All rights reserved.

Notes

Copyright © 2008, 2004, 2000, 1995, 1990 by Saunders, an imprint of Elsevier Inc. All rights reserved.

Name ______________________________ Date ______________

PRETEST

True or False

_____ 1. Blood enters the right atrium from the superior and inferior vena cava.

_____ 2. The cardiac cycle represents one complete heartbeat.

_____ 3. A standard electrocardiogram consists of 10 leads.

_____ 4. An electrolyte facilitates the transmission of electrical impulses.

_____ 5. Leads V1 through V6 are known as the augmented leads.

_____ 6. Electrodes that are too loose can cause an alternating current artifact.

_____ 7. When running an ECG, the medical assistant should work on the left side of the patient.

_____ 8. An ECG that is within normal limits is said to have a normal sinus rhythm.

_____ 9. The most serious cardiac dysrhythmia is atrial fibrillation.

_____ 10. The purpose of a pulmonary function test is to assess cardiac functioning.

POSTTEST

True or False

_____ 1. An electrocardiogram is a recording of the electrical activity of the heart.

_____ 2. The AV node sets the pace of the heart.

_____ 3. The P wave represents the contraction of the ventricles.

_____ 4. If the electrocardiograph is standardized, the standardization mark will be 20 mm high.

_____ 5. Electrocardiograms are normally recorded with the paper moving at a speed of 25 mm/second.

_____ 6. A muscle artifact can be identified by its fuzzy, irregular baseline.

_____ 7. The patient is permitted to shower while wearing a Holter monitor.

_____ 8. A patient with a PAT dysrhythmia often experiences weakness and acute apprehension.

_____ 9. A spirometer measures how much air is exhaled by the lungs and how fast it is exhaled.

_____ 10. Spirometry can be used to assess a patient with emphysema.

Copyright © 2008, 2004, 2000, 1995, 1990 by Saunders, an imprint of Elsevier Inc. All rights reserved.

KEY TERM ASSESSMENT

Directions: Match each medical term with its definition.

_____ 1. Artifact

_____ 2. Atherosclerosis

_____ 3. Baseline

_____ 4. Cardiac cycle

_____ 5. Dysrhythmia

_____ 6. ECG cycle

_____ 7. Electrocardiogram

_____ 8. Electrocardiograph

_____ 9. Electrode

_____ 10. Electrolyte

_____ 11. Interval

_____ 12. Ischemia

_____ 13. Normal sinus rhythm

_____ 14. Segment

_____ 15. Spirometer

A. A chemical substance that promotes conduction of an electrical current
B. The flat horizontal line that separates the various waves of the ECG cycle
C. The instrument used to record the electrical activity of the heart
D. Additional electrical activity picked up by the electrocardiograph that interferes with the normal appearance of the ECG cycles
E. Refers to an electrocardiogram that is within normal limits
F. One complete heartbeat
G. The graphic representation of the electrical activity of the heart
H. The length of a wave or the length of a wave with a segment
I. The graphic representation of a heartbeat
J. A conductor of electricity, which is used to promote contact between the body and the electrocardiograph
K. The portion of the ECG between two waves
L. Deficiency of blood in a body part
M. An instrument for measuring air taken into and expelled from the lungs
N. Buildup of fibrous plaques of fatty deposits and cholesterol on the inner walls of the coronary arteries
O. An irregular heart rhythm

Copyright © 2008, 2004, 2000, 1995, 1990 by Saunders, an imprint of Elsevier Inc. All rights reserved.

Notes

Copyright © 2008, 2004, 2000, 1995, 1990 by Saunders, an imprint of Elsevier Inc. All rights reserved.

EVALUATION OF LEARNING

Directions: Fill in each blank with the correct answer.

1. What is the purpose of electrocardiography?

____

____

____

2. Trace the path blood takes through the heart, starting with the right atrium.

____

____

____

3. What is the function of the SA node?

____

____

4. Why is the impulse (initiated by the SA node) delayed momentarily by the AV node?

____

5. What is the cardiac cycle?

____

6. Label the following on the ECG cycle:

P wave	P-R segment
QRS complex	S-T segment
T wave	P-R interval
Q-T interval	

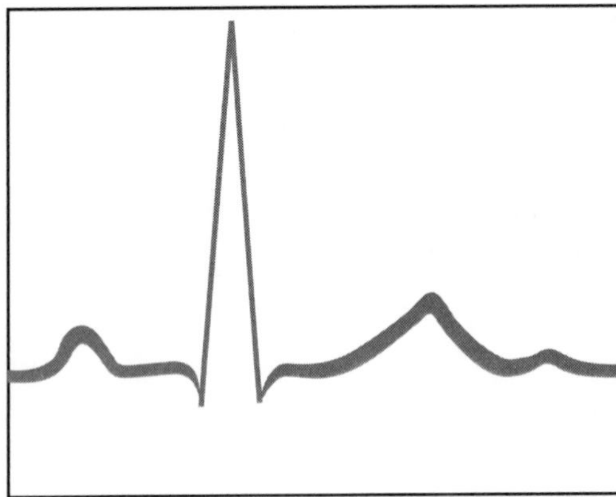

Copyright © 2008, 2004, 2000, 1995, 1990 by Saunders, an imprint of Elsevier Inc. All rights reserved.

7. Explain what each component of the ECG cycle represents.

   P wave ______

   QRS complex ______

   T wave ______

   P-R segment ______

   S-T segment ______

   P-R interval ______

   Q-T interval ______

8. What is the purpose of standardizing the electrocardiograph?

   ______

9. How high should the standardization mark be when the ECG is standardized?

   ______

10. What is the function of an electrode?

    ______

11. Why must an electrolyte be used when recording an ECG?

    ______

12. Diagram the bipolar leads on the following illustration:

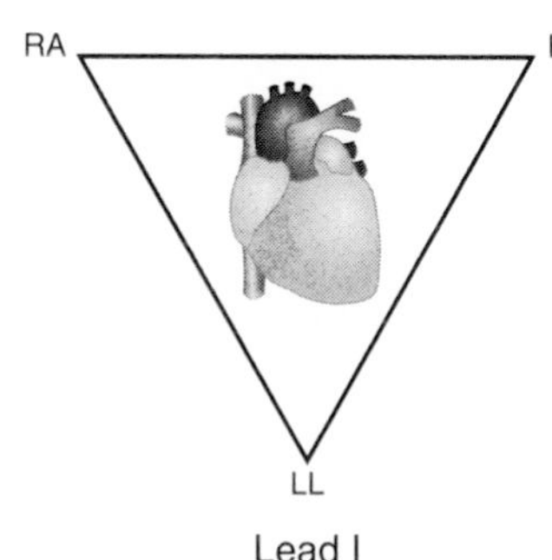

Lead I

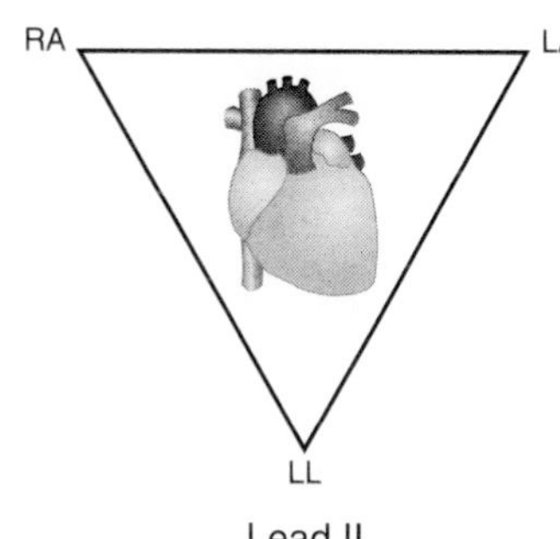

Lead II

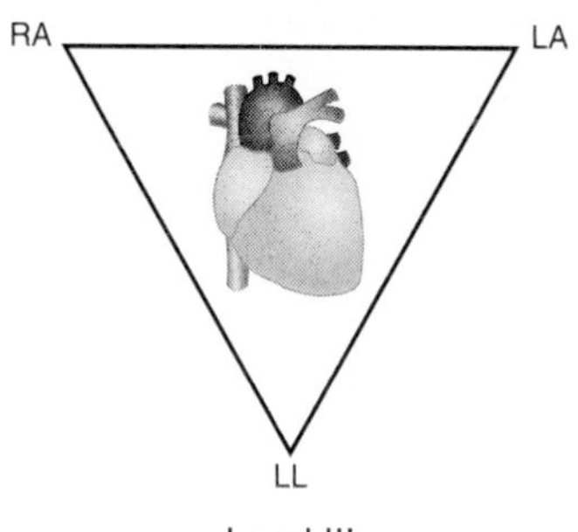

Lead III

Copyright © 2008, 2004, 2000, 1995, 1990 by Saunders, an imprint of Elsevier Inc. All rights reserved.

13. Locate and label the location of the chest leads on the following illustration:

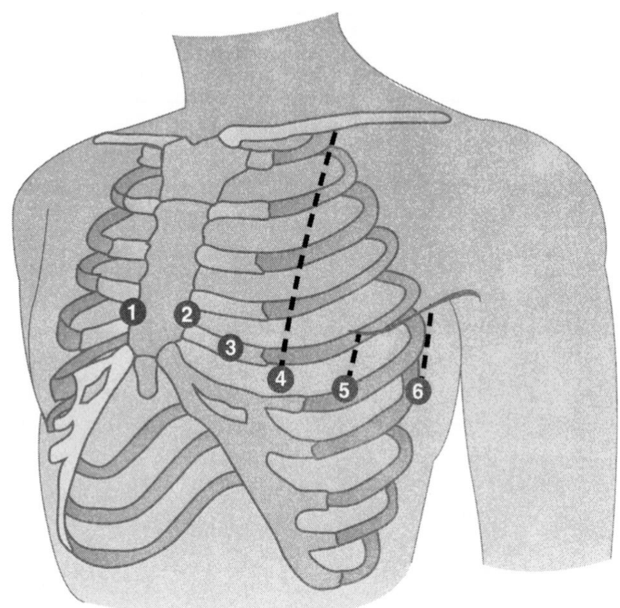

14. A normal ECG is recorded with the paper moving at a speed of:

____

15. What is the difference between a three-channel and a single-channel electrocardiograph?

____

____

____

16. What is the purpose of each of the following electrocardiograph capabilities?

    a. Teletransmission

    ____

    ____

    b. Interpretive capability

    ____

    ____

17. Why should artifacts be eliminated if they occur in an ECG recording?

____

____

____

18. What is the function of an artifact filter?

____

Copyright © 2008, 2004, 2000, 1995, 1990 by Saunders, an imprint of Elsevier Inc. All rights reserved.

19. List three possible causes of muscle artifacts.

20. List two possible causes of wandering baseline.

21. List three possible causes of AC artifacts.

22. List three uses of Holter monitor electrocardiography.

23. Explain the use of the patient activity diary in Holter monitor electrocardiography.

24. List five guidelines that should be relayed to the patient undergoing Holter monitor electrocardiography.

25. List the distinguishing characteristics of each of the following cardiac arrhythmias.

Paroxysmal atrial tachycardia

Atrial flutter

Premature ventricular contraction

Ventricular fibrillation

Copyright © 2008, 2004, 2000, 1995, 1990 by Saunders, an imprint of Elsevier Inc. All rights reserved.

26. What is the purpose of a pulmonary function test?

27. What are the indications for performing spirometry?

28. What is forced vital capacity?

29. What patient preparation is required for spirometry?

30. What is the purpose of postbronchodilator spirometry?

CRITICAL THINKING ACTIVITIES

A. CHEST LEADS

Practice locating the six chest leads on five different individuals. Try to select individuals of both sexes of various ages and body contours. Record each individual's name here after you have successfully located the chest leads. Also record any problems you encountered locating the leads.

1.
2.
3.
4.
5.

Copyright © 2008, 2004, 2000, 1995, 1990 by Saunders, an imprint of Elsevier Inc. All rights reserved.

B. ECG CYCLE

Attach part of an ECG from a recording. Identify and label the various waves, intervals, and segments making up an ECG cycle on two of the leads.

Copyright © 2008, 2004, 2000, 1995, 1990 by Saunders, an imprint of Elsevier Inc. All rights reserved.

C. GO TO! GAME

Object: To demonstrate your knowledge of locating the waves, intervals, and segments on an ECG cycle and to answer questions relating to the ECG cycle.

Needed: **GO TO!** game board
Game cards
A small token for each player (such as a button or coin)
Score card

Directions:

1. Cut out the **GO TO!** game cards.
2. Review the components of the ECG cycle.
3. Get into a group of three players.
4. Place one complete set of the game cards on the game board with the **GO TO!** question facing up and the answer facing down.
5. In turn, a player selects a game card and goes to the site indicated on the card.
6. If the player goes to the correct site, he or she is awarded 5 points. If there is a question regarding the correct site, consult your instructor.
7. The player then answers the question on the game card. If answered correctly, the player is awarded another 5 points.
8. Keep track of your points on the score card provided.
9. Continue playing until all the game cards have been used.
10. Calculate your points and determine the knowledge level you attained.
11. If time permits, shuffle the game cards and play the game again.

GO TO!
SCORE CARD

Name: ______________________________

Recording Points:
Cross off a number each time you go to a site correctly. Cross off another number each time you answer a question correctly. Your total points will be equal to the last number you crossed off. Record this number in the space provided and determine the knowledge level you attained.

Points:	
5	75
10	80
15	85
20	90
25	95
30	100
35	105
40	110
45	115
50	120
55	125
60	130
65	135
70	140

TOTAL POINTS: _______

LEVEL:

- ☐ 95 points and above: **Sheer genius!**
- ☐ 75 to 90 points: **Shows great promise**
- ☐ 55 to 70 points: **Time to study**
- ☐ 50 points and below: **Brain freeze**

Copyright © 2008, 2004, 2000, 1995, 1990 by Saunders, an imprint of Elsevier Inc. All rights reserved.

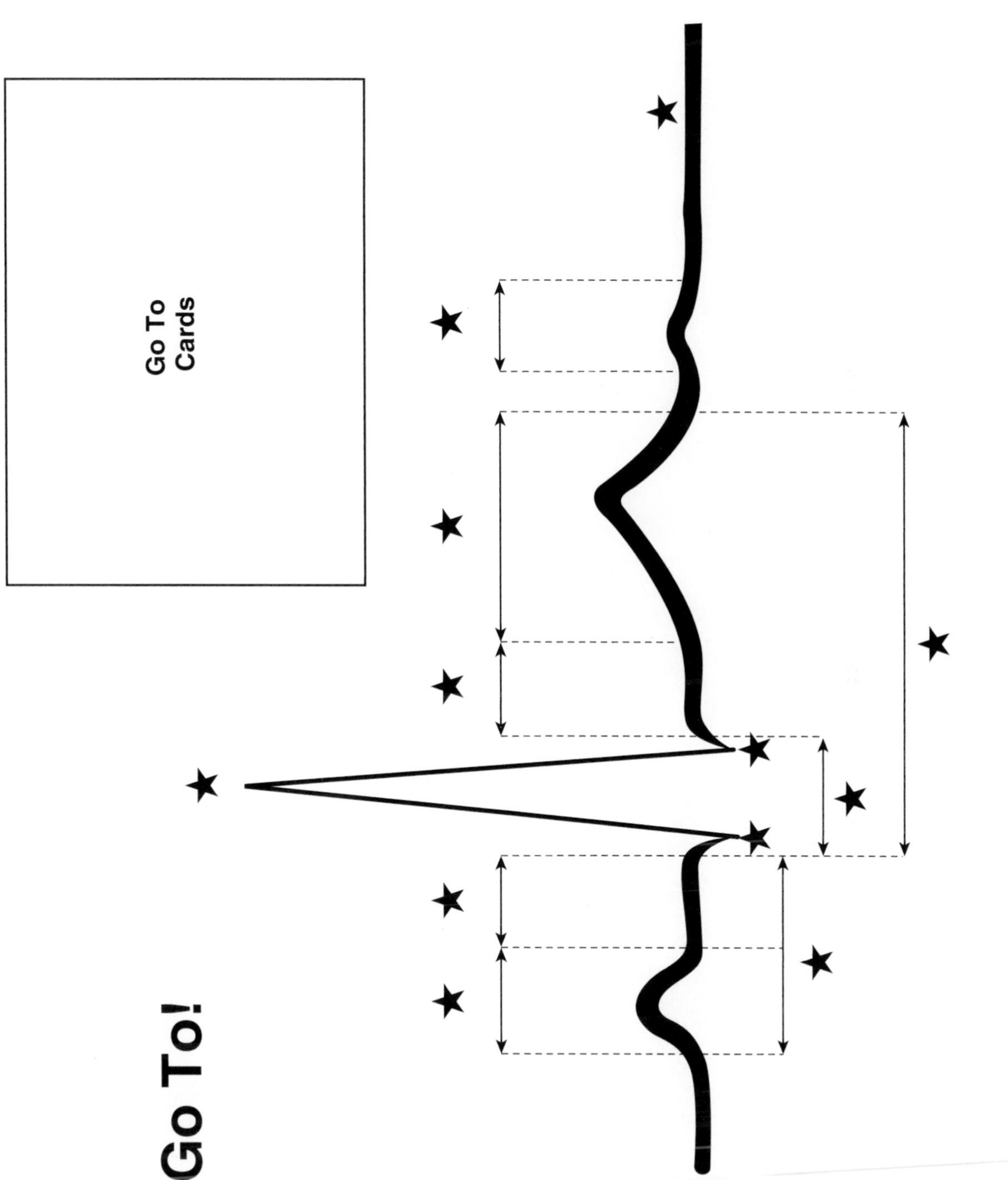

Copyright © 2008, 2004, 2000, 1995, 1990 by Saunders, an imprint of Elsevier Inc. All rights reserved.

Notes

Copyright © 2008, 2004, 2000, 1995, 1990 by Saunders, an imprint of Elsevier Inc. All rights reserved.

GO TO:

P-WAVE

Q: What are the cuspid valves doing right now?

GO TO:

Q-WAVE

Q: Which heart chamber pumps blood from the heart and out into the body?

GO TO:

R-WAVE

You're on top of the world. Answer your question and take another turn.

Q: State the location of V_5.

GO TO:

S-WAVE

Q: State the location of V_2.

GO TO:

T-WAVE

Q: What is happening in the heart during this time?

GO TO:

U-WAVE

Q: State the location of V_1.

GO TO:

P-R SEGMENT

Q: What does this time lapse represent?

GO TO:

P-R INTERVAL

Q: What does this time lapse represent?

A: Left ventricle

A: The cuspid valves are open.

A: Fourth intercostal space at left margin of sternum

A: At horizontal level of V_4 at left anterior axillary line

A: Fourth intercostal space at right margin of sternum.

A: The muscle cells of the heart are recovering in preparation for another impulse.

A: The time interval from the beginning of the atrial depolarization to the beginning of ventricular depolarization

A: The time interval from the end of the atrial depolarization to the beginning of ventricular depolarization

GO TO:

QRS COMPLEX

Q: What are the atria doing right now?

GO TO:

S-T SEGMENT

Q: What does this time interval represent?

GO TO:

Q-T INTERVAL

Q: What does this time interval represent?

GO TO:

WHERE THE ATRIA ARE CONTRACTING

Q: What are the semilunar valves doing right now?

GO TO:

WHERE THE IMPULSE IS BEING DELAYED AT THE AV NODE

Q: Why is the impulse being delayed at the AV Node?

GO TO:

WHERE THE VENTRICLES ARE CONTRACTING

Q: What are the cuspid valves doing right now?

GO TO:

VENTRICLES ARE RECOVERING

Q: State the location of V_3.

GO TO:

Where the heart rests. Take a rest. Answer this question, but you lose your next turn.

Q: State the location of V_4.

A: The time interval from the end of the ventricular depolarization to the beginning of repolarization of the ventricles

A: The atria are resting.

A: The semilunar valves are closed.

A: The time interval from the beginning of the ventricular depolarization to the end of repolarization of the ventricles

A: The cuspid valves are closed.

A: To give the ventricles a chance to fill with blood from the atria

A: Fifth intercostal space at junction of the left midclavicular line

A: Midway between V_2 and V_4

D. ARTIFACTS

If possible, attach examples of the following types of artifacts here:

1. Muscle artifact

2. Wandering baseline

3. Alternating current artifact

E. MYOCARDIAL INFARCTION

You are working for a cardiologist. Your physician is concerned about the increase in the numbers of patients having heart attacks. He asks you to design a colorful, creative, and informative brochure on heart attacks using the brochure provided on the following page. This brochure will be published and placed in the waiting room to provide patients with education on heart attacks. The heart disease Internet sites listed under **On the Web** at the end of Chapter 12 in your textbook can be used to complete this activity.

Copyright © 2008, 2004, 2000, 1995, 1990 by Saunders, an imprint of Elsevier Inc. All rights reserved.

Notes

Copyright © 2008, 2004, 2000, 1995, 1990 by Saunders, an imprint of Elsevier Inc. All rights reserved.

FAQ on:

Q:

A:

Q:

A:

Q:

A:

Q:

A:

Illustration

F. CROSSWORD PUZZLE
Cardiopulmonary Procedures

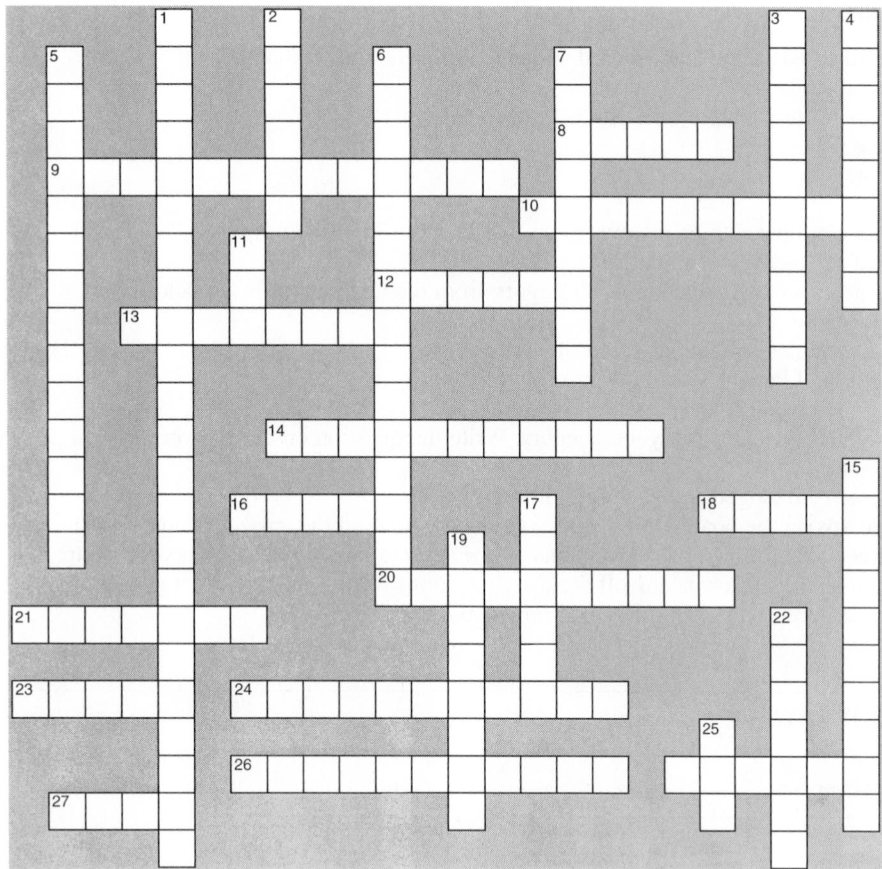

Directions: Complete the crossword puzzle using the clues presented below.

ACROSS

8 Atria contract
9 Drug for angina
10 Heart muscle layer
12 Natural pacemaker
13 Keep this blanket away from a Holter
14 Rhythm not normal
16 Get your oxygen here!
18 The ventricles are recovering
20 "How well can you breathe" test
21 Leads I, II, III
23 Mighty big artery
24 Long recording of lead II
26 "Too loose" electrodes cause this
27 Fourth intercostal to the left

DOWN

1 Serious rhythm disturbance
2 Artifact from a moving patient
3 Small straight spiked lines
4 Not enough blood
5 Drug that opens air passages
6 Coronary artery plaque condition
7 Damaged alveoli disease
11 Take a deep breath and blow it all out!
15 Lower heart chambers
17 Not with a Holter on
19 Left side heart valve
22 Primary cause of COPD
25 ECG std mark in mm

Copyright © 2008, 2004, 2000, 1995, 1990 by Saunders, an imprint of Elsevier Inc. All rights reserved.

G. ROAD TO RECOVERY
Cardiopulmonary Procedures

Object: The object of the game is to lead your "patient" to recovery by correctly answering questions relating to cardiopulmonary procedures.

Needed: **Road to Recovery** game board (located at the end of this manual)
Game cards
A token for each player (such as a button or coin)
Dice (1)
Score card

Directions:

1. Select three other classmates to be in your group (total of four in each group).
2. Cut out the **Road to Recovery** game cards.
3. Each person in the group selects a different category from the textbook as listed below:
   A. Electrocardiography
   B. Cardiac Dysrhythmias and Highlight on Stress Testing
   C. Holter Monitor and Patient Teaching for Angina
   D. Pulmonary Function Tests and Highlight on Smoking Cessation
4. Make up 16 true/false questions for your category. Write the question on one side of the card and the answer on the opposite side (T or F).
5. Put all of the game cards together and shuffle them.
6. Place the game cards on the board with the question facing up (and the answer facing down).
7. Play **Road to Recovery** following the directions on the reverse side of the game board. (Note: It is alright to answer a question from your own card.) If there are questions regarding the correct answer, consult your instructor.
8. Keep track of your points using the score card provided below.

ROAD TO RECOVERY
SCORE CARD

Name: ____

Recording Points:
Using the Game Card Points box, cross off a number each time you answer a game card correctly (starting with 5 and continuing in sequence). Your total game card points will be equal to the last number you crossed off. Record this number in the space provided (1). Record any extra points you were awarded during the game (2), and any points that were deducted (3). To determine your total points, add (1) and (2) together and deduct (3). Record this number in the Total Points Earned space provided. Compare your score with the other players and determine where you placed. Place a check mark next to the level of recovery your patient attained.

Game Card Points:

5	75	145	215
10	80	150	220
15	85	155	225
20	90	160	230
25	95	165	235
30	100	170	240
35	105	175	245
40	110	180	250
45	115	185	255
50	120	190	260
55	125	195	265
60	130	200	270
65	135	205	275
70	140	210	280

Calculation of Points:

(1) Total Game Card Points: ________

(2) Additional Points Awarded: ________

(3) Deducted Points: ________

TOTAL POINTS EARNED: ________

LEVEL OF RECOVERY:

Patient's Name: ____________________
☐ First Place: **Fully Recovered**
☐ Second Place: **Almost Recovered**
☐ Third Place: **Still Recovering**
☐ Fourth Place: **Gasping for Air**

Copyright © 2008, 2004, 2000, 1995, 1990 by Saunders, an imprint of Elsevier Inc. All rights reserved.

Question:	Question:	Question:	Question:
Question:	Question:	Question:	Question:
Question:	Question:	Question:	Question:
Question:	Question:	Question:	Question:

Answer:	Answer:	Answer:	Answer:
Answer:	Answer:	Answer:	Answer:
Answer:	Answer:	Answer:	Answer:
Answer:	Answer:	Answer:	Answer:

PRACTICE FOR COMPETENCY

Procedure 12-1: 12-Lead Electrocardiogram. Practice the procedure for running a 12-lead electrocardiogram and record the procedure in the chart provided.

Procedure 12-2: Holter Monitor

1. **Activity Diary.** Complete the patient information section on the Holter Activity Diary on the following page.
2. **Holter Monitor.** Practice the procedure for applying the Holter monitor and record the procedure in the chart provided.

Procedure 12-3: Spirometry. Practice the procedure for performing a spirometry test and record the procedure in the chart provided.

CHART	
Date	

Copyright © 2008, 2004, 2000, 1995, 1990 by Saunders, an imprint of Elsevier Inc. All rights reserved.

HOLTER MONITOR

PATIENT ACTIVITY DIARY

☐ 10 Hr. ☐ 12 Hr. ☐ 24 Hr. ☐ 26 Hr.

Patient's Name: ______________________________

Patient's Address: ______________________________

____

Age: ____ **Sex:** ____ **Phone:** ___________________

Date of Birth: ________ **Soc. Sec. #:** _____________

Medication: ___________________________________

Doctor: __________________ **Phone:** ____________

Hospital: ______________________ **Room:** _______

Date or Recording: ________ **Started:** ________ **AM PM**

Serial Numbers

Recorder: _________________________________

Battery: __________________________________

Connected by: ______________________________

____

Copyright © 2008, 2004, 2000, 1995, 1990 by Saunders, an imprint of Elsevier Inc. All rights reserved.

EVALUATION OF COMPETENCY

Procedure 12-1: Running a 12-Lead, Three-Channel Electrocardiogram

Name: ______________________________ Date: ______________

Evaluated By: ______________________________ Score: ______________

Performance Objective

Outcome:	Record a 12-lead electrocardiogram.
Conditions:	Using a three-channel electrocardiograph.
	Given ECG paper and disposable electrodes.
Standards:	Time: 15 minutes. Student completed procedure in ____ minutes.
	Accuracy: Satisfactory score on the Performance Evaluation Checklist.

Performance Evaluation Checklist

Trial 1	*Trial 2*	*Point Value*	*Performance Standards*
		•	Worked in a quiet atmosphere away from sources of electrical interference.
		•	Sanitized hands.
		•	Greeted the patient and introduced yourself.
		•	Identified the patient and explained the procedure.
		•	Instructed patient that he/she will need to lie still and not talk during the procedure.
		▷	Explained why the patient should lie still and not talk.
		•	Asked patient to remove appropriate clothing.
		•	Assisted patient into a supine position on the table.
		•	Made sure that patient's arms and legs were adequately supported on the table.
		•	Draped patient properly.
		•	Positioned the electrocardiograph with the power cord pointing away from patient and not passing under the table.
		•	Worked on the left side of the patient.
		•	Prepared the patient's skin for application of the disposable electrodes.
		▷	Explained why the patient's skin must be prepared properly.
		•	Applied the limb electrodes.
		•	Properly located each chest position and applied the chest electrodes.
		▷	Explained why the tabs of the electrodes should be positioned correctly.
		•	Connected the lead wires to the electrodes.
		•	Arranged lead wires to follow body contour.

Copyright © 2008, 2004, 2000, 1995, 1990 by Saunders, an imprint of Elsevier Inc. All rights reserved.

Trial 1	*Trial 2*	*Point Value*	*Performance Standards*
		▷	Explained why the lead wires should follow body contour.
		•	Plugged the patient cable into machine and properly supported the cable.
		•	Turned on the electrocardiograph.
		•	Entered patient data using the soft-touch keypad.
		▷	Stated the purpose of entering patient data.
		•	Reminded patient to lie still and pressed the AUTO button to run the recording.
		•	Checked to make sure the standardization mark is 10 mm high.
		•	Checked to make sure the R wave has a positive deflection.
		▷	Stated what would cause the R wave to have a negative deflection.
		•	Checked the recording for artifacts and corrected them if they occurred.
		•	Informed the patient he or she can move and talk.
		•	Turned off the electrocardiograph.
		•	Disconnected the lead wires.
		•	Removed and discarded the disposable electrodes.
		•	Assisted patient from the table.
		•	Sanitized hands.
		•	Charted the procedure correctly.
		•	Placed the recording in the appropriate place to be reviewed by physician.
		•	Returned equipment to proper place.
		*	Completed the procedure within 15 minutes.
			TOTALS

CHART	
Date	

Copyright © 2008, 2004, 2000, 1995, 1990 by Saunders, an imprint of Elsevier Inc. All rights reserved.

Evaluation of Student Performance

EVALUATION CRITERIA			COMMENTS
Symbol	Category	Point Value	
*	Critical Step	16 points	
•	Essential Step	6 points	
▷	Theory Question	2 points	
Score calculation: 100 points – ____ points missed ____ Score Satisfactory score: 85 or above			

AAMA/CAAHEP Competency Achieved:

☑ III. C. 3. b. (3) (a): Perform electrocardiography.

Copyright © 2008, 2004, 2000, 1995, 1990 by Saunders, an imprint of Elsevier Inc. All rights reserved.

Notes

Copyright © 2008, 2004, 2000, 1995, 1990 by Saunders, an imprint of Elsevier Inc. All rights reserved.

EVALUATION OF COMPETENCY

Procedure 12-2: Applying a Holter Monitor

Name: ______________________________ Date: ____________

Evaluated By: ______________________________ Score: ____________

Performance Objective

Outcome: Apply a Holter monitor.

Conditions: Using a Holter monitor.

Given the following: blank cassette tape, battery, carrying case, belt or shoulder strap, disposable electrodes, alcohol swabs, gauze, razor, nonallergenic tape, patient diary, and a liquid skin abrasive.

Standards: Time: 20 minutes. Student completed procedure in ____ minutes.

Accuracy: Satisfactory score on the Performance Evaluation Checklist.

Performance Evaluation Checklist

Trial 1	Trial 2	Point Value	*Performance Standards*
		•	Assembled equipment.
		•	Installed a new battery.
		•	Inserted a cassette tape or flash memory card into recorder.
		•	Sanitized hands.
		•	Greeted the patient and introduced yourself.
		•	Identified the patient and explained procedure.
		•	Instructed patient in the guidelines for wearing a Holter monitor.
		•	Asked patient to remove clothing from waist up.
		•	Positioned patient in a sitting position.
		•	Located electrode placement sites.
		•	Shaved patient's chest at each electrode site, if needed.
		•	Swabbed skin with alcohol and allowed it to dry.
		•	Slightly abraded skin.
		▷	Explained why skin should be abraded.
		•	Properly applied electrodes.
		▷	Explained why electrodes should be firmly attached.
		•	Attached the lead wires to electrodes.
		•	Formed a loop in each lead wire.

Copyright © 2008, 2004, 2000, 1995, 1990 by Saunders, an imprint of Elsevier Inc. All rights reserved.

Trial 1	*Trial 2*	*Point Value*	*Performance Standards*
		•	Attached the loop to the patient with tape.
		•	Placed tape over each electrode.
		▷	Explained why tape should be applied over electrodes.
		•	Connected the lead wires to patient cable.
		•	Checked the recorder's effectiveness, using the test cable connected to an ECG machine and running a short baseline recording.
		▷	Explained why recorder should be checked.
		•	Instructed patient to dress and properly positioned patient cable.
		•	Inserted recorder into its carrying case and strapped it over the patient's clothing.
		•	Made sure that strap was properly adjusted.
		•	Plugged electrode cable into the recorder.
		•	Turned on the recorder.
		•	Recorded the starting time in the diary.
		▷	Stated why the starting time should be recorded.
		•	Completed patient information section of the diary.
		•	Provided patient with instructions on completing the diary.
		•	Instructed patient when to return for removal of monitor.
		•	Sanitized hands.
		•	Charted the procedure correctly.
		*	Completed the procedure within 20 minutes.
			TOTALS

CHART	
Date	

Copyright © 2008, 2004, 2000, 1995, 1990 by Saunders, an imprint of Elsevier Inc. All rights reserved.

Evaluation of Student Performance

EVALUATION CRITERIA			COMMENTS
Symbol	Category	Point Value	
✶	Critical Step	16 points	
●	Essential Step	6 points	
▷	Theory Question	2 points	
Score calculation: 100 points – ______ points missed ____ Score Satisfactory score: 85 or above			

AAMA/CAAHEP Competency Achieved:

☑ III. C. 3. b. (3) (a): Perform electrocardiography.

Copyright © 2008, 2004, 2000, 1995, 1990 by Saunders, an imprint of Elsevier Inc. All rights reserved.

Notes

Copyright © 2008, 2004, 2000, 1995, 1990 by Saunders, an imprint of Elsevier Inc. All rights reserved.

EVALUATION OF COMPETENCY

Procedure 12-3: Spirometry Testing

Name: ______________________________ Date: ______________

Evaluated By: ______________________________ Score: ______________

Performance Objective

Outcome:	Perform a spirometry test.
Conditions:	Using a spirometer.
	Given the following: disposable tubing, disposable mouthpiece, disposable nose clips, waste container
Standards:	Time: 20 minutes. Student completed procedure in ____ minutes.
	Accuracy: Satisfactory score on the Performance Evaluation Checklist.

Performance Evaluation Checklist

Trial 1	*Trial 2*	*Point Value*	*Performance Standards*
		•	Sanitized hands.
		•	Assembled and prepared equipment.
		•	Calibrated the spirometer.
		▷	Stated the reason for calibrating the spirometer.
		•	Applied a disposable mouthpiece to the mouthpiece holder.
		•	Greeted the patient and introduced yourself.
		•	Identified the patient and explained the procedure.
		•	Asked the patient if he or she prepared properly.
		•	Asked the patient to remove heavy or restricting clothing and to loosen tight clothing.
		▷	Explained why tight clothing should be loosened.
		•	Measured the patient's weight and height.
		▷	Explained the reason for measuring weight and height.
		•	Asked the patient to sit near the machine.
		•	Entered patient data into the computer database of the spirometer.
			Described and demonstrated the breathing maneuver:
		•	Relax and take the deepest breath possible.
		•	Place the mouthpiece in your mouth and seal your lips tightly around it.
		•	Blow out as hard as you can for as long as possible.

Copyright © 2008, 2004, 2000, 1995, 1990 by Saunders, an imprint of Elsevier Inc. All rights reserved.

Trial 1	Trial 2	Point Value	*Performance Standards*
		•	Do not block the opening of the mouthpiece with your tongue.
		•	Remove the mouthpiece from your mouth.
		▷	Explained why the lips should be tightly sealed around the mouthpiece.
		•	Told the patient the instructions would be repeated during the test.
		•	Encouraged the patient to remain calm.
		•	Gently applied the nose clips.
		▷	Stated the purpose of the nose clips.
		•	Handed mouthpiece to patient.
		•	Began the test and actively coached the patient.
		•	Informed patient of modifications needed if breathing maneuver was not performed correctly.
		•	Continued the test until three acceptable efforts were obtained.
		•	Gently removed the nose clips from patient's nose.
		•	Removed the mouthpiece from its holder.
		•	Disposed of nose clips and mouthpiece in a waste container.
		•	Allowed the patient to remain seated for a few minutes.
		•	Sanitized your hands.
		•	Printed the report and labeled it.
		•	Charted the procedure correctly.
		•	Placed the spirometry report in appropriate location for review by the physician.
		•	Cleaned the spirometer.
		*	Completed the procedure within 20 minutes.
			TOTALS

CHART	
Date	

Copyright © 2008, 2004, 2000, 1995, 1990 by Saunders, an imprint of Elsevier Inc. All rights reserved.

Evaluation of Student Performance

EVALUATION CRITERIA			COMMENTS
Symbol	**Category**	**Point Value**	
✶	Critical Step	16 points	
•	Essential Step	6 points	
▷	Theory Question	2 points	
Score calculation: 100 points – ______ points missed ____ Score Satisfactory score: 85 or above			

AAMA/CAAHEP Competency Achieved:

☑ III. C. 3. b. (3) (b): Perform respiratory testing.
☑ III. C. 3. c. (3) (b): Instruct individuals according to their needs.
☑ III. C. 3. c. (3) (c): Provide instruction for health maintenance and disease prevention.

Copyright © 2008, 2004, 2000, 1995, 1990 by Saunders, an imprint of Elsevier Inc. All rights reserved.

Notes

Copyright © 2008, 2004, 2000, 1995, 1990 by Saunders, an imprint of Elsevier Inc. All rights reserved.

13

Colon Procedures and Male Reproductive Health

CHAPTER ASSIGNMENTS

√ After Completing	Date Due	Textbook Page(s)	TEXTBOOK ASSIGNMENTS	Possible Points	Points You Earned
		526-542	Read Chapter 13: Colon Procedures and Male Reproductive Health		
		529 539	Read Case Study 1 Case Study 1 questions	 5	
		536 539	Read Case Study 2 Case Study 2 questions	 5	
		537 539-540	Read Case Study 3 Case Study 3 questions	 5	
		540-541	Apply Your Knowledge questions	12	
			TOTAL POINTS		
√ After Completing	**Date Due**	**Study Guide Page(s)**	**STUDY GUIDE ASSIGNMENTS (CTA: Critical Thinking Activity)**	**Possible Points**	**Points You Earned**
		603	Pretest	10	
		604	Key Term Assessment	9	
		606-608	Evaluation of Learning questions	25	
		608	CTA A: FOBT Patient Preparation	10	
		608	CTA B: Sigmoidoscopy	10	
		609	CTA C: FOBT Diet/Medication Modifications Game (Record points earned)		
		615	CTA D: Dear Gabby	10	
		616	CTA E: Crossword Puzzle	24	

Copyright © 2008, 2004, 2000, 1995, 1990 by Saunders, an imprint of Elsevier Inc. All rights reserved.

√ After Completing	Date Due	Study Guide Page(s)	STUDY GUIDE ASSIGNMENTS (CTA: Critical Thinking Activity)	Possible Points	Points You Earned
			CD Activity: Chapter 13 Animations	20	
		603	Posttest	10	
			ADDITIONAL ASSIGNMENTS		
			TOTAL POINTS		

Copyright © 2008, 2004, 2000, 1995, 1990 by Saunders, an imprint of Elsevier Inc. All rights reserved.

√ When Assigned By Your Instructor	Study Guide Page(s)	Practices Required	LABORATORY ASSIGNMENTS (Procedure Number and Name)	*Score
	617-618	5	DVD **Practice for Competency** 13-1 and 13-2: Fecal Occult Blood Testing: Guaiac Slide Test Method and Developing the Hemoccult Slide Test Textbook reference: pp. 530-533	
	619-621		**Evaluation of Competency** 13-1 and 13-2: Fecal Occult Blood Testing: Guaiac Slide Test Method and Developing the Hemoccult Slide Test	*
	617-618	3	**Practice for Competency** 13-3: Assisting with a Flexible Sigmoidoscopy Textbook reference: pp. 535-536	
	623-624		**Evaluation of Competency** 13-3: Assisting with a Flexible Sigmoidoscopy	*
			ADDITIONAL ASSIGNMENTS	

Copyright © 2008, 2004, 2000, 1995, 1990 by Saunders, an imprint of Elsevier Inc. All rights reserved.

Notes

Copyright © 2008, 2004, 2000, 1995, 1990 by Saunders, an imprint of Elsevier Inc. All rights reserved.

Name ______________________________ Date ______________

PRETEST

True or False

_____ 1. Hemorrhoids can cause visible red blood to appear on the outside of the stool.

_____ 2. Nonvisible blood in the stool is termed occult blood.

_____ 3. Colorectal cancer is a common form of cancer in individuals over 40 years of age.

_____ 4. A blue color appearing on a Hemoccult test result is interpreted as a negative reaction.

_____ 5. If a Hemoccult test is positive, the physician may order a colonoscopy.

_____ 6. The patient is placed in the prone position for a flexible sigmoidoscopy.

_____ 7. The function of the prostate gland is to produce sperm.

_____ 8. Prostate screening is recommended once a year for men over the age of 50.

_____ 9. A normal prostate gland feels firm and hard.

_____ 10. The most common sign of testicular cancer is a small, hard, painless lump on the testicle.

POSTTEST

True or False

_____ 1. Melena means that the stool appears hard and dry.

_____ 2. Consuming red meat may cause a false-positive result on a Hemoccult test.

_____ 3. Aspirin should be avoided for 7 days before beginning a fecal occult blood test.

_____ 4. The Hemoccult test should be stored in the refrigerator after applying a stool specimen to it.

_____ 5. Patient preparation for a sigmoidoscopy includes a high fiber diet.

_____ 6. A flexible sigmoidoscopy can be used to diagnose colorectal cancer.

_____ 7. After use, a sigmoidoscope must be autoclaved for 20 minutes.

_____ 8. There are often no symptoms in the early stages of prostate cancer.

_____ 9. A PSA level of 20 is within normal range.

_____ 10. Testicular cancer occurs most commonly between the ages of 15 and 34.

Copyright © 2008, 2004, 2000, 1995, 1990 by Saunders, an imprint of Elsevier Inc. All rights reserved.

KEY TERM ASSESSMENT

Directions: Match each medical term with its definition.

_____ 1. Biopsy

_____ 2. Colonoscopy

_____ 3. Endoscope

_____ 4. Insufflate

_____ 5. Melena

_____ 6. Occult blood

_____ 7. Peroxidase

_____ 8. Sigmoidoscope

_____ 9. Sigmoidoscopy

A. The visualization of the entire colon using a colonoscope
B. Blood occurring in such a small amount that it is not visually detectable by the unaided eye
C. The surgical removal and examination of tissue from the living body
D. The visual examination of the rectum and sigmoid colon using a sigmoidoscope
E. The darkening of the stool caused by the presence of blood in an amount of 50 ml or greater
F. An instrument that consists of a tube and an optical system that is used for direct visual inspection of organs or cavities
G. A substance that is able to transfer oxygen from hydrogen peroxide to oxidize guaiac, causing the guaiac to turn blue
H. An endoscope that is specially designed for passage through the anus to permit visualization of the rectum and sigmoid colon
I. To blow a powder, vapor, or gas (such as air) into a body cavity

Copyright © 2008, 2004, 2000, 1995, 1990 by Saunders, an imprint of Elsevier Inc. All rights reserved.

Notes

Copyright © 2008, 2004, 2000, 1995, 1990 by Saunders, an imprint of Elsevier Inc. All rights reserved.

EVALUATION OF LEARNING

Fill in each blank with the correct answer.

1. List five causes of blood in the stool.

2. Define the term melena and explain what causes it.

3. What is the primary reason for screening patients for the presence of fecal occult blood?

4. Why must three stool specimens be obtained for the fecal occult guaiac slide test?

5. List two reasons for placing the patient on a high-fiber diet when testing for fecal occult blood.

6. List examples of medications that must be discontinued prior to guaiac slide testing.

7. List two factors that could cause false-positive test results on a guaiac slide test.

8. List three examples of diagnostic tests that may be performed if the guaiac slide test is positive.

9. Why is it important to perform quality control methods when developing the guaiac slide test?

Copyright © 2008, 2004, 2000, 1995, 1990 by Saunders, an imprint of Elsevier Inc. All rights reserved.

10. What is the purpose of performing a sigmoidoscopy?

11. Describe the advance patient preparation that may be required for a sigmoidoscopy.

12. What is the purpose of the digital rectal examination?

13. What is the purpose of insufflating air into the colon during a sigmoidoscopy?

14. What is the purpose of suctioning during sigmoidoscopy?

15. What is the recommended patient position for flexible fiberoptic sigmoidoscopy?

16. How can the medical assistant help the patient relax during the sigmoidoscopy?

17. Where is the prostate gland located?

18. What are the symptoms of prostate cancer?

19. How is the digital rectal examination used for the early detection of prostate cancer?

Copyright © 2008, 2004, 2000, 1995, 1990 by Saunders, an imprint of Elsevier Inc. All rights reserved.

20. What is the purpose of the PSA test?

____

____

21. What is the PSA level for each of the following:

A. Normal range ____________________

B. Slightly elevated range ____________________

C. Moderately elevated range ____________________

D. Highly elevated ____________________

22. What patient preparation is required for a PSA test?

____

____

23. What tests may be ordered by the physician if the patient has positive prostate screening results?

____

____

24. What are the risk factors for testicular cancer?

____

____

____

25. What is the most common sign of testicular cancer?

____

____

CRITICAL THINKING ACTIVITIES

A. FOBT PATIENT PREPARATION

Frank Morrison has been given a Hemoccult slide kit for fecal occult blood testing. In the space provided, plan breakfast, lunch, and dinner for him following the FOBT patient preparation guidelines on page 530 of your textbook.

____

____

____

____

____

____

B. SIGMOIDOSCOPY

Ken Hofmann has been scheduled to have a sigmoidoscopy. He asks for your help in planning a light evening meal containing low-residue foods. In the space provided, plan a balanced evening meal for Mr. Hofmann.

____

____

____

____

____

Copyright © 2008, 2004, 2000, 1995, 1990 by Saunders, an imprint of Elsevier Inc. All rights reserved.

C. FOBT DIET/MEDICATION MODIFICATIONS

Object: To demonstrate your knowledge of foods and medications that are permitted and not permitted before and during a fecal occult blood test using a guaiac slide test.

Needed: Game cards

Directions:

1. Cut out the game cards.
2. Determine if each food and medication is permitted or not permitted before and during fecal occult blood testing using the guaiac slide test.
3. On the reverse side of the card, indicate if it is permitted by placing a **P** on the card. If it is not permitted, place an **NP** on the reverse side of the card.
4. Choose a partner and place one complete set of game cards on a flat surface between both players with the food or medication facing up.
5. Taking turns, select a game card and indicate if the food/medication is permitted or not permitted before and during a FOBT.
6. If the player gives the correct answer, he or she is awarded 5 points. If there is a question regarding an answer, consult your instructor.
7. Keep track of your points on the score card provided. Continue playing until all the game cards have been used.
8. Calculate your points and determine the knowledge level you attained.
9. If time permits, shuffle the game cards and play the game again.

FOBT
SCORE CARD

Name: ______________________________

Recording Points:
Cross off a number each time you go to a site correctly. Cross off another number each time you answer a question correctly. Your points will be equal to the last number you crossed off. Record this number in the space provided and determine the knowledge level you attained.

Points:	
5	75
10	80
15	85
20	90
25	95
30	100
35	105
40	110
45	115
50	120
55	125
60	130
65	135
70	140

TOTAL POINTS: ______

LEVEL OF KNOWLEDGE:

☐ 75 points and above: **Sheer genius!**
☐ 55 to 70 points: **Shows great promise**
☐ 35 to 50 points: **Time to study**
☐ Below 35 points: **Brain freeze**

Copyright © 2008, 2004, 2000, 1995, 1990 by Saunders, an imprint of Elsevier Inc. All rights reserved.

Notes

Copyright © 2008, 2004, 2000, 1995, 1990 by Saunders, an imprint of Elsevier Inc. All rights reserved.

Popcorn	Aspirin	Iron Supplement	Vitamin C
Horseradish	Pear	Bran Cereal	Corticosteroid
Calcium Supplement	Vitamin A	Green Beans	Turnip
Lamb	Carrots	Oatmeal	Bacon

Red Meat	Liver	Fish	Chicken
Lettuce	Spinach	Corn	Celery
Broccoli	Cauliflower	Radish	Apple
Banana	Peach	Melon	Whole Wheat Bread

D. DEAR GABBY

Dear Gabby broke her wrist while ice skating and wants you to fill in for her. In the space provided, respond to the following letter using the knowledge you have acquired in this chapter.

Dear Gabby:

I am 15 years old, and my mom just took me to a new doctor for a sports physical examination. I am going to play football this fall at my high school. Before this, I had always gone to the doctor I had since I was little, but I had to switch since I am getting older. After the doctor did my physical, he told me that I needed to examine my testicles every month and that the medical assistant would be in to explain how this is done.

Gabby, I was totally shocked, and you can bet I got out of that office before she had a chance to do that. I am too embarrassed to ask my parents about this. Gabby, what is going on? I am only 15 years old. Are my parents taking me to a quack, and should I report this to someone?

Signed,

Don't Know What to Do

Copyright © 2008, 2004, 2000, 1995, 1990 by Saunders, an imprint of Elsevier Inc. All rights reserved.

E. CROSSWORD PUZZLE

Colon Procedures and Male Reproductive Health

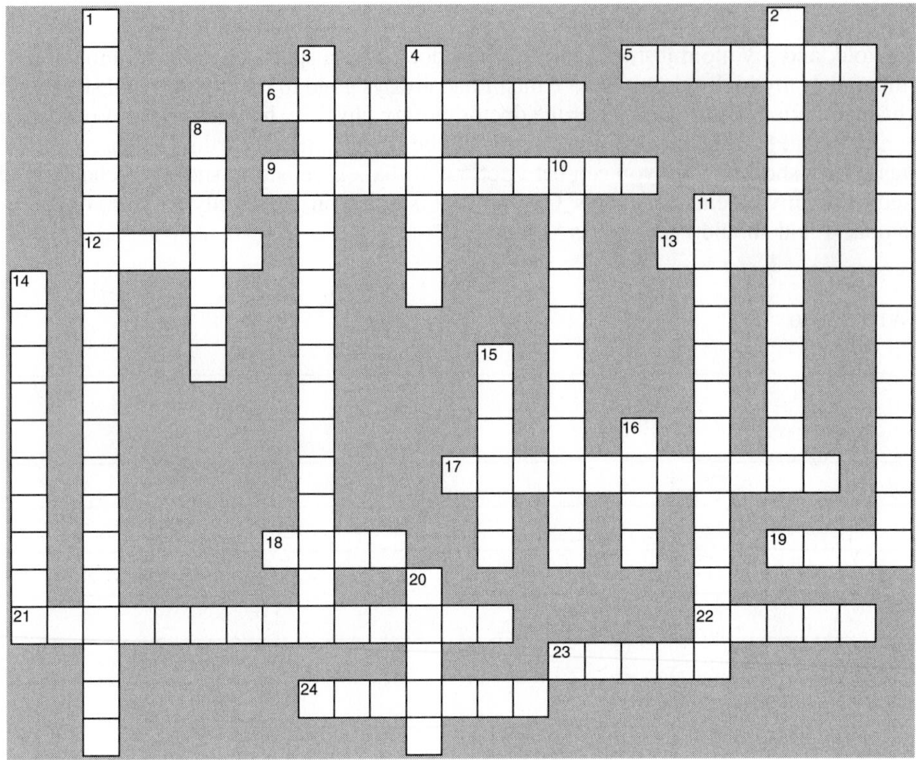

Directions: Complete the crossword puzzle using the clues presented below.

ACROSS

5 Med to avoid during FOBT
6 How to clean sigmoidoscope
9 Visualization of colon
12 Pt prep for flex sigmoid
13 Age to start TSE
17 Can cause blood in the stool
18 Pt position for flex sig
19 Color of + Hemoccult
21 Symptom of CRC
22 CRC often starts from this
23 CRC increases after this age
24 Prostate CA screening test

DOWN

1 Testicular CA risk factor
2 Secretes fluid that transports sperm
3 Increases PSA level
4 Cause of CRC
7 Increases risk of CRC
8 Can cause false + on FOBT
10 Nonvisible blood
11 May be done after a + FOBT
14 Leading cause of CA deaths
15 Black and tarlike stool
16 May be done after elevated PSA
20 Prostate CA increases after this age

Copyright © 2008, 2004, 2000, 1995, 1990 by Saunders, an imprint of Elsevier Inc. All rights reserved.

PRACTICE FOR COMPETENCY

Procedure 13-1: Hemoccult Slide Test

1. **Patient Instructions.** Instruct an individual in the specimen collection procedure for a Hemoccult slide test. Record patient instructions in the chart provided.
2. **Developing the Test.** Develop a Hemoccult test and record the results in the chart provided.

Procedure 13-2: Sigmoidoscopy. Practice the procedure for assisting with a sigmoidoscopy. Record advance patient preparation instructions in the chart provided.

CHART	
Date	

Copyright © 2008, 2004, 2000, 1995, 1990 by Saunders, an imprint of Elsevier Inc. All rights reserved.

Chart	
Date	

Copyright © 2008, 2004, 2000, 1995, 1990 by Saunders, an imprint of Elsevier Inc. All rights reserved.

EVALUATION OF COMPETENCY

Procedures 13-1 and 13-2: Fecal Occult Blood Testing: Guaiac Slide Test Method and Developing the Hemoccult Slide Test

Name: ______________________ Date: ____________

Evaluated By: ______________________ Score: ____________

Performance Objective

Outcome:	Instruct an individual in the specimen collection procedure for a Hemoccult slide test and develop the test.
Conditions:	Given the following: Hemoccult slide testing kit, developing solution, reference card, and a waste container.
Standards:	Time: 15 minutes. Student completed procedure(s) in ____ minutes.
	Accuracy: Satisfactory score in the Performance Evaluation Checklist.

Performance Evaluation Checklist

Trial 1	*Trial 2*	*Point Value*	*Performance Standards*
			Instructions for the Hemoccult Slide Test
		•	Obtained the Hemoccult slide testing kit.
		•	Checked expiration date on the slides.
		▷	Described what might occur if the slides are outdated.
		•	Greeted the patient and introduced yourself.
		•	Identified the patient and explained purpose of the test.
		•	Informed patient when the test should not be performed.
		•	Instructed patient in the proper preparation required for the test.
		•	Encouraged patient to adhere to the diet modifications.
		▷	Explained why the patient should follow the diet modifications.
		•	Provided patient with the Hemoccult slide test kit.
		•	Instructed patient in completion of the information on the front flap of each card.
		•	Provided instructions on the proper care and storage of the slides.
		▷	Explained why the slides must be stored properly.
			Instructed the patient in the initiation of the test by:
		•	Beginning the diet modifications.
		•	Collecting a stool specimen from the first bowel movement after the 3-day preparatory period.

Copyright © 2008, 2004, 2000, 1995, 1990 by Saunders, an imprint of Elsevier Inc. All rights reserved.

Trial 1	*Trial 2*	*Point Value*	*Performance Standards*
			Instructed the patient in the collection of the stool specimen:
		•	Fill in the collection date on the front flap.
		•	Use a clean dry container to collect the stool specimen.
		•	Collect the stool sample before it comes in contact with toilet bowel water.
		•	Use the wooden applicator to obtain specimen from one part of the stool.
		•	Open the front flap of the first cardboard slide.
		•	Spread a thin smear of the specimen over the filter paper in the square labeled "A."
		•	Obtain another specimen from a different area of the stool, using the other end of the applicator.
		•	Spread a thin smear of the specimen over the filter paper in the square labeled "B."
		•	Close the front flap of the cardboard slide and fill in the date.
		•	Discard the applicator in a waste container.
		▷	Explained why a sample is collected from two different parts of the stool.
		•	Instructed patient to place slides in a regular envelope to air-dry overnight.
		•	Instructed the patient to continue the testing period on 3 different days until all three specimens have been obtained.
		•	Instructed patient to place the cardboard slides in the foil envelope and return them to the medical office.
		•	Provided patient with an opportunity to ask questions.
		•	Made sure the patient understood the instructions.
		•	Charted the procedure correctly.
			Developing the Hemoccult Slide Test
		•	Assembled equipment.
		•	Checked expiration date on the developing solution bottle.
		▷	Explained how the solution should be stored.
		•	Sanitized hands and applied gloves.
		•	Opened the back flap of the cardboard slides.
		•	Applied 2 drops of the developing solution to the guaiac test paper underlying the back of each smear.
		•	Did not allow the developing solution to come in contact with skin or eyes.
		•	Read results within 60 seconds.
		*	The results were identical to the evaluator's results.
		▷	Explained why the slides should be read within 60 seconds.
		•	Performed the quality-control procedure on each slide.
		•	Read the quality-control results after 10 seconds.

Copyright © 2008, 2004, 2000, 1995, 1990 by Saunders, an imprint of Elsevier Inc. All rights reserved.

Trial 1	*Trial 2*	*Point Value*	*Performance Standards*
		▷	Described what is observed during a normal positive and negative control reaction.
		▷	Stated the purpose of the quality-control procedure.
		●	Properly disposed of the slides in a regular waste container.
		●	Removed gloves and sanitized hands.
		●	Charted the results correctly.
		✶	Completed the procedure within 15 minutes.
			TOTALS

CHART	
Date	

Evaluation of Student Performance

EVALUATION CRITERIA			COMMENTS
Symbol	Category	Point Value	
✶	Critical Step	16 points	
●	Essential Step	6 points	
▷	Theory Question	2 points	
Score calculation: 100 points			
– ______ points missed			
______ Score			
Satisfactory score: 85 or above			

AAMA/CAAHEP Competency Achieved:

☑ III. C. 3. b. (2) (e): Instruct patients in the collection of fecal specimens.
☑ III. C. 3. c. (3) (b): Instruct individuals according to their needs.
☑ III. C. 3. c. (3) (c): Provide instruction for health maintenance and disease prevention.
☑ III. C. 3. c. (4) (d): Use methods of quality control.

Copyright © 2008, 2004, 2000, 1995, 1990 by Saunders, an imprint of Elsevier Inc. All rights reserved.

Notes

Copyright © 2008, 2004, 2000, 1995, 1990 by Saunders, an imprint of Elsevier Inc. All rights reserved.

EVALUATION OF COMPETENCY

Procedure 13-3: Assisting with a Flexible Sigmoidoscopy

Name: ______________________________ Date: ____________

Evaluated By: ______________________________ Score: ____________

Performance Objective

Outcome:	Assist with a sigmoidoscopy.
Conditions:	Given the following: disposable gloves, flexible sigmoidoscope, lubricant, a drape, biopsy forceps, sterile specimen container with a preservative, tissue wipes, and a waste container.
Standards:	Time: 15 minutes. Student completed procedure in ____ minutes.
	Accuracy: Satisfactory score in the Performance Evaluation Checklist.

Performance Evaluation Checklist

Trial 1	*Trial 2*	*Point Value*	*Performance Standards*
		•	Sanitized hands.
		•	Assembled equipment.
		•	Checked to make sure that light source is working.
		•	Labeled specimen container.
		•	Greeted the patient and introduced yourself.
		•	Identified the patient and explained the procedure.
		•	Asked patient if he or she needs to empty bladder.
		▷	Explained why the patient should have an empty bladder.
		•	Instructed and prepared patient for the examination.
		•	Assisted patient onto examining table.
		•	Assisted patient into the Sim's position.
		•	Properly draped patient.
		•	Reassured patient and helped him or her to relax during the examination.
			Assisted physician during the examination:
		•	Lubricated physician's gloved finger for the digital rectal examination.
		•	Placed lubricant on the end of the insertion tube of the sigmoidoscope.
		•	Assisted with the suction equipment as required.
		▷	Stated the purpose of the suctioning equipment.
		•	Assisted with the collection of a biopsy.
		•	After the examination, applied gloves and cleaned patient's anal region of excess lubricant.

Copyright © 2008, 2004, 2000, 1995, 1990 by Saunders, an imprint of Elsevier Inc. All rights reserved.

Trial 1	Trial 2	Point Value	*Performance Standards*
		•	Removed gloves and sanitized hands.
		•	Assisted patient from examining table and instructed patient to get dressed.
		•	Prepared biopsy specimen for transport to the laboratory.
		•	Transported any specimens to laboratory, along with a completed laboratory request form.
		•	Charted date of transport of specimen to lab.
		•	Cleaned the examining room.
		•	Sanitized and disinfected the sigmoidoscope according to the manufacturer's instructions.
		✶	Completed the procedure within 15 minutes.
			TOTALS

Evaluation of Student Performance

EVALUATION CRITERIA			COMMENTS
Symbol	Category	Point Value	
✶	Critical Step	16 points	
•	Essential Step	6 points	
▷	Theory Question	2 points	
Score calculation: 100 points – ____ points missed ____ Score Satisfactory score: 85 or above			

AAMA/CAAHEP Competency Achieved:

☑ III. C. 3. b. (4) (d): Prepare and maintain examination and treatment areas.
☑ III. C. 3. b. (4) (e): Prepare patient for and assist with routine and specialty examinations.

Copyright © 2008, 2004, 2000, 1995, 1990 by Saunders, an imprint of Elsevier Inc. All rights reserved.

14

Radiology and Diagnostic Imaging

CHAPTER ASSIGNMENTS

√ After Completing	Date Due	Textbook Page(s)	TEXTBOOK ASSIGNMENTS	Possible Points	Points You Earned
		543-558	Read Chapter 14: Radiology and Diagnostic Imaging		
		545 555	Read Case Study 1 Case Study 1 questions	5	
		550 555	Read Case Study 2 Case Study 2 questions	5	
		553 555-556	Read Case Study 3 Case Study 3 questions	5	
		556-557	Apply Your Knowledge questions	10	
			TOTAL POINTS		

√ After Completing	Date Due	Study Guide Page(s)	STUDY GUIDE ASSIGNMENTS (CTA: Critical Thinking Activity)	Possible Points	Points You Earned
		629	Pretest	10	
		630	Key Term Assessment	13	
		631-633	Evaluation of Learning questions	24	
		633	CTA A: Lower GI	5	
		634	CTA B: Intravenous Pyelogram (IVP)	5	
		634-635	CTA C: Magnetic Resonance Imaging	7	
		636	CTA D: Crossword Puzzle	21	
			CD Activity: Chapter 14 Animations	20	
		629	Posttest	10	
			ADDITIONAL ASSIGNMENTS		
			TOTAL POINTS		

Copyright © 2008, 2004, 2000, 1995, 1990 by Saunders, an imprint of Elsevier Inc. All rights reserved.

Notes

Copyright © 2008, 2004, 2000, 1995, 1990 by Saunders, an imprint of Elsevier Inc. All rights reserved.

√ When Assigned By Your Instructor	Study Guide Page(s)	Practices Required	LABORATORY ASSIGNMENTS (Procedure Number and Name)	*Score
	637-638	3	**Practice for Competency** 14-A: Preparation for Radiology Examinations Textbook reference: p. 546-549	
	639-640		**Evaluation of Competency** 14-A: Preparation for Radiology Examinations	*
	637-638	3	**Practice for Competency** 14-B: Preparation for Diagnostic Imaging Procedures Textbook reference: p. 550-554	
	641-642		**Evaluation of Competency** 14-B: Preparation for Diagnostic Imaging Procedures	*
			ADDITIONAL ASSIGNMENTS	

Copyright © 2008, 2004, 2000, 1995, 1990 by Saunders, an imprint of Elsevier Inc. All rights reserved.

Notes

Copyright © 2008, 2004, 2000, 1995, 1990 by Saunders, an imprint of Elsevier Inc. All rights reserved.

Name ____ Date ______________

PRETEST

True or False

_____ 1. A radiologist is a medical doctor specializing in the diagnosis and treatment of disease using radiant energy.

_____ 2. The permanent record of the picture produced on x-ray film is a sonogram.

_____ 3. The purpose of a contrast medium is to make a structure visible on a radiograph.

_____ 4. With an anteroposterior view, the x-rays are directed from the back towards the front of the body.

_____ 5. Mammography can be used to detect breast calcifications.

_____ 6. An upper GI examination assists in diagnosing kidney stones.

_____ 7. An IVP is a radiograph of the kidneys and urinary tract.

_____ 8. Ultrasonography allows for continuous viewing of a structure.

_____ 9. Obstetric ultrasound can be used to determine gestational age.

_____ 10. A patient must remove all metal before having an MRI.

POSTTEST

True or False

_____ 1. Wilhelm Roentgen discovered x-rays in 1895.

_____ 2. Bone is an example of a radiolucent structure.

_____ 3. An instrument used to view internal organs directly is a fluoroscope.

_____ 4. The patient should be instructed not to move during a radiographic exam to prevent confusing shadows on the film.

_____ 5. The breasts are compressed during mammography to prevent radiation burns.

_____ 6. After an upper GI is performed, the barium will cause the stool to be loose and watery.

_____ 7. Gas must be removed from the colon before a lower GI study to prevent blurring of the radiograph.

_____ 8. Before performing an IVP, the patient must be asked if he or she is allergic to penicillin.

_____ 9. Computed tomography produces a series of cross-sectional images.

_____ 10. A radioactive material is introduced into the body before a nuclear medicine imaging procedure is performed.

Copyright © 2008, 2004, 2000, 1995, 1990 by Saunders, an imprint of Elsevier Inc. All rights reserved.

KEY TERM ASSESSMENT

Directions: Match each medical term with its definition.

_____ 1. Contrast medium

_____ 2. Echocardiogram

_____ 3. Enema

_____ 4. Fluoroscope

_____ 5. Fluoroscopy

_____ 6. Radiograph

_____ 7. Radiography

_____ 8. Radiologist

_____ 9. Radiology

_____ 10. Radiolucent

_____ 11. Radiopaque

_____ 12. Sonogram

_____ 13. Ultrasonography

A. A permanent record of a picture of an internal body organ or structure produced on radiographic film
B. A medical doctor who specializes in the diagnosis and treatment of disease using radiant energy such as x-rays, radium, and radioactive material
C. A substance used to make a particular structure visible on a radiograph
D. The record obtained with ultrasonography
E. An injection of fluid into the rectum to aid in the elimination of feces from the colon
F. The branch of medicine that deals with the use of radiant energy in the diagnosis and treatment of disease
G. An instrument used to view internal organs and structures directly
H. Describing a structure that obstructs the passage of x-rays
I. The taking of permanent records of internal body organs and structures by passing x-rays through the body to act on a specially sensitized film
J. Describing a structure that permits the passage of x-rays
K. Examination of a patient with a fluoroscope
L. An ultrasound examination of the heart
M. The use of high-frequency sound waves to produce an image of an organ or tissue

Copyright © 2008, 2004, 2000, 1995, 1990 by Saunders, an imprint of Elsevier Inc. All rights reserved.

EVALUATION OF LEARNING

Directions: Fill in each blank with the correct answer.

1. Who discovered x-rays?

2. What is the function of x-rays?

3. Why is it so important for a patient to prepare properly for a radiographic examination?

4. What is the function of a radiopaque contrast medium?

5. How is a patient positioned to obtain an anteroposterior view?

6. What is the purpose of mammography?

7. Why must the breasts be compressed during mammography?

8. What is the purpose of the upper gastrointestinal (GI) radiographic examination?

9. Why must the GI tract be free of food and fluid before an upper GI radiographic examination is performed?

10. A lower GI radiographic examination assists in the diagnosis of what conditions?

Copyright © 2008, 2004, 2000, 1995, 1990 by Saunders, an imprint of Elsevier Inc. All rights reserved.

11. Why is it important to remove gas and fecal material from the colon before a lower GI radiographic examination is performed?

____

____

12. What is an intravenous pyelogram (IVP)?

____

____

13. What type of patient preparation is required for an IVP?

____

____

____

____

14. Define the following:

a. Angiocardiogram

____

____

b. Bronchogram

____

____

c. Coronary angiogram

____

____

d. Cerebral angiogram

____

____

e. Cystogram

____

____

15. What are the primary uses of ultrasonography?

____

____

16. What are the advantages of ultrasonography?

____

____

____

17. What is the purpose of performing an obstetric ultrasound?

____

____

____

Copyright © 2008, 2004, 2000, 1995, 1990 by Saunders, an imprint of Elsevier Inc. All rights reserved.

18. What are the primary uses of computed tomography?

19. What type of image is produced by computed tomography?

20. What type of patient preparation is required for computed tomography?

21. What are the primary uses of magnetic resonance imaging?

22. What material is used with a nuclear medicine diagnostic imaging procedure?

23. What are the most common nuclear medicine diagnostic imagining procedures?

24. What are the advantages of digital imaging technology?

CRITICAL THINKING ACTIVITIES

A. LOWER GI

Trent Douglas has been having pain in his lower abdomen and occult blood in his stool. Dr. Hartman tells you to schedule him for a lower GI radiographic examination at Grant Hospital. In the space provided, explain how you would instruct Mr. Douglas to prepare for this examination. Include both the patient preparation and the reason for each of the measures.

Copyright © 2008, 2004, 2000, 1995, 1990 by Saunders, an imprint of Elsevier Inc. All rights reserved.

B. INTRAVENOUS PYELOGRAM (IVP)

Dr. Tristen instructs you to schedule Ellie Ray for an intravenous pyelogram (IVP) at Grant Hospital. After you have explained to Ms. Ray the instructions for preparing for the examination, she asks you the following questions. Respond to them in the space provided.

1. What body structures will be x-rayed during the exam?

____

____

____

2. Why must gas and fecal material be removed from the intestines?

____

____

____

3. Why will iodine be injected into my veins?

____

____

____

4. Will I feel anything when the iodine is injected?

____

____

____

5. What is done if an individual is allergic to iodine?

____

____

C. MAGNETIC RESONANCE IMAGING

Jason Zindra, a college baseball player, has been experiencing pain in his left shoulder joint. Dr. Baker schedules him for magnetic resonance imaging of the left shoulder. Jason asks you the following questions regarding this procedure. Respond to them in the space provided.

1. Is this a safe procedure?

____

____

2. Will there be any pain involved with this procedure?

____

____

3. Will I be exposed to x-rays?

____

____

Copyright © 2008, 2004, 2000, 1995, 1990 by Saunders, an imprint of Elsevier Inc. All rights reserved.

4. What should I wear to the test?

____

____

5. May I wear my watch during the procedure to keep track of the time?

____

____

6. Does the MRI machine make any noise?

____

____

7. Will the technician be in the room with me?

____

____

Copyright © 2008, 2004, 2000, 1995, 1990 by Saunders, an imprint of Elsevier Inc. All rights reserved.

D. CROSSWORD PUZZLE

Radiology and Diagnostic Imaging

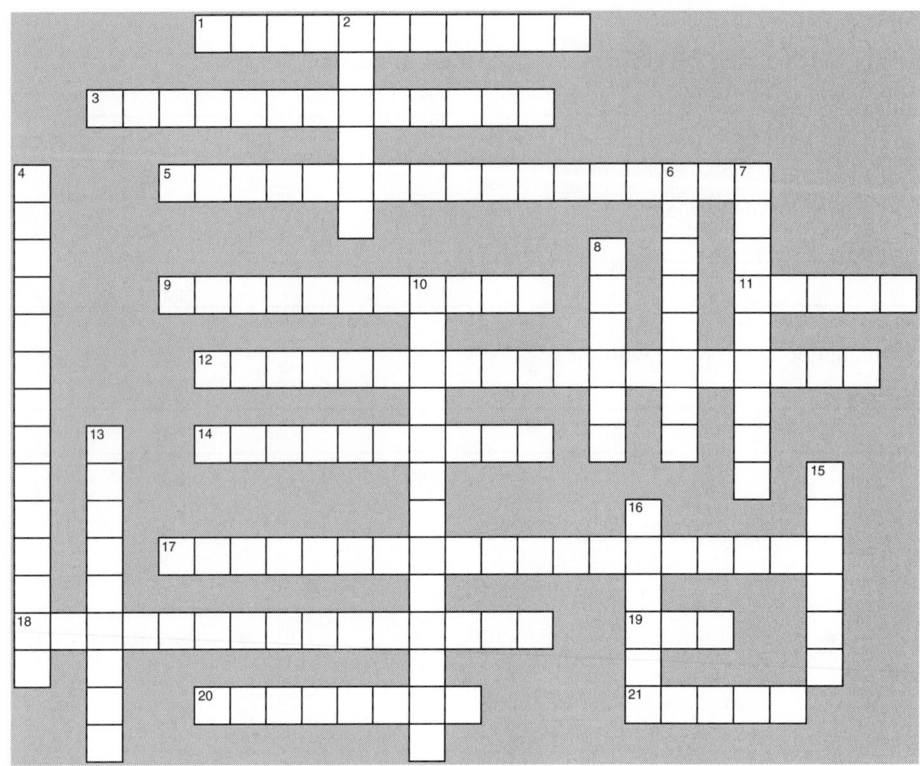

Directions: Complete the crossword puzzle using the clues provided below.

ACROSS

1 Radiograph of the lungs
3 Gallbladder inflammation
5 Radiograph of coronary arteries
9 For direct viewing of internal organs
11 Remove during an MRI
12 Radiograph of uterus and fallopian tubes
14 Obstructs x-rays
17 Can tell if it is twins
18 Radiograph of the heart
19 Used to dx kidney stones
20 US recording
21 Color of radiolucent structure

DOWN

2 Produces cross-sectional images
4 US of heart
6 Discovered x-rays
7 Breast radiograph
8 Lower GI contrast medium
10 Radiograph of bile ducts
13 Radiograph of urinary bladder
15 IVP contrast medium
16 X-rays directed from back to front

Copyright © 2008, 2004, 2000, 1995, 1990 by Saunders, an imprint of Elsevier Inc. All rights reserved.

PRACTICE FOR COMPETENCY

Procedure 14-A: Radiology Examinations. Instruct a patient in the proper preparation required for each of the following types of radiographic examinations: Mammogram, Upper GI, Lower GI, and Intravenous Pyelogram. Record the procedure in the chart provided.

Procedure 14-B: Diagnostic Imaging Procedures. Instruct a patient in the proper preparation required for each of the following types of diagnostic imaging procedures: Ultrasonography, Computed Tomography, Magnetic Resonance Imaging, and Nuclear Medicine. Record the procedure in the chart provided.

CHART	
Date	

Copyright © 2008, 2004, 2000, 1995, 1990 by Saunders, an imprint of Elsevier Inc. All rights reserved.

CHART	
Date	

Copyright © 2008, 2004, 2000, 1995, 1990 by Saunders, an imprint of Elsevier Inc. All rights reserved.

EVALUATION OF COMPETENCY

Procedure 14-A: Preparation for Radiology Examinations

Name: ______________________________ Date: ______________

Evaluated By: ______________________________ Score: ______________

Performance Objective

Outcome:	Instruct a patient in the proper preparation required for each of the following radiographic examinations: mammogram, upper GI, lower GI, and intravenous pyelogram.
Conditions:	Given the following: a patient instruction sheet for each radiographic examination.
Standards:	Time: 15 minutes. Student completed procedure in ____ minutes.
	Accuracy: Satisfactory score in the Performance Evaluation Checklist.

Performance Evaluation Checklist

Trial 1	*Trial 2*	*Point Value*	*Performance Standards*
		•	Greeted and identified patient.
		•	Introduced yourself.
			Instructed patient in the proper preparation for each of the following radiographic examinations:
		•	Mammogram
		•	Upper GI
		•	Lower GI
		•	Intravenous pyelogram
		•	Charted the procedure correctly.
		*	Completed the procedure within 15 minutes.
			TOTALS

CHART	
Date	

Copyright © 2008, 2004, 2000, 1995, 1990 by Saunders, an imprint of Elsevier Inc. All rights reserved.

Evaluation of Student Performance

EVALUATION CRITERIA			COMMENTS
Symbol	Category	Point Value	
*	Critical Step	16 points	
●	Essential Step	6 points	
▷	Theory Question	2 points	
Score calculation: 100 points – ____ points missed ____ Score Satisfactory score: 85 or above			

AAMA/CAAHEP Competency Achieved:

☑ III. C. 3. c. (3) (b): Instruct individuals according to their needs.
☑ III. C. 3. c. (3) (c): Provide instructions for health maintenance and disease prevention.

Copyright © 2008, 2004, 2000, 1995, 1990 by Saunders, an imprint of Elsevier Inc. All rights reserved.

EVALUATION OF COMPETENCY

Procedure 14-B: Preparation for Diagnostic Imaging Procedures

Name: ______________________________ Date: ______________

Evaluated By: ______________________________ Score: ______________

Performance Objective

Outcome:	Instruct a patient in the proper preparation required for each of the following diagnostic imaging procedures: ultrasonography, computed tomography, magnetic resonance imaging, and nuclear medicine.
Conditions:	Given the following: a patient instruction sheet for each diagnostic imaging procedure.
Standards:	Time: 15 minutes. Student completed procedure in ____ minutes.
	Accuracy: Satisfactory score in the Performance Evaluation Checklist.

Performance Evaluation Checklist

Trial 1	Trial 2	Point Value	*Performance Standards*
		•	Greeted and identified patient.
		•	Introduced yourself.
			Instructed patient in the proper preparation for each of the following diagnostic imaging procedures:
		•	Ultrasonography
		•	Computed tomography
		•	Magnetic resonance imaging
		•	Nuclear medicine
		•	Charted the procedure correctly.
		*	Completed the procedure within 15 minutes.
			TOTALS

CHART	
Date	

Copyright © 2008, 2004, 2000, 1995, 1990 by Saunders, an imprint of Elsevier Inc. All rights reserved.

Evaluation of Student Performance

EVALUATION CRITERIA			COMMENTS
Symbol	Category	Point Value	
*	Critical Step	16 points	
•	Essential Step	6 points	
▷	Theory Question	2 points	
Score calculation: 100 points – ______ points missed ____ Score Satisfactory score: 85 or above			

AAMA/CAAHEP Competency Achieved:

☑ III. C. 3. c. (3) (b): Instruct individuals according to their needs.
☑ III. C. 3. c. (3) (c): Provide instructions for health maintenance and disease prevention.

Copyright © 2008, 2004, 2000, 1995, 1990 by Saunders, an imprint of Elsevier Inc. All rights reserved.

15

Introduction to the Clinical Laboratory

CHAPTER ASSIGNMENTS

√ After Completing	Date Due	Textbook Page(s)	TEXTBOOK ASSIGNMENTS	Possible Points	Points You Earned
		559-583	Read Chapter 15: Introduction to the Clinical Laboratory		
		565 579	Read Case Study 1 Case Study 1 questions	5	
		569 579-580	Read Case Study 2 Case Study 2 questions	5	
		570 580	Read Case Study 3 Case Study 3 questions	5	
		580-581	Apply Your Knowledge questions	10	
			TOTAL POINTS		
√ After Completing	Date Due	Study Guide Page(s)	STUDY GUIDE ASSIGNMENTS (CTA: Critical Thinking Activity)	Possible Points	Points You Earned
		647	Pretest	10	
		648	Key Term Assessment	11	
		649-652	Evaluation of Learning questions	20	
		652	CTA A: Laboratory Directory Information	10	
		652-653	CTA B: Specimen Requirements	15	
		653	CTA C: Identifying Abnormal Values	10	
		653	CTA D: Laboratory Report	25	
		654	CTA E: Crossword Puzzle	23	

Copyright © 2008, 2004, 2000, 1995, 1990 by Saunders, an imprint of Elsevier Inc. All rights reserved.

√ After Completing	Date Due	Study Guide Page(s)	STUDY GUIDE ASSIGNMENTS (CTA: Critical Thinking Activity)	Possible Points	Points You Earned
		656	CTA F: Road to Recovery Game Laboratory Test Categories (Team Players) (Record points earned)		
			CD Activity: Chapter 15 Road to Recovery Game: Laboratory Test Categories (Individual Player) (Record points earned)		
		647	Posttest	10	
			ADDITIONAL ASSIGNMENTS		
			TOTAL POINTS		

Copyright © 2008, 2004, 2000, 1995, 1990 by Saunders, an imprint of Elsevier Inc. All rights reserved.

√ When Assigned By Your Instructor	Study Guide Page(s)	Practices Required	LABORATORY ASSIGNMENTS (Procedure Number and Name)	*Score
	665	3	**Practice for Competency** 15-1: Collecting a Specimen for Transport to an Outside Laboratory Textbook reference: p. 572-574	
	667-668		**Evaluation of Competency** 15-1: Collecting a Specimen for Transport to an Outside Laboratory	*
			ADDITIONAL ASSIGNMENTS	

Copyright © 2008, 2004, 2000, 1995, 1990 by Saunders, an imprint of Elsevier Inc. All rights reserved.

Notes

Copyright © 2008, 2004, 2000, 1995, 1990 by Saunders, an imprint of Elsevier Inc. All rights reserved.

Name ______________________________ Date ______________

PRETEST

True or False

_____ 1. When the body is in homeostasis, an imbalance exists in the body.

_____ 2. A routine test is performed to assist in the early detection of disease.

_____ 3. The laboratory request form provides the outside laboratory with information needed to test the specimen.

_____ 4. The clinical diagnosis is indicated on a laboratory request to correlate laboratory data with the needs of the physician.

_____ 5. The purpose of a laboratory report is to indicate the patient's diagnosis.

_____ 6. A patient who is fasting in preparation for a lab test is permitted to drink diet soda.

_____ 7. A small sample taken from the body to represent the nature of the whole is known as a specimen.

_____ 8. A laboratory report marked QNS means that the patient did not prepare properly.

_____ 9. Fecal occult blood testing is an example of a CLIA-waived test.

_____ 10. The purpose of quality control is to prevent accidents in the laboratory.

POSTTEST

True or False

_____ 1. Laboratory tests are most frequently ordered by the physician to assist in the diagnosis of pathologic conditions.

_____ 2. A laboratory directory indicates the patient preparation required for laboratory tests.

_____ 3. Laboratory tests termed profiles contain a number of different tests.

_____ 4. A lipid profile includes a test for glucose.

_____ 5. The purpose of patient preparation for a laboratory test is to ensure the test results fall within normal range.

_____ 6. A comprehensive metabolic profile requires that the patient fast.

_____ 7. Antibiotics taken by the patient prior to the collection of a throat specimen for culture may result in a falsely-positive result.

_____ 8. The purpose of CLIA is to prevent exposure of employees to bloodborne pathogens.

_____ 9. If a POL is performing moderate-complexity tests, CLIA requires that two levels of controls be run daily.

_____ 10. The study of blood and blood-forming tissues is known as serology.

Copyright © 2008, 2004, 2000, 1995, 1990 by Saunders, an imprint of Elsevier Inc. All rights reserved.

KEY TERM ASSESSMENT

Directions: Match each medical term with its definition.

_____ 1. Fasting

_____ 2. Homeostasis

_____ 3. In vivo

_____ 4. Laboratory test

_____ 5. Normal range

_____ 6. Plasma

_____ 7. Profile

_____ 8. Quality control

_____ 9. Routine test

_____ 10. Serum

_____ 11. Specimen

A. A certain established and acceptable parameter or reference range within which the laboratory test results of a healthy individual are expected to fall

B. The clear, straw-colored part of the blood (plasma) that remains after the solid elements and the clotting factor fibrinogen have been separated out of it

C. The state in which body systems are functioning normally and the internal environment of the body is in equilibrium

D. A number of laboratory tests providing related or complementary information used to determine the health of a patient

E. Abstaining from food or fluids (except water) for a specified amount of time before the collection of a specimen

F. The clinical analysis and study of materials, fluids, or tissues obtained from patients to assist in diagnosing and treating disease

G. Occurring in the living body or organism

H. Laboratory test performed routinely on apparently healthy patients to assist in the early detection of disease

I. The liquid part of the blood, consisting of a clear, yellowish fluid that makes up approximately 55% of the blood volume

J. A small sample of something taken to show the nature of the whole

K. The application of methods to ensure that test results are reliable and valid and errors are detected and eliminated

Copyright © 2008, 2004, 2000, 1995, 1990 by Saunders, an imprint of Elsevier Inc. All rights reserved.

EVALUATION OF LEARNING

Directions: Fill in each blank with the correct answer.

1. What is the general purpose of a laboratory test?

2. List five specific uses of laboratory test results.

3. What is the purpose of performing a routine test?

4. What information is included in a laboratory directory?

5. What is the purpose of a laboratory request?

6. What is the reason for indicating the following information on the laboratory request form?

   a. Patient's age and gender

   b. Date and time of collection of the specimen

   c. Source of the specimen

   d. Physician's clinical diagnosis

   e. Any medications the patient is taking

Copyright © 2008, 2004, 2000, 1995, 1990 by Saunders, an imprint of Elsevier Inc. All rights reserved.

7. What tests are included in the following profiles?
   a. Comprehensive Metabolic Profile

   ____

   ____

   b. Hepatic Profile

   ____

   ____

   c. Prenatal Profile

   ____

   ____

   d. Lipid Profile

   ____

   ____

8. What information is included on laboratory reports?

   ____

   ____

   ____

   ____

9. Why must the test results of specimens tested by an outside laboratory be compared with the normal ranges supplied by the laboratory?

   ____

   ____

10. Why do some laboratory tests require advance patient preparation?

    ____

    ____

11. Why is it important to explain the reason for the advance preparation to the patient?

    ____

    ____

12. What is a specimen?

    ____

    ____

13. List 10 examples of specimens.

    ____

    ____

    ____

    ____

    ____

Copyright © 2008, 2004, 2000, 1995, 1990 by Saunders, an imprint of Elsevier Inc. All rights reserved.

14. List and explain five guidelines that should be followed during specimen collection and handling.

15. Why must a specimen be properly handled and stored?

16. Define each of the following categories of laboratory tests based on function.
    a. Hematology
    b. Clinical Chemistry
    c. Serology and Blood Banking
    d. Urinalysis
    e. Microbiology

17. What are the six basic steps involved in testing a specimen?

Copyright © 2008, 2004, 2000, 1995, 1990 by Saunders, an imprint of Elsevier Inc. All rights reserved.

18. What is the purpose of quality control?

____

____

____

19. List four quality control methods that should be employed in testing a specimen.

____

____

____

____

20. List 10 laboratory safety guidelines that should be followed in the medical office to prevent accidents from occurring.

____

____

____

____

____

CRITICAL THINKING ACTIVITIES

A. LABORATORY DIRECTORY INFORMATION

Look at a laboratory directory (from an outside medical laboratory) and list the categories of information included in it (e.g., normal range of lab tests).

____

____

____

____

____

____

B. SPECIMEN REQUIREMENTS

Refer to Table 15-1 in your textbook and list the specimen requirements for each of the following tests:

1. Albumin, serum ________________________
2. ALT ________________________
3. Bilirubin, total ________________________
4. Blood group (ABO) ________________________
5. BUN, serum ________________________
6. Calcium ________________________
7. CBC (with differential) ________________________
8. CPK ________________________
9. Glucose, plasma ________________________
10. LD ________________________
11. Sedimentation rate (ESR) ________________________

Copyright © 2008, 2004, 2000, 1995, 1990 by Saunders, an imprint of Elsevier Inc. All rights reserved.

12. Thyroxine (T_4) ____________________
13. Triglycerides ____________________
14. Uric acid, serum ____________________
15. Urinalysis ____________________

C. IDENTIFYING ABNORMAL VALUES

Refer to the laboratory report in your textbook (Figure 15-2), and circle any abnormal values using a red pen.

D. LABORATORY REPORT

Refer to the laboratory report in your textbook (Figure 15-2). Using the normal values listed on this report, determine if the following tests fall within normal range or if they are high or low. Mark each test according to the following: **N** = normal, **H** = high, **L** = low. Your patient is an adult female.

1. Glucose: 140 mg/dL ____________________
2. BUN: 15 mg/dL ____________________
3. Creatinine: 1.7 mg/dL ____________________
4. Calcium: 10.2 mg/dL ____________________
5. Magnesium: 0.4 mmol/L ____________________
6. Sodium: 156 mmol/L ____________________
7. Potassium: 5.5 mmol/L ____________________
8. Chloride: 84 mmol/L ____________________
9. Carbon dioxide: 18 mmol/L ____________________
10. Uric acid: 5.2 mg/dL____________________
11. Total protein: 4.0 g/dL ____________________
12. Albumin: 3.5 g/dL ____________________
13. Total bilirubin: 0.8 mg/dL ____________________
14. Alkaline phosphatase: 80 U/L____________________
15. LD: 132 U/L ____________________
16. AST: 24 U/L____________________
17. ALT: 44 U/L____________________
18. Total cholesterol: 260 mg/dL ____________________
19. HDL cholesterol: 57 mg/dL ____________________
20. LDL cholesterol: 165 mg/dL____________________
21. WBC: 15.5 (X $10^3/mm^3$) ____________________
22. Hemoglobin: 10.4 g/dL ____________________
23. Hematocrit: 34% ____________________
24. Prothrombin time: 10 seconds ____________________
25. Neutrophils: 84% ____________________

Copyright © 2008, 2004, 2000, 1995, 1990 by Saunders, an imprint of Elsevier Inc. All rights reserved.

E. CROSSWORD PUZZLE
Introduction to the Clinical Laboratory

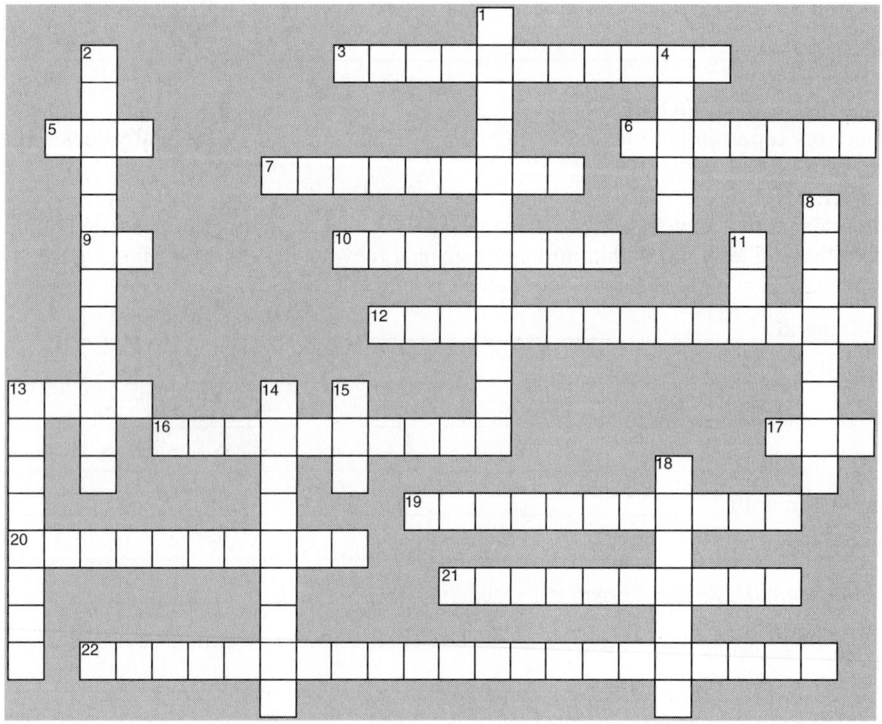

Directions: Complete the crossword puzzle using the clues presented below.

ACROSS

3 Detects disease early
5 Syphilis test
6 More than one lab test
7 Study of tissues
9 CLIA requires three times per year
10 Sample of the body
12 Accurate and reliable test results
13 To improve quality of lab testing
16 Study of blood
17 Hemoglobin abbreviation
19 Healthy body
20 Order a lab test
21 Exempt from CLIA
22 Which disease is it?

DOWN

1 Study of MOs
2 CHD tests
4 Plasma minus fibrinogen
8 Study of antigen-antibody reactions
11 Hematocrit abbreviation
13 Pap test (ex)
14 What are the results?
15 In-house lab
18 No food or fluid

Copyright © 2008, 2004, 2000, 1995, 1990 by Saunders, an imprint of Elsevier Inc. All rights reserved.

Notes

Copyright © 2008, 2004, 2000, 1995, 1990 by Saunders, an imprint of Elsevier Inc. All rights reserved.

F. ROAD TO RECOVERY
Lab Test Categories

Object: The object of the game is to lead your "patient" to recovery by correctly determining the category to which a particular test belongs.

Needed: **Road to Recovery** game board
Game cards
A token for each player (such as a button or coin)
Dice (1)
Score card

Directions:

1. Cut out the game cards on the following pages. On the reverse side of each card, write the lab category for that test. Use Table 15-4 in your textbook to complete this assignment.
2. Using the game cards as flash cards, learn the appropriate category for each test.
3. Get into your playing groups.
4. Place one complete set of cards on the game board with the lab test facing up (and the lab category facing down).
5. Play **Road to Recovery** following the directions on the reverse side of the game board. A player should pick up a card and state the category for the lab test. Turn your card over to determine if you answered correctly. If you did, award yourself 5 points. If you answered incorrectly, you receive 0 points.
6. Keep track of your points using the score card provided below.

ROAD TO RECOVERY
SCORE CARD

Name: ______________________________

Recording Points:
Using the Game Card Points box, cross off a number each time you answer a game card correctly (starting with 5 and continuing in sequence). Your total game card points will be equal to the last number you crossed off. Record this number in the space provided (1). Record any extra points you were awarded during the game (2), and any points that were deducted (3). To determine your total points, add (1) and (2) together and deduct (3). Record this number in the Total Points Earned space provided. Compare your score with the other players and determine where you placed. Place a check mark next to the level of recovery your patient attained.

Game Card Points:

5	75	145	215
10	80	150	220
15	85	155	225
20	90	160	230
25	95	165	235
30	100	170	240
35	105	175	245
40	110	180	250
45	115	185	255
50	120	190	260
55	125	195	265
60	130	200	270
65	135	205	275
70	140	210	280

Calculation of Points:

(1) Total Game Card Points: ________

(2) Additional Points Awarded: ________

(3) Deducted Points: ________

TOTAL POINTS EARNED: ________

LEVEL OF RECOVERY:

Patient's Name: ______________________

☐ First Place: **Fully Recovered**
☐ Second Place: **Almost Recovered**
☐ Third Place: **Still Recovering**
☐ Fourth Place: **Gasping for Air**

Copyright © 2008, 2004, 2000, 1995, 1990 by Saunders, an imprint of Elsevier Inc. All rights reserved.

White Blood Count	Red Blood Count	Differential White Blood Count	Hemoglobin
Hematocrit	Prothrombin Time	Erythrocyte Sedimentation Rate	Platelet Count
Serum Glucose	Blood Urea Nitrogen	Creatinine	Total Serum Protein
Albumin	Globulin	Calcium	Phosphorus

Chloride	Sodium	Potassium	Serum Bilirubin
Cholesterol	Triglycerides	Uric Acid	Lactase Dehydrogenase (LD)
Aspartate Aminotransferase (AST)	Alkaline Aminotransferase (ALT)	Alkaline Phosphatase (ALP)	Amylase
Carbon Dioxide	Thyroxine (T_4)	T_3 uptake	Creatine Phosphokinase (CPK)

Gonorrhea	Meningitis	Pneumonia	Streptococcal Sore Throat
Tuberculosis	Hookworms	Malaria	Pinworms
Tapeworms	Trichinosis	Trichomoniasis	Scabies
Chromosome Studies	Pap Test	Tissue Analysis	Biopsy Studies

VDRL	RPR	C-reactive Protein (CRP)	ABO Blood Typing
Rh Typing	Rh Antibody Test	Antinuclear Antibody (ANA)	Rheumatoid Factor
Mono Test	Hepatitis Tests	HIV Tests	Antistreptolysin O (ASO)
Serum Pregnancy Test	Candidiasis	Chlamydia	Diphtheria

PRACTICE FOR COMPETENCY

Procedure 15-1: Collecting Specimen for Transport to an Outside Laboratory

1. **Laboratory Requisition.** Complete the Laboratory Request Form on the following page using a classmate as a patient. The tests that have been ordered by the physician include the following: CBC (with differential), total cholesterol, HDL cholesterol, and plasma glucose.
2. **Specimen Collection.** Practice the procedure for collecting a specimen for transport to an outside laboratory and record the procedure in the chart provided.

CHART	
Date	

Copyright © 2008, 2004, 2000, 1995, 1990 by Saunders, an imprint of Elsevier Inc. All rights reserved.

LABORATORY REQUISITION

Biomedical Laboratories, Inc.
100 Main Street
Athens, Georgia 45760

☐ Fax Send additional copy of report to: ( )
☐ Call Client Number/Physician's Name Phone/Fax number
☐ Mail Physician's Address City, State, Zip

Patient's Name (Last) (First) (MI) Sex Date of Birth MO | DAY | YEAR Collection Time : AM PM Fasting YES NO Collection Date MO | DAY | YEAR

NPI/UPIN | Physician's ID # | Patient's SS # | Patient's ID # | Urine hrs/vol hrs_____ vol_____

Physician's Name (Last, First) Physician's Signature

Medicare # (Include prefix/suffix) ☐ Primary ☐ Secondary

Medicaid # State Physician's Provider #

Diagnosis/Signs/Symptoms in ICD-9 Format (Highest Specificity)

REQUIRED

PATIENT

Patient's Address Phone

City State ZIP

RESP. PARTY

Name of Responsible Party (if different from patient)

Address of Responsible Party (if different from patient) APT #

City State ZIP

INSURANCE

Patient's Relationship to Responsible Party ■ 1–Self ■ 2–Spouse ■ 3–Child ■ 4–Other

Insurance Company Name | Plan | Carrier Code

Subscriber/Member # | Location | Group #

Insurance Address | Physician's Provider #

City | State | ZIP

Employer's Name or Number | Insured SS # (If not patient) | Worker's Comp ☐ Yes ☐ No

Performance Lab ☐ | Carrier | Group # | Employee # | Mem

I hereby authorize the release of medical information related to the service subscribed herein and authorize payment directed to LabCorp.

X ____________________ __________
Patient's Signature Date

MEDICARE ADVANCE BENEFICIARY NOTICE

I have read the ABN on the reverse. If Medicare denies payment, I agree to pay for the identified test(s).

X ____________________ __________
Patient's Signature Date

NOTE: WHEN ORDERING TESTS FOR WHICH MEDICARE OR MEDICAID REIMBURSEMENT WILL BE SOUGHT, PHYSICIANS SHOULD ONLY ORDER TESTS THAT ARE MEDICALLY NECESSARY FOR THE DIAGNOSIS OR TREATMENT OF THE PATIENT. COMPONENTS OF THE ORGAN OR DISEASE PANELS/COMBINATIONS PRINTED BELOW ARE SHOWN ON THE REVERSE SIDE AND MAY ALSO BE ORDERED INDIVIDUALLY BELOW. COMPONENTS MAY BE BILLED SEPARATELY PER CARRIER POLICY.

PROFILES (See reverse for components)

Code	Test	Container
80049	Basic Metabolic Profile	SST
80054	Comp Metabolic Profile	SST
80051	Electrolyte Profile	SST
80058	Hepatic Profile	SST
80059	Hepatitis Profile	SST
80061	Lipid Profile	
80091	Thyroid Profile	SST
80055	Prenatal Profile	RED LAV
80072	Rheumatoid Profile	SST

HEMATOLOGY

Code	Test	Container
85025	CBC w Diff	
85027	CBC w/o Diff	LAV
85014	Hematocrit	LAV
85018	Hemoglobin	LAV
85595	Platelet Count	LAV
85041	RBC Count	LAV
85048	WBC Count	LAV
85007	WBC Differential	LAV
89190	Nasal Smear, Eosin	Nasal Smear
85060	Pathologist Consult–Peripheral Smear	LAV

ALPHABETICAL/COMBINATION TESTS

Code	Test	Container
86900 86901	ABO and Rh	LAV
82040	Albumin	SST
84075	Alkaline Phosphatase	SST
84460	ALT (SGPT)	SST
82150	Amylase, Serum	SST
86038	Antinuclear Antibodies	SST
84450	AST (SGOT)	SST
82607 82746	B_{12} and Folate	SST
82250	Bilirubin, Total	SST

ALPHABETICAL TESTS CON'T

Code	Test	Container
84520	BUN	SST
82310	Calcium	SST
80156	Carbamazepine (Tegretol®)	SER
82378	CEA	SST
82465	Cholesterol, Total	SST
82565	Creatinine	SST
80162	Digoxin	SER
82670	Estradiol	SST
82728	Ferritin, Serum	SST
82985	Fructosamine	SST
83001	FSH	SST
83001 83002	FSH and LH	SST
82977	GGT	SST
82947	Glucose, Plasma	GRY
82947	Glucose, Serum	SST
82950	Glucose, 2-hr. PP	SST
83036	Glycohemoglobin, Total	LAV
84703	hCG, Beta Subunit, Qual	SST
84702	hCG, Beta Subunit, Quant	SST
83718	HDL Cholesterol	SST
86677	*Helicobacter pylori*, IgG	SST
86706	Hep B Surface Antibody	SST
87340	Hep B Surface Antigen	SST
86803	Hep C Antibody	SST
83036	Hemoglobin A_{1C}	LAV
86701	HIV Antibodies	SST
83540	Iron, Total	SST
83540 83550	Iron and IBC	SST
83615	LDH	SST

ALPHABETICAL TESTS CON'T

Code	Test	Container
83002	LH	SST
83690	Lipase	SER
80178	Lithium (Eskalith®)	SER
83735	Magnesium, Serum	SST
80184	Phenobarbital (Luminal®)	SER
80185	Phenytoin (Dilantin®)	SER
84132	Potassium	SST
84146	Prolactin, Serum	SST
84153	Prostate-Specific Antigen	SST
84066	Prostatic Acid Phos	SST
84155	Protein, Total	SST
85610	Prothrombin Time (PT)	BLU
85610 85730	PT and PTT Activated	BLU
85730	PTT Activated	BLU
86431	Rheumatoid Arthritis Factor	SST
86592	RPR	SST
86762	Rubella Antibodies, IgG	SST
85651	Sed Rate	LAV
84295	Sodium	SST
84403	Testosterone	SST
80198	Theophylline	SER
84436	Thyroxine (T_4)	SST
84478	Triglycerides	SST
84480	Triiodothyronine (T_3)	SST
84443	TSH, High Sensitivity	SST
84550	Uric Acid	SST
81003	Urinalysis Microscopic on Positives	URN
81001	Urinalysis with Microscopic	URN
80164	Valproic Acid (Depakene®)	SER

MICROBIOLOGY See Reverse Side

■ ENDOCERVICAL ■ THROAT ■ URINE
■ STOOL ■ URETHRAL INDICATE SOURCE

Code	Test	Container
87070	Aerobic Bacterial Culture	Bact Trnspt
87490 87590	*Chlamydia/GC* DNA Probe w/ Confirmation on Positives	Probe Trnspt
87490 87590	*Chlamydia/GC* DNA Probe Without Confirmation	Probe Trnspt
87490	*Chlamydia* DNA Probe	Probe Trnspt
87081	Genital, *Beta-Hemolytic Strep Cult, Group B*	Bact Trnspt
87070	Genital Culture, Routine	Bact Trnspt
87070	Lower Respiratory Culture	Steril Trnspt
87590	*N. gonorrhoeae* DNA Probe	Probe Trnspt
87015 87211	Ova and Parasites	O & P Kit
87081 X2 87045	Stool Culture	Fecal Trnspt
87081	Throat, *Beta-Hemolytic Strep Cult, Group A*	Bact Trnspt
87060	Upper Respiratory Culture, Routine	Bact Trnspt
87086	Urine Culture, Routine	Urn Cul Trnspt

Clinical Information/Comments

OTHER TESTS/INDIVIDUAL COMPONENTS

TEST #	TEST NAMES

LAB USE ONLY	STAT	VENIPUNCTURE	TRAVEL	NON LABCORP	VERBAL ORDER	CHART ORDER	HANDWRITTEN	24 HR TUV	PST/PSC #
	☐998074	☐998085	☐998096	☐998239	☐998250	☐998261	☐998272	☐998283	

CONTAINERS RECEIVED →

SST	USST	SER	FRZ	RED	LAV	SLD	BLU	GRY	GRN	RYB	YEL	PLS	URN	24U	TA-U	FL	OT	BACT TRNSP	O & P KIT	PROBE TRNSP	URN CULT TRNSP	STERIL TRNSP	FECAL TRNSP	VIRAL TRNSP
SPUN	UNSPUN	SERUM TRNSPT	FRZ TRNS	RED	LAVENDER	SLIDE	LT. BLUE	GREY	GREEN	RYL BLU	ACD	PLASMA	URINE	24 HR URINE	TART. ACID	FLUID	OTHER							

300-0384

Copyright © 2008, 2004, 2000, 1995, 1990 by Saunders, an imprint of Elsevier Inc. All rights reserved.

EVALUATION OF COMPETENCY

Procedure 15-1: Collecting a Specimen for Transport to an Outside Laboratory

Name: ______________________ Date: ____________

Evaluated By: ______________________ Score: ____________

Performance Objective

Outcome: Collect a specimen for transport to an outside laboratory.

Conditions: Given the appropriate supplies for the specimen collection and transport (will be based upon the type of specimen collected).

Standards: Time: 10 minutes. Student completed procedure in ____ minutes.

Accuracy: Satisfactory score in the Performance Evaluation Checklist.

Performance Evaluation Checklist

Trial 1	Trial 2	Point Value	*Performance Standards*
		•	Informed patient of any advance preparation or special instructions.
		▷	Explained why patient should prepare properly.
		•	Reviewed requirements in the laboratory directory for the collection and handling of the specimen.
		•	Completed laboratory request form.
		•	Sanitized hands.
		•	Assembled equipment and supplies.
		•	Labeled the tubes and containers with patient's name, date, and initials.
		•	Greeted patient and introduced yourself. Identified patient and explained procedure.
		▷	Stated why it is important to correctly identify patient. Detertermined if patient prepared properly for test.
			Collected specimen incorporating the following guidelines:
		•	Followed the OSHA Standard.
		•	Collected specimen using proper technique.
		•	Collected the proper type and amount of specimen required for the test.
		•	Processed specimen further if required by the outside laboratory.
		•	Placed the lid tightly on specimen container.
			Prepared specimen for transport:
		•	Placed specimen in biohazard specimen bag.
		•	Placed lab request in outside pocket of bag.
		•	Properly handled and stored specimen.
		•	Charted the procedure correctly.

Copyright © 2008, 2004, 2000, 1995, 1990 by Saunders, an imprint of Elsevier Inc. All rights reserved.

Trial 1	Trial 2	Point Value	Performance Standards
			Processed laboratory report:
		•	Reviewed laboratory report when it was returned.
		•	Notified physician of any abnormal results.
		•	Filed laboratory report in patient's chart after review by physician.
		*	Completed the procedure within 10 minutes.
			TOTALS

CHART	
Date	

Evaluation of Student Performance

EVALUATION CRITERIA			COMMENTS
Symbol	Category	Point Value	
*	Critical Step	16 points	
•	Essential Step	6 points	
▷	Theory Question	2 points	
Score calculation: 100 points – ______ points missed ____ Score Satisfactory score: 85 or above			

AAMA/CAAHEP Competency Achieved:

☑ III. C. 3. b. (4) (i): Screen and follow-up test results.
☑ III. C. 3. c. (4) (d): Use methods of quality control.

Copyright © 2008, 2004, 2000, 1995, 1990 by Saunders, an imprint of Elsevier Inc. All rights reserved.

16

Urinalysis

CHAPTER ASSIGNMENTS

√ After Completing	Date Due	Textbook Page(s)	TEXTBOOK ASSIGNMENTS	Possible Points	Points You Earned
		584-627	Read Chapter 16: Urinalysis		
		586 624	Read Case Study 1 Case Study 1 questions	5	
		595 624	Read Case Study 2 Case Study 2 questions	5	
		621 624	Read Case Study 3 Case Study 3 questions	5	
		625	Apply Your Knowledge questions	10	
			TOTAL POINTS		

√ After Completing	Date Due	Study Guide Page(s)	STUDY GUIDE ASSIGNMENTS (CTA: Critical Thinking Activity)	Possible Points	Points You Earned
		673	Pretest	10	
		674	Key Term Assessment	17	
		675-678	Evaluation of Learning questions	37	
		678	CTA A: First-Voided Specimen	2	
		678	CTA B: Clean-Catch Specimen	4	
		678-679	CTA C: Urine Testing Kit Instructions	6	
			CD Activity: Chapter 16 Gotta Go Right Now (Record points earned)		
		680	CTA D: Crossword Puzzle	21	
		682	CTA E: Road to Recovery: Urinalysis Terminology (Team Players) (Record points earned)		

Copyright © 2008, 2004, 2000, 1995, 1990 by Saunders, an imprint of Elsevier Inc. All rights reserved.

√ After Completing	Date Due	Study Guide Page(s)	STUDY GUIDE ASSIGNMENTS (CTA: Critical Thinking Activity)	Possible Points	Points You Earned
			CD Activity: Road to Recovery: Urinalysis Terminology (Individual Player) (Record points earned)		
			CD Activity: Chapter 16 Animations	20	
		673	Posttest	10	
			ADDITIONAL ASSIGNMENTS		
			TOTAL POINTS		

Copyright © 2008, 2004, 2000, 1995, 1990 by Saunders, an imprint of Elsevier Inc. All rights reserved.

√ When Assigned By Your Instructor	Study Guide Page(s)	Practices Required	LABORATORY ASSIGNMENTS (Procedure Number and Name)	*Score
	687-688	3	**Practice for Competency** 16-1: Clean-Catch Midstream Specimen Collection Instructions Textbook reference: pp. 589-590	
	691-693		**Evaluation of Competency** 16-1: Clean-Catch Midstream Specimen Collection Instructions	*
	687-688	3	**Practice for Competency** 16-2: Collection of a 24-Hour Urine Specimen Textbook reference: pp. 590-591	
	695-696		**Evaluation of Competency** 16-2: Collection of a 24-Hour Urine Specimen	*
	687-688	5	**Practice for Competency** 16-A: Assessing Color and Appearance of a Urine Specimen Textbook reference: p. 592	
	697-698		**Evaluation of Competency** 16-A: Assessing Color and Appearance of a Urine Specimen	*
	687-688	3	**Practice for Competency** 16-3 and 16-4: Measuring Specific Gravity of Urine: Refractometer Method and Quality Control: Calibration of the Refractometer Textbook reference: pp. 593-595	
	699-700		**Evaluation of Competency** 16-3 and 16-4: Measuring Specific Gravity of Urine: Refractometer Method and Quality Control: Calibration of the Refractometer	*
	687-688	5	**Practice for Competency** 16-5: Chemical Testing of Urine with the Multistix 10 SG Reagent Strip Textbook reference: pp. 603-604	
	701-702		**Evaluation of Competency** 16-5: Chemical Testing of Urine with the Multistix 10 SG Reagent Strip	*
	687-688	2	**Practice for Competency** 16-6: Microscopic Examination of Urine: Kova Method Textbook reference: pp. 616-618	
	705-707		**Evaluation of Competency** 16-6: Microscopic Examination of Urine: Kova Method	*

Copyright © 2008, 2004, 2000, 1995, 1990 by Saunders, an imprint of Elsevier Inc. All rights reserved.

√ When Assigned By Your Instructor	Study Guide Page(s)	Practices Required	LABORATORY ASSIGNMENTS (Procedure Number and Name)	*Score
	687-688		**Practice for Competency** 16-7: Performing a Rapid Urine Culture Test Textbook reference: pp. 619-620	
	709-710	2	**Evaluation of Competency** 16-7: Performing a Rapid Urine Culture Test	*
	687-688		DVD **Practice for Competency** 16-8: Performing a Urine Pregnancy Test Textbook reference: pp. 622-623	
	711-712	2	**Evaluation of Competency** 16-8: Performing a Urine Pregnancy Test	*
			ADDITIONAL ASSIGNMENTS	

Copyright © 2008, 2004, 2000, 1995, 1990 by Saunders, an imprint of Elsevier Inc. All rights reserved.

Name ______________________________ Date ______________

PRETEST

True or False

_____ 1. The urinary system functions to regulate the fluid balance of the body.

_____ 2. The functional unit of the kidney is the nephron.

_____ 3. An excessive increase in urine output is termed polyuria.

_____ 4. A clean-catch midstream urine specimen is required for a urine culture.

_____ 5. Urinalysis consists of a physical, chemical, and microscopic examination of urine.

_____ 6. A urine specimen that is light yellow in color indicates that bacteria are present in the specimen.

_____ 7. The pH of most urine specimens is neutral.

_____ 8. Blood may normally be present in the urine due to menstruation.

_____ 9. Hematuria refers to the presence of blood in the urine.

_____ 10. HCG is a hormone that is present in the urine and blood of a pregnant woman.

POSTTEST

True or False

_____ 1. The external opening of the urethra is known as the external os.

_____ 2. A normal adult excretes approximately 250 ml of urine each day.

_____ 3. Vomiting can result in oliguria.

_____ 4. The distal urethra normally contains microorganisms.

_____ 5. A 24-hour urine specimen may be collected to assist in the diagnosis of a UTI.

_____ 6. If a urine specimen is allowed to stand for more than 1 hour at room temperature, the pH becomes more acidic.

_____ 7. If a freshly voided specimen is cloudy, this may mean that a urinary tract infection is present.

_____ 8. The normal specific gravity of urine ranges from 1.003 to 1.030.

_____ 9. Dysuria is the inability to control urination at night.

_____ 10. Casts are formed in the urinary bladder.

Copyright © 2008, 2004, 2000, 1995, 1990 by Saunders, an imprint of Elsevier Inc. All rights reserved.

KEY TERM ASSESSMENT

Directions: Match each medical term with its definition.

_____ 1. Bilirubinuria
_____ 2. Glycosuria
_____ 3. Ketonuria
_____ 4. Ketosis
_____ 5. Micturition
_____ 6. Nephron
_____ 7. Oliguria
_____ 8. pH
_____ 9. Polyuria
_____ 10. Proteinuria
_____ 11. Refractive index
_____ 12. Refractometer
_____ 13. Renal threshold
_____ 14. Specific gravity
_____ 15. Supernatant
_____ 16. Urinalysis
_____ 17. Void

A. Decreased or scanty output of urine
B. The presence of protein in the urine
C. The clear liquid that remains at the top after a precipitate settles
D. The presence of bilirubin in the urine
E. Increased output of urine
F. The concentration at which a substance in the blood that is not normally excreted by the kidneys begins to appear in the urine
G. The presence of sugar in the urine
H. The physical, chemical, and microscopic analysis of urine
I. The presence of ketone bodies in the urine
J. The act of voiding urine
K. An accumulation of large amounts of ketone bodies in the tissues and body fluids
L. The weight of a substance compared with the weight of an equal volume of a substance known as the standard
M. The unit that describes the acidity or alkalinity of a solution
N. The functional unit of the kidney
O. An instrument used to measure the refractive index of urine, which is an indirect measurement of the specific gravity of urine
P. The ratio of the velocity of light in air to the velocity of light in a solution
Q. To empty the bladder

Copyright © 2008, 2004, 2000, 1995, 1990 by Saunders, an imprint of Elsevier Inc. All rights reserved.

EVALUATION OF LEARNING

Directions: Fill in each blank with the correct answer.

1. List two functions of the urinary system.

____

____

2. What is the function of the urinary bladder?

____

____

3. How does the function of the urethra differ in the male and female?

____

____

4. What is the urinary meatus?

____

____

5. Most of the urine (95%) is composed of what substance?

____

____

6. List two conditions that may cause polyuria.

____

____

7. List two conditions that may cause oliguria.

____

____

8. What is the term used to describe painful urination?

____

9. What is the term used to describe a condition of frequent urination?

____

10. What is the term used to describe excessive (voluntary) urination during the night?

____

11. The inability to retain urine is known as:

____

12. What type of urine specimen is required for the detection of a urinary tract infection (UTI)?

____

Copyright © 2008, 2004, 2000, 1995, 1990 by Saunders, an imprint of Elsevier Inc. All rights reserved.

13. List three changes that may take place in a urine specimen if it is allowed to stand at room temperature for more than 1 hour.

14. Why is a first-voided morning specimen often preferred for urine testing?

15. What condition is a 24-hour urine specimen often used to diagnose?

16. Why does concentrated urine tend to be dark yellow in color?

17. List two factors that may cause a urine specimen to become cloudy.

18. A urine specimen that has been allowed to stand at room temperature for a long period of time will have what type of odor?

19. What is the purpose of testing the specific gravity of urine?

20. What is the normal range for the specific gravity of urine?

21. What is the difference between a qualitative test and a quantitative test?

22. What may cause an increase in the pH of urine?

23. Why does urine become more alkaline if it is not preserved?

24. What may cause glycosuria?

Copyright © 2008, 2004, 2000, 1995, 1990 by Saunders, an imprint of Elsevier Inc. All rights reserved.

25. What may cause ketosis?

26. What may cause blood to appear in the urine?

27. Why should a nitrite test not be performed on a urine specimen that has been left standing at room temperature?

28. How should urine reagent strips be stored?

29. What is the purpose of performing a microscopic examination of the urine?

30. Why is a first-voided urine specimen recommended for a microscopic examination of the urine?

31. What effect does concentrated urine have on red blood cells present in it?

32. What is a urinary cast?

33. List one condition that may cause yeast cells to appear in the urine.

34. List two reasons for performing a urine culture test.

35. List three reasons for performing a pregnancy test.

36. What is the name of the hormone that is present only in the urine and blood of a pregnant woman?

Copyright © 2008, 2004, 2000, 1995, 1990 by Saunders, an imprint of Elsevier Inc. All rights reserved.

37. List five guidelines that should be followed when performing a pregnancy test.

CRITICAL THINKING ACTIVITIES

A. FIRST-VOIDED SPECIMEN

You have instructed Jim Pratt to collect a first-voided morning urine specimen, to be brought to the medical office for testing. Mr. Pratt asks the following questions. Respond to them in the spaces provided.

1. Why is a first-voided specimen desired?

2. Why must the specimen be preserved until it is brought to the medical office?

B. CLEAN-CATCH SPECIMEN

You have just instructed Ann Berger to obtain a clean-catch midstream specimen at the medical office. Mrs. Berger asks the following questions. Respond to them in the spaces provided.

1. What is the purpose of cleansing the urinary meatus?

2. Why must a front-to-back motion be used to clean the urinary meatus?

3. Why must a small amount of urine first be voided into the toilet?

4. Why should the inside of the specimen cup not be touched?

C. URINE TESTING KIT INSTRUCTIONS

Obtain the package insert instructions that come with any type of commercially prepared diagnostic kit for the chemical testing of urine (e.g., Multistix 10 SG). Using the instructions, answer the following questions in the spaces provided. (Note: A package insert for Multistix 10 SG can be obtained on the Internet by following these steps: 1. Go to http://diagnostics.siemens.com; 2. Click on Products [at the top of the page]; 3. Under the Urinalysis category, click on Multistix 10 SG Reagent Strips; 4. Click on Multistix 10 SG Package Insert; 5. Print out the package insert for Multistix 10 SG.)

1. What is the brand name of the test?

Copyright © 2008, 2004, 2000, 1995, 1990 by Saunders, an imprint of Elsevier Inc. All rights reserved.

2. This test assists in the diagnosis of what conditions?

3. What type of urine specimen is recommended for this test?

4. This test is used to detect the presence of what substances?

5. Explain the proper storage and handling of this test.

6. List any substances or techniques that may interfere with obtaining an accurate reading (for example, not reading the test at the prescribed time).

Copyright © 2008, 2004, 2000, 1995, 1990 by Saunders, an imprint of Elsevier Inc. All rights reserved.

D. CROSSWORD PUZZLE
Urinalysis

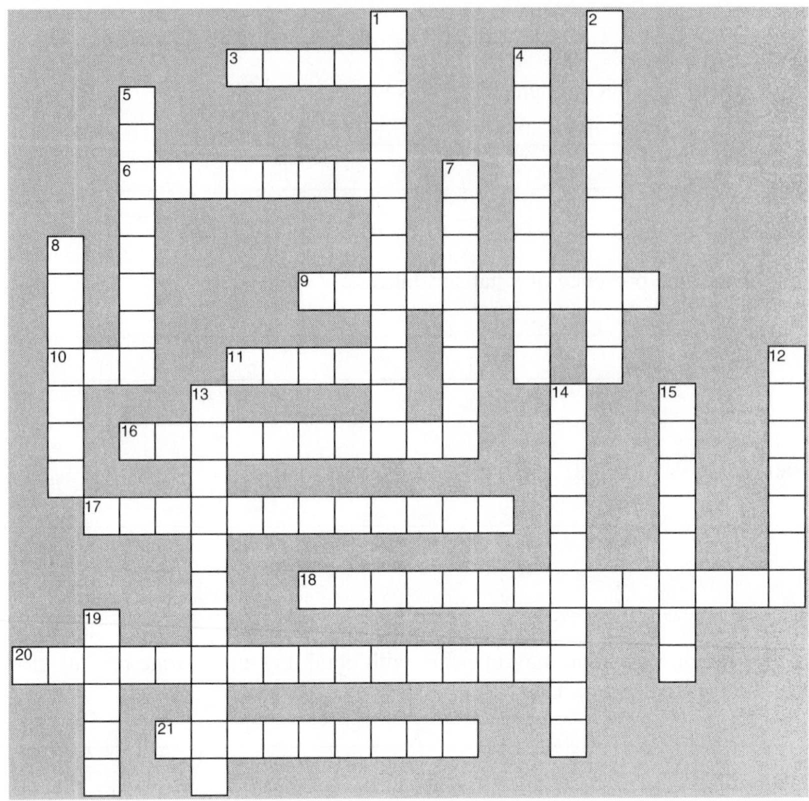

Directions: Complete the crossword puzzle using the clues presented below.

ACROSS

3 UTI bacteria
6 Deteriorates urine strips
9 Tx for UTI
10 Makes preg test +
11 Neutral pH
16 Physical, chemical, and microscopic
17 Normal cause of hematuria
18 Security for drug testing
20 Exactly!
21 Cause of bilirubinuria

DOWN

1 24-hour spec dx can cause this
2 Cause of ketonuria
4 Yellow urine pigment
5 Cause of oliguria
7 Cause of glycosuria
8 Kidney unit
12 Sym of UTI
13 Spec for preg test
14 Spec for C & S
15 This drug causes polyuria
19 Most of urine

Copyright © 2008, 2004, 2000, 1995, 1990 by Saunders, an imprint of Elsevier Inc. All rights reserved.

Notes

Copyright © 2008, 2004, 2000, 1995, 1990 by Saunders, an imprint of Elsevier Inc. All rights reserved.

E. ROAD TO RECOVERY
Urinalysis

Object: The object of the game is to lead your "patient" to recovery by correctly providing the definition to medical terms relating to urinalysis.

Needed: **Road to Recovery** game board (located at the end of this manual)
Game cards
A token for each player (such as a button or coin)
Dice (1)
Score card

Directions:

1. Cut out the terminology game cards on the following pages.
2. Study the terms/definitions in preparation for the game.
3. Place one complete set of terms on the game board with the definitions facing up (and the medical terms facing down).
4. Play **Road to Recovery** following the directions on the reverse side of the game board.
5. Place the set of cards on the game board again with the medical terms face-up and the definitions face-down, and continue playing the game until all the cards have been used.
6. Keep track of your points using the score card provided.

ROAD TO RECOVERY
SCORE CARD

Name: ______________________________

Recording Points:
Using the Game Card Points box, cross off a number each time you answer a game card correctly (starting with 5 and continuing in sequence). Your total game card points will be equal to the last number you crossed off. Record this number in the space provided (1). Record any extra points you were awarded during the game (2), and any points that were deducted (3). To determine your total points, add (1) and (2) together and deduct (3). Record this number in the Total Points Earned space provided. Compare your score with the other players and determine where you placed. Place a check mark next to the level of recovery your patient attained.

Game Card Points:

5	75	145	215
10	80	150	220
15	85	155	225
20	90	160	230
25	95	165	235
30	100	170	240
35	105	175	245
40	110	180	250
45	115	185	255
50	120	190	260
55	125	195	265
60	130	200	270
65	135	205	275
70	140	210	280

Calculation of Points:

(1) Total Game Card Points: ________

(2) Additional Points Awarded: ________

(3) Deducted Points: ________

TOTAL POINTS EARNED: ________

LEVEL OF RECOVERY:

Patient's Name: ______________________
☐ First Place: **Fully Recovered**
☐ Second Place: **Almost Recovered**
☐ Third Place: **Still Recovering**
☐ Fourth Place: **Gasping for Air**

Copyright © 2008, 2004, 2000, 1995, 1990 by Saunders, an imprint of Elsevier Inc. All rights reserved.

Anuria	Diuresis	Dysuria	Frequency
Hematuria	Nocturia	Nocturnal Enuresis	Proteinuria
Pyuria	Retention	Urgency	Urinary Incontinence
Qualitative	Quantitative	Leukocyturia	Supernatant

The condition of having to urinate often	Difficult or painful urination	Secretion and passage of large amounts of urine	Failure of the kidneys to produce urine
The presence of protein in the urine	The inability of the patient to control urination at night during sleep (bed wetting)	Excessive (voluntary) urination during the night	Blood present in the urine
The inability to retain urine	The immediate need to urinate	The inability to empty the bladder—urine is being produced normally but is not being voided	Pus present in the urine
The clear liquid that remains at the top after a precipitate settles	The presence of leukocytes in the urine	A test that indicates the exact amount of a substance that is present	A test that provides an approximate indication of whether or not a substance is present in abnormal quantities

Ureter	**Urinary Bladder**	**Urethra**	**Urinary Meatus**
Bilirubinuria	**Glycosuria**	**Ketonuria**	**Ketosis**
Micturition	**Nephron**	**Oliguria**	**pH**
Polyuria	**Specific Gravity**	**Urinalysis**	**Void**

The external opening of the urethra	Tube that extends from the urinary bladder to the outside of the body	A hollow muscular sac that stores and expels urine	A tube that drains urine from the kidneys and into the urinary bladder
An accumulation of large amounts of ketone bodies in the tissues and body fluids	The presence of ketone bodies in the urine	The presence of sugar in the urine	The presence of bilirubin in the urine
The unit that describes the acidity or alkalinity of a solution	Decreased or scanty output of urine	The functional unit of the kidney	The act of voiding urine
To empty the bladder	The physical, chemical, and microscopic analysis of urine	The measurement of the amount of dissolved substances present in the urine	Increased output of urine

PRACTICE FOR COMPETENCY

Procedure 16-1: Clean-Catch Midstream Urine Specimen. Collection Instructions. Instruct an individual in the procedure for collecting a clean-catch midstream specimen and record the procedure in the chart provided.

Procedure 16-2: 24-Hour Urine Specimen. Instruct an individual in the procedure for collecting a 24-hour urine specimen and record the procedure in the chart provided.

Procedure 16-A: Color and Appearance of a Urine Specimen. Assess the color and appearance of a urine specimen and record the results in the chart provided.

Procedure 16-3 and 16-4: Specific Gravity of Urine: Refractometer Method. Measure the specific gravity of a urine specimen using a refractometer. Record the results in the chart provided.

Procedure 16-5: Chemical Testing of Urine Using the Multistix 10 SG Reagent Strip. Perform a chemical assessment of a urine specimen using a Multistix 10 SG reagent strip. Record the results on the laboratory report form provided. Circle any abnormal results.

Procedure 16-6: Microscopic Examination of Urine. Practice the procedure for preparing a urine specimen for a microscopic analysis of the urine sediment. Examine the specimen and record the results in the chart provided.

Procedure 16-7: Rapid Urine Culture Test. Perform a rapid urine culture test and record the results in the chart provided.

Procedure 16-8: Urine Pregnancy Test. Perform a urine pregnancy test and record results in the chart provided.

CHART	
Date	

Copyright © 2008, 2004, 2000, 1995, 1990 by Saunders, an imprint of Elsevier Inc. All rights reserved.

Chart	
Date	

Copyright © 2008, 2004, 2000, 1995, 1990 by Saunders, an imprint of Elsevier Inc. All rights reserved.

CHARTING EXAMPLE

Multistix® 10 SG Reagent Strips for Urinalysis

PATIENT

DATE TIME

LEUKOCYTES	NEGATIVE ☐		TRACE ☐	SMALL + ☐	MODERATE ++ ☐	LARGE +++ ☐	
NITRITE	NEGATIVE ☐		POSITIVE ☐	POSITIVE ☐	(Any degree of uniform pink color is found)		
UROBILINOGEN	NORMAL 0.2 ☐	NORMAL 1 ☐	mg/dL 2 ☐	4 ☐	8 ☐	(1mg = approx. 1 BU)	
PROTEIN	NEGATIVE ☐	TRACE ☐	mg/dL 30 * ☐	100 ++ ☐	300 +++ ☐	2000 OR MORE ☐	
pH	5.0 ☐	6.0 ☐	6.5 ☐	7.0 ☐	7.5 ☐	8.0 ☐	8.5 ☐
BLOOD	NEGATIVE ☐	NON-HEMOLYZED TRACE ☐	NON-HEMOLYZED MODERATE ☐	HEMOLYZED TRACE ☐	SMALL + ☐	MODERATE ++ ☐	LARGE +++ ☐
SPECIFIC GRAVITY	1.000 ☐	1.006 ☐	1.010 ☐	1.015 ☐	1.020 ☐	1.025 ☐	1.030 ☐
KETONE	NEGATIVE ☐	mg/dL	TRACE 5 ☐	SMALL 15 ☐	MODERATE 40 ☐	LARGE 80 ☐	LARGE 160 ☐
BILIRUBIN	NEGATIVE ☐		SMALL + ☐	MODERATE ++ ☐	LARGE +++ ☐		
GLUCOSE	NEGATIVE ☐	g/L (%) mg/dL	1/10 tr.) 100 ☐	1/6 250 ☐	1/2 500 ☐	1 1000 ☐	2 or more 2000 or more ☐

(Modified and printed by permission of Siemens Medical Solutions Diagnostic, Tarrytown, NY, 10591.)

CHARTING EXAMPLE

Multistix® 10 SG Reagent Strips for Urinalysis

PATIENT

DATE TIME

LEUKOCYTES	NEGATIVE ☐		TRACE ☐	SMALL + ☐	MODERATE ++ ☐	LARGE +++ ☐	
NITRITE	NEGATIVE ☐		POSITIVE ☐	POSITIVE ☐	(Any degree of uniform pink color is found)		
UROBILINOGEN	NORMAL 0.2 ☐	NORMAL 1 ☐	mg/dL 2 ☐	4 ☐	8 ☐	(1mg = approx. 1 BU)	
PROTEIN	NEGATIVE ☐	TRACE ☐	mg/dL 30 * ☐	100 ++ ☐	300 +++ ☐	2000 OR MORE ☐	
pH	5.0 ☐	6.0 ☐	6.5 ☐	7.0 ☐	7.5 ☐	8.0 ☐	8.5 ☐
BLOOD	NEGATIVE ☐	NON-HEMOLYZED TRACE ☐	NON-HEMOLYZED MODERATE ☐	HEMOLYZED TRACE ☐	SMALL + ☐	MODERATE ++ ☐	LARGE +++ ☐
SPECIFIC GRAVITY	1.000 ☐	1.006 ☐	1.010 ☐	1.015 ☐	1.020 ☐	1.025 ☐	1.030 ☐
KETONE	NEGATIVE ☐	mg/dL	TRACE 5 ☐	SMALL 15 ☐	MODERATE 40 ☐	LARGE 80 ☐	LARGE 160 ☐
BILIRUBIN	NEGATIVE ☐		SMALL + ☐	MODERATE ++ ☐	LARGE +++ ☐		
GLUCOSE	NEGATIVE ☐	g/L (%) mg/dL	1/10 tr.) 100 ☐	1/6 250 ☐	1/2 500 ☐	1 1000 ☐	2 or more 2000 or more ☐

(Modified and printed by permission of Siemens Medical Solutions Diagnostic, Tarrytown, NY, 10591.)

Copyright © 2008, 2004, 2000, 1995, 1990 by Saunders, an imprint of Elsevier Inc. All rights reserved.

CHARTING EXAMPLE

Multistix® 10 SG Reagent Strips for Urinalysis

PATIENT

DATE TIME

LEUKOCYTES	NEGATIVE ☐		TRACE ☐	SMALL + ☐	MODERATE ++ ☐	LARGE +++ ☐	
NITRITE	NEGATIVE ☐		POSITIVE ☐	POSITIVE ☐	(Any degree of uniform pink color is found)		
UROBILINOGEN	NORMAL 0.2 ☐	NORMAL 1 ☐	mg/dL 2 ☐	4 ☐	8 ☐	(1mg = approx. 1 BU)	
PROTEIN	NEGATIVE ☐	TRACE ☐	mg/dL 30 * ☐	100 ++ ☐	300 +++ ☐	2000 OR MORE ☐	
pH	5.0 ☐	6.0 ☐	6.5 ☐	7.0 ☐	7.5 ☐	8.0 ☐	8.5 ☐
BLOOD	NEGATIVE ☐	NON-HEMOLYZED TRACE ☐	NON-HEMOLYZED MODERATE ☐	HEMOLYZED TRACE ☐	SMALL + ☐	MODERATE ++ ☐	LARGE +++ ☐
SPECIFIC GRAVITY	1.000 ☐	1.006 ☐	1.010 ☐	1.015 ☐	1.020 ☐	1.025 ☐	1.030 ☐
KETONE	NEGATIVE ☐	mg/dL	TRACE 5 ☐	SMALL 15 ☐	MODERATE 40 ☐	LARGE 80 ☐	LARGE 160 ☐
BILIRUBIN	NEGATIVE ☐		SMALL + ☐	MODERATE ++ ☐	LARGE +++ ☐		
GLUCOSE	NEGATIVE ☐	g/L (%) mg/dL	1/10 tr.) 100 ☐	1/6 250 ☐	1/2 500 ☐	1 1000 ☐	2 or more 2000 or more ☐

(Modified and printed by permission of Siemens Medical Solutions Diagnostic, Tarrytown, NY, 10591.)

CHARTING EXAMPLE

Multistix® 10 SG Reagent Strips for Urinalysis

PATIENT

DATE TIME

LEUKOCYTES	NEGATIVE ☐		TRACE ☐	SMALL + ☐	MODERATE ++ ☐	LARGE +++ ☐	
NITRITE	NEGATIVE ☐		POSITIVE ☐	POSITIVE ☐	(Any degree of uniform pink color is found)		
UROBILINOGEN	NORMAL 0.2 ☐	NORMAL 1 ☐	mg/dL 2 ☐	4 ☐	8 ☐	(1mg = approx. 1 BU)	
PROTEIN	NEGATIVE ☐	TRACE ☐	mg/dL 30 * ☐	100 ++ ☐	300 +++ ☐	2000 OR MORE ☐	
pH	5.0 ☐	6.0 ☐	6.5 ☐	7.0 ☐	7.5 ☐	8.0 ☐	8.5 ☐
BLOOD	NEGATIVE ☐	NON-HEMOLYZED TRACE ☐	NON-HEMOLYZED MODERATE ☐	HEMOLYZED TRACE ☐	SMALL + ☐	MODERATE ++ ☐	LARGE +++ ☐
SPECIFIC GRAVITY	1.000 ☐	1.006 ☐	1.010 ☐	1.015 ☐	1.020 ☐	1.025 ☐	1.030 ☐
KETONE	NEGATIVE ☐	mg/dL	TRACE 5 ☐	SMALL 15 ☐	MODERATE 40 ☐	LARGE 80 ☐	LARGE 160 ☐
BILIRUBIN	NEGATIVE ☐		SMALL + ☐	MODERATE ++ ☐	LARGE +++ ☐		
GLUCOSE	NEGATIVE ☐	g/L (%) mg/dL	1/10 tr.) 100 ☐	1/6 250 ☐	1/2 500 ☐	1 1000 ☐	2 or more 2000 or more ☐

(Modified and printed by permission of Siemens Medical Solutions Diagnostic, Tarrytown, NY, 10591.)

Copyright © 2008, 2004, 2000, 1995, 1990 by Saunders, an imprint of Elsevier Inc. All rights reserved.

EVALUATION OF COMPETENCY

Procedure 16-1: Clean-Catch Midstream Specimen Collection Instructions

Name: ______________________________ Date: ____________

Evaluated By: ______________________________ Score: ____________

Performance Objective

Outcome:	Instruct a patient in the procedure for collecting a clean-catch midstream urine specimen.
Conditions:	Given the following: sterile specimen container and personal antiseptic towelettes, and tissues.
Standards:	Time: 10 minutes. Student completed procedure in ____ minutes.
	Accuracy: Satisfactory score on the Performance Evaluation Checklist.

Performance Evaluation Checklist

Trial 1	Trial 2	Point Value	*Performance Standards*
		•	Sanitized hands.
		•	Greeted the patient and introduced yourself.
		•	Identified the patient and explained the procedure.
		•	Assembled equipment.
		•	Labeled specimen container.
			Instructed the female patient by telling her to:
		•	Wash hands and open antiseptic towelettes.
		•	Remove lid from specimen container without touching inside of container or lid.
		•	Pull down undergarments and sit on the toilet.
		•	Expose the urinary meatus by spreading the labia apart with one hand.
		•	Cleanse each side of the urinary meatus with a front-to-back motion using a separate towelette on each side of the meatus.
		▷	Explained why a front-to-back motion should be used.
		•	After use, discard each towelette in toilet.
		•	Cleanse directly across the meatus using a third towelette and discard it.
		•	Void a small amount of urine into the toilet, while continuing to hold the labia apart.
		▷	Explained the purpose of voiding into the toilet.
		•	Collect the next amount of urine by voiding into the sterile container without touching the inside of the container.
		•	Fill container approximately half full with urine.
		•	Void the last amount of urine into the toilet.
		•	Replace specimen container lid.

Copyright © 2008, 2004, 2000, 1995, 1990 by Saunders, an imprint of Elsevier Inc. All rights reserved.

Trial 1	*Trial 2*	*Point Value*	*Performance Standards*
		•	Wipe area dry with a tissue, flush the toilet, and wash hands.
			Instructed the male patient by telling him to:
		•	Wash hands and open antiseptic towelettes, and remove lid from specimen container.
		•	Pull down undergarments and stand in front of toilet.
		•	Retract the foreskin of the penis if uncircumcised.
		•	Cleanse area around the meatus and the urethral opening by wiping each side of the meatus with a separate antiseptic towelette.
		•	Cleanse directly across the meatus using a third antiseptic towelette.
		•	Discard each towelette in the toilet after use.
		•	Void a small amount of urine into the toilet.
		•	Collect the next amount of urine by voiding into the sterile container without touching the inside of the container.
		•	Fill container approximately half full with urine.
		•	Void the last amount of urine into the toilet.
		•	Replace lid on specimen container.
		•	Wipe area dry with a tissue and wash hands.
			Performed the following:
		•	Provided patient with instructions on what to do with specimen.
		•	Completed a laboratory requisition, if required.
		•	Charted the procedure correctly.
		•	Tested specimen or prepared it for transport to an outside laboratory.
		*	Completed the procedure within 10 minutes.
			TOTALS

CHART	
Date	

Copyright © 2008, 2004, 2000, 1995, 1990 by Saunders, an imprint of Elsevier Inc. All rights reserved.

Evaluation of Student Performance

EVALUATION CRITERIA			COMMENTS
Symbol	Category	Point Value	
*	Critical Step	16 points	
•	Essential Step	6 points	
▷	Theory Question	2 points	
Score calculation: 100 points – ______ points missed ____ Score Satisfactory score: 85 or above			

AAMA/CAAHEP Competency Achieved:

☑ III. C. 3. b. (2) (d): Instruct patients in the collection of a clean-catch midstream urine specimen.

Copyright © 2008, 2004, 2000, 1995, 1990 by Saunders, an imprint of Elsevier Inc. All rights reserved.

Notes

Copyright © 2008, 2004, 2000, 1995, 1990 by Saunders, an imprint of Elsevier Inc. All rights reserved.

EVALUATION OF COMPETENCY

Procedure 16-2: Collection of a 24-Hour Urine Specimen

Name: ______________________________ Date: ______________

Evaluated By: ______________________________ Score: ______________

Performance Objective

Outcome:	Instruct a patient in the procedure for collecting a 24-hour urine specimen.
Conditions:	Given a large urine collection container, written instructions, and a laboratory requisition.
Standards:	Time: 5 minutes. Student completed procedure in ____ minutes.
	Accuracy: Satisfactory score on the Performance Evaluation Checklist.

Performance Evaluation Checklist

Trial 1	*Trial 2*	*Point Value*	*Performance Standards*
		•	Sanitized hands.
		•	Assembled equipment.
		•	Greeted and introduced yourself.
		•	Identified patient and explained the procedure.
		•	Assembled equipment.
		•	Labeled specimen container.
			Instructed the patient in the collection of the specimen:
		•	Empty your bladder when you get up in the morning.
		•	Make a note of what time it is and write it down.
		•	The next time you need to urinate, void the urine into the plastic container.
		•	Tightly screw the lid onto the container.
		•	Store the container in the refrigerator or in an ice chest.
		•	Repeat these steps each time you urinate.
		•	Collect all of your urine in a 24-hour period.
		▷	Stated when the patient must start the collection process again from the beginning.
		•	On the following morning, get up at the same time.
		•	Void into the container for the last time.
		•	Put the lid on the container tightly.
		•	Return the urine collection container to the office the same morning as completing the test.

Copyright © 2008, 2004, 2000, 1995, 1990 by Saunders, an imprint of Elsevier Inc. All rights reserved.

Trial 1	Trial 2	Point Value	*Performance Standards*
		•	Provided the patient with the collection container and written instructions.
		•	Charted instructions given to the patient in his or her medical record.
			Processing the specimen:
		•	Asked the patient if there were any problems when he or she returned the collection container.
		▷	Explained what should be done if the specimen was undercollected or overcollected.
		•	Prepared the specimen for transport to the laboratory.
		•	Completed a laboratory request form.
		•	Charted the results correctly.
		*	Completed the procedure within 5 minutes.
			TOTALS

CHART	
Date	

Evaluation of Student Performance

EVALUATION CRITERIA			COMMENTS
Symbol	Category	Point Value	
*	Critical Step	16 points	
•	Essential Step	6 points	
▷	Theory Question	2 points	

Score calculation: 100 points
– ____ points missed
____ Score
Satisfactory score: 85 or above

AAMA/CAAHEP Competency Achieved:

☑ III. C. 3. c. (3) (b): Instruct individuals according to their needs.

Copyright © 2008, 2004, 2000, 1995, 1990 by Saunders, an imprint of Elsevier Inc. All rights reserved.

EVALUATION OF COMPETENCY

Procedure 16-A: Assessing Color and Appearance of a Urine Specimen

Name: ______________________________ Date: ______________

Evaluated By: ______________________________ Score: ______________

Performance Objective

Outcome:	Assess the color and appearance of a urine specimen.
Conditions:	Given a transparent container and a urine specimen.
Standards:	Time: 5 minutes. Student completed procedure in ____ minutes.
	Accuracy: Satisfactory score on the Performance Evaluation Checklist.

Performance Evaluation Checklist

Trial 1	*Trial 2*	*Point Value*	*Performance Standards*
			Color
		•	Sanitized hands and applied gloves.
		•	Transferred urine specimen to a transparent container.
		•	Assessed the color of the urine specimen.
		*	The assessment was identical to the evaluator's assessment.
		•	Charted the results correctly.
			Appearance
		•	Assessed the appearance of the urine specimen in the transparent container.
		*	Confirmed that the assessment was identical to the evaluator's assessment.
		•	Charted the results correctly.
		•	Properly disposed of urine specimen.
		•	Sanitized hands and removed gloves.
		*	Completed the procedure within 5 minutes.
			TOTALS

CHART	
Date	

Copyright © 2008, 2004, 2000, 1995, 1990 by Saunders, an imprint of Elsevier Inc. All rights reserved.

Evaluation of Student Performance

EVALUATION CRITERIA			COMMENTS
Symbol	Category	Point Value	
*	Critical Step	16 points	
•	Essential Step	6 points	
▷	Theory Question	2 points	
Score calculation: 100 points – ______ points missed ____ Score Satisfactory score: 85 or above			

AAMA/CAAHEP Competency Achieved:

☑ III. C. 3. b. (3) (c) (i): Perform urinalysis.

Copyright © 2008, 2004, 2000, 1995, 1990 by Saunders, an imprint of Elsevier Inc. All rights reserved.

EVALUATION OF COMPETENCY

Procedures 16-3 and 16-4: Measuring Specific Gravity of Urine: Refractometer Method and Quality Control: Calibration of the Refractometer

Name: ______________________________ Date: ______________

Evaluated By: ______________________________ Score: ______________

Performance Objective

Outcome:	Calibrate the refractometer and measure the specific gravity of a urine specimen.
Conditions:	Given the following: disposable gloves, refractometer, urine specimen, disposable pipet, lint-free tissues, antiseptic wipe, distilled water, and a waste container.
Standards:	Time: 5 minutes. Student completed procedure(s) in ____ minutes.
	Accuracy: Satisfactory score on the Performance Evaluation Checklist.

Performance Evaluation Checklist

Trial 1	*Trial 2*	*Point Value*	*Performance Standards*
			Measuring Specific Gravity
		•	Sanitized hands.
		•	Assembled equipment.
		•	Calibrated the refractometer.
		•	Applied gloves.
		•	Prepared the urine specimen.
		•	Mixed the urine specimen with the pipet.
		▷	Explained why the specimen must be well mixed.
		•	Withdrew a small amount of urine into the pipet.
		•	Held the pipet in a vertical position.
		•	Placed drop of urine on the surface of the prism of the refractometer.
		•	Pointed the refractometer toward a light source.
		•	Rotated eyepiece to bring the calibrated scale clearly into view.
		•	Read the value on the scale at the boundary line between the light and dark areas.
		*	The reading was within ± 0.002 of the evaluator's reading.
		•	Cleaned the prism with a lint-free tissue.
		•	Disinfected the prism surface with an alcohol wipe.
		•	Removed gloves and sanitized hands.
		•	Charted results correctly.

Copyright © 2008, 2004, 2000, 1995, 1990 by Saunders, an imprint of Elsevier Inc. All rights reserved.

Trial 1	Trial 2	Point Value	Performance Standards
			Calibration of the Refractometer
		•	Placed a drop of distilled water on the surface of the prism.
		•	Pointed the refractometer toward a light source.
		•	Rotated the eyepiece to bring the calibrated scale clearly into view.
		•	Read the value on the scale at the boundary line between the light and dark areas.
		•	Determined if the calibration is correct.
		▷	Stated the value of the correct calibration.
		•	Corrected the calibration if necessary.
		▷	Explained how the calibration is corrected.
		•	Cleaned prism surface with a lint-free tissue.
		✶	Completed the procedure within 5 minutes.
			TOTALS

CHART	
Date	

Evaluation of Student Performance

EVALUATION CRITERIA			COMMENTS
Symbol	Category	Point Value	
✶	Critical Step	16 points	
•	Essential Step	6 points	
▷	Theory Question	2 points	
Score calculation: 100 points – ____ points missed ____ Score Satisfactory score: 85 or above			

AAMA/CAAHEP Competency Achieved:

☑ III. C. 3. b. (3) (c) (i): Perform urinalysis.
☑ III. C. 3. c. (4) (d): Use methods of quality control.

Copyright © 2008, 2004, 2000, 1995, 1990 by Saunders, an imprint of Elsevier Inc. All rights reserved.

EVALUATION OF COMPETENCY

Procedure 16-5: Chemical Testing of Urine with the Multistix 10 SG Reagent Strip

Name: ______________________________ Date: ______________

Evaluated By: ______________________________ Score: ______________

Performance Objective

Outcome: Perform a chemical assessment of a urine specimen.

Conditions: Given the following: disposable gloves, Multistix 10 SG reagent strips, urine container, laboratory report form, and a waste container.

Standards: Time: 5 minutes. Student completed procedure in ____ minutes.

Accuracy: Satisfactory score on the Performance Evaluation Checklist.

Performance Evaluation Checklist

Trial 1	*Trial 2*	*Point Value*	*Performance Standards*
		•	If necessary, performed a quality control procedure.
		▷	Stated when a quality control procedure should be performed.
		•	Obtained a freshly voided urine specimen from patient.
		▷	Explained why the container used to collect specimen should be clean.
		•	Sanitized hands.
		•	Assembled equipment.
		•	Checked expiration date of the reagent strips.
		▷	Stated why expiration date should be checked.
		•	Applied gloves.
		•	Removed a reagent strip from container and recapped immediately.
		▷	Explained why container should be recapped immediately.
		•	Did not touch the test areas with fingers.
		•	Explained why the test areas should not be touched with fingers.
		•	Mixed the urine specimen thoroughly.
		•	Removed the lid and completely immersed the reagent strip in urine specimen.
		•	Removed the strip immediately and ran the edge against the rim of urine container. Started the timer.
		▷	Explained why excess urine should be removed from the strip.
		•	Held the reagent strip in a horizontal position and placed it as close as possible to the corresponding color blocks on color chart.
		▷	Explained why the strip should be held in a horizontal position.

Copyright © 2008, 2004, 2000, 1995, 1990 by Saunders, an imprint of Elsevier Inc. All rights reserved.

Trial 1	Trial 2	Point Value	Performance Standards
		•	Read the results at the exact reading times specified on color chart.
		▷	Explained why the results must be read at specified times.
		✶	The results were identical to the evaluator's results.
		•	Disposed of the strip in a regular waste container.
		•	Removed gloves and sanitized hands.
		•	Charted the results correctly.
		✶	Completed the procedure within 5 minutes.
			TOTALS

CHART	
Date	

Evaluation of Student Performance

EVALUATION CRITERIA			COMMENTS
Symbol	Category	Point Value	
✶	Critical Step	16 points	
•	Essential Step	6 points	
▷	Theory Question	2 points	
Score calculation: 100 points – ____ points missed ____ Score Satisfactory score: 85 or above			

AAMA/CAAHEP Competency Achieved:

☑ III. C. 3. b. (3) (c) (i): Perform urinalysis.
☑ III. C. 3. c. (4) (d): Use methods of quality control.

Copyright © 2008, 2004, 2000, 1995, 1990 by Saunders, an imprint of Elsevier Inc. All rights reserved.

CHARTING EXAMPLE

Multistix® 10 SG Reageant Strips for Urinalysis

PATIENT

DATE TIME

LEUKOCYTES	NEGATIVE ☐		TRACE ☐	SMALL + ☐	MODERATE ++ ☐	LARGE +++ ☐	
NITRITE	NEGATIVE ☐		POSITIVE ☐	POSITIVE ☐	(Any degree of uniform pink color is found)		
UROBILINOGEN	NORMAL 0.2 ☐	NORMAL 1 ☐	mg/dL 2 ☐	4 ☐	8 ☐ (1mg = approx. 1 BU)		
PROTEIN	NEGATIVE ☐	TRACE ☐	mg/dL 30 + ☐	100 ++ ☐	300 +++ ☐	2000 OR MORE ☐	
pH	5.0 ☐	6.0 ☐	6.5 ☐	7.0 ☐	7.5 ☐	8.0 ☐	8.5 ☐
BLOOD	NEGATIVE ☐	NON-HEMOLYZED TRACE ☐	NON-HEMOLYZED MODERATE ☐	HEMOLYZED TRACE ☐	SMALL + ☐	MODERATE ++ ☐	LARGE +++ ☐
SPECIFIC GRAVITY	1.000 ☐	1.006 ☐	1.010 ☐	1.015 ☐	1.020 ☐	1.025 ☐	1.030 ☐
KETONE	NEGATIVE ☐	mg/dL	TRACE 5 ☐	SMALL 15 ☐	MODERATE 40 ☐	LARGE 80 ☐	LARGE 160 ☐
BILIRUBIN	NEGATIVE ☐		SMALL + ☐	MODERATE ++ ☐	LARGE +++ ☐		
GLUCOSE	NEGATIVE ☐	g/L (%) mg/dL	1/10 tr.) 100 ☐	1/6 250 ☐	1/2 500 ☐	1 1000 ☐	2 or more 2000 or more ☐

(Modified and printed by permission of Siemens Medical Solutions Diagnostic, Tarrytown, NY, 10591.)

CHARTING EXAMPLE

Multistix® 10 SG Reageant Strips for Urinalysis

PATIENT

DATE TIME

LEUKOCYTES	NEGATIVE ☐		TRACE ☐	SMALL + ☐	MODERATE ++ ☐	LARGE +++ ☐	
NITRITE	NEGATIVE ☐		POSITIVE ☐	POSITIVE ☐	(Any degree of uniform pink color is found)		
UROBILINOGEN	NORMAL 0.2 ☐	NORMAL 1 ☐	mg/dL 2 ☐	4 ☐	8 ☐ (1mg = approx. 1 BU)		
PROTEIN	NEGATIVE ☐	TRACE ☐	mg/dL 30 + ☐	100 ++ ☐	300 +++ ☐	2000 OR MORE ☐	
pH	5.0 ☐	6.0 ☐	6.5 ☐	7.0 ☐	7.5 ☐	8.0 ☐	8.5 ☐
BLOOD	NEGATIVE ☐	NON-HEMOLYZED TRACE ☐	NON-HEMOLYZED MODERATE ☐	HEMOLYZED TRACE ☐	SMALL + ☐	MODERATE ++ ☐	LARGE +++ ☐
SPECIFIC GRAVITY	1.000 ☐	1.006 ☐	1.010 ☐	1.015 ☐	1.020 ☐	1.025 ☐	1.030 ☐
KETONE	NEGATIVE ☐	mg/dL	TRACE 5 ☐	SMALL 15 ☐	MODERATE 40 ☐	LARGE 80 ☐	LARGE 160 ☐
BILIRUBIN	NEGATIVE ☐		SMALL + ☐	MODERATE ++ ☐	LARGE +++ ☐		
GLUCOSE	NEGATIVE ☐	g/L (%) mg/dL	1/10 tr.) 100 ☐	1/6 250 ☐	1/2 500 ☐	1 1000 ☐	2 or more 2000 or more ☐

(Modified and printed by permission of Siemens Medical Solutions Diagnostic, Tarrytown, NY, 10591.)

Copyright © 2008, 2004, 2000, 1995, 1990 by Saunders, an imprint of Elsevier Inc. All rights reserved.

Notes

Copyright © 2008, 2004, 2000, 1995, 1990 by Saunders, an imprint of Elsevier Inc. All rights reserved.

EVALUATION OF COMPETENCY

Procedure 16-6: Microscopic Examination of Urine: Kova Method

Name: ______________________________ Date: ______________

Evaluated By: ______________________________ Score: ______________

Performance Objective

Outcome:	Prepare a urine specimen for microscopic analysis and examine the specimen under the microscope.
Conditions:	Given the following: disposable gloves; first-voided morning urine specimen; Kova urine centrifuge tube, cap, pipet, slide, and stain; test tube rack; urine centrifuge; mechanical stage microscope; and waste container.
Standards:	Time: 15 minutes. Student completed procedure in ____ minutes. Accuracy: Satisfactory score on the Performance Evaluation Checklist.

Performance Evaluation Checklist

Trial 1	Trial 2	Point Value	*Performance Standards*
		•	Sanitized hands.
		•	Assembled equipment.
		•	Applied gloves.
		•	Mixed urine specimen with pipet.
		▷	Stated the purpose of mixing the specimen.
		•	Poured urine specimen into urine centrifuge tube to the 12 ml mark.
		•	Capped the tube.
		•	Centrifuged specimen for 5 minutes.
		▷	Stated the purpose of centrifuging the specimen.
		•	Removed the tube from the centrifuge without disturbing the sediment.
		•	Removed the cap.
		•	Inserted Kova pipet into the urine tube and seated it firmly.
		•	Poured off the supernatant fluid.
		•	Removed pipet from the tube.
		•	Added one drop of Kova stain to the tube.
		▷	Stated the purpose of the stain.
		•	Placed pipet back in tube and mixed specimen thoroughly.
		•	Placed urine tube in test tube rack.
		•	Transferred a sample of the specimen to the Kova slide.

Copyright © 2008, 2004, 2000, 1995, 1990 by Saunders, an imprint of Elsevier Inc. All rights reserved.

Trial 1	Trial 2	Point Value	Performance Standards
		•	Did not overfill or underfill the well of the Kova slide.
		•	Placed pipet in the urine tube.
		•	Allowed specimen to sit for 1 minute.
		▷	Explained the purpose of allowing the specimen to sit 1 minute.
		•	Properly focused the specimen under low power.
		•	Examined the sediment under low power to scan for the presence of casts.
		•	Properly focused the specimen under high power.
		•	Examined the urine sediment with the high-power objective.
		•	Identified the specific type of casts (if present).
		•	Examined the sediment for the presence of smaller structures (red blood cells, white blood cells, bacteria, or crystals).
		•	Examined 10 to 15 high-power fields.
		•	Calculated an average of the high-power fields.
		*	The calculation was performed without a mathematical error.
		•	Turned off the light source.
		•	Removed the slide from the stage.
		•	Disposed of the slide and pipet in a regular waste container.
		•	Flushed the remaining urine down the sink.
		•	Capped the empty urine tube and disposed of it in a regular waste container.
		•	Removed gloves and sanitized hands.
		•	Charted the results correctly.
		*	Completed the procedure within 15 minutes.
			TOTALS

CHART	
Date	

Copyright © 2008, 2004, 2000, 1995, 1990 by Saunders, an imprint of Elsevier Inc. All rights reserved.

Evaluation of Student Performance

EVALUATION CRITERIA			COMMENTS
Symbol	Category	Point Value	
✶	Critical Step	16 points	
•	Essential Step	6 points	
▷	Theory Question	2 points	
Score calculation: 100 points – _____ points missed ____ Score Satisfactory score: 85 or above			

AAMA/CAAHEP Competency Achieved:

☑ III. C. 3. b. (3) (c) (i): Perform urinalysis.
☑ III. C. 3. c. (4) (d): Use methods of quality control.

Copyright © 2008, 2004, 2000, 1995, 1990 by Saunders, an imprint of Elsevier Inc. All rights reserved.

Notes

Copyright © 2008, 2004, 2000, 1995, 1990 by Saunders, an imprint of Elsevier Inc. All rights reserved.

EVALUATION OF COMPETENCY

Procedure 16-7: Performing a Rapid Urine Culture Test

Name: ______________________________ Date: ______________

Evaluated By: ______________________________ Score: ______________

Performance Objective

Outcome:	Perform a rapid urine culture test.
Conditions:	Given the following: disposable gloves, rapid urine culture kit, clean-catch midstream urine specimen, incubator, biohazard waste container.
Standards:	Time: 5 minutes. Student completed procedure in ____ minutes.
	Accuracy: Satisfactory score on the Performance Evaluation Checklist.

Performance Evaluation Checklist

Trial 1	*Trial 2*	*Point Value*	*Performance Standards*
			Preparing the Specimen
		•	Sanitized hands.
		•	Assembled equipment.
		•	Checked the expiration date on the rapid culture test.
		•	Labeled the vial with the patient's name and date and time of inoculation.
		•	Applied gloves.
		•	Removed the slide from the vial.
		•	Did not touch the culture media.
		•	Completely immersed the slide in urine specimen.
		•	Allowed excess urine to drain from the slide.
		•	Immediately replaced the slide in the vial.
		•	Screwed the cap on loosely.
		•	Placed the vial upright in an incubator.
		▷	Explained why the slide should not remain in the incubator for more than 24 hours.
			Reading Test Results
		•	Applied gloves.
		•	Removed the vial from the incubator.
		•	Removed the slide from the vial.
		•	Compared the slide with the reference chart.
		•	Read and interpreted the results.

Copyright © 2008, 2004, 2000, 1995, 1990 by Saunders, an imprint of Elsevier Inc. All rights reserved.

Trial 1	Trial 2	Point Value	Performance Standards
		✶	The results were identical to the evaluator's results.
		•	Returned the slide to the vial and screwed on the cap.
		•	Disposed of the test in a biohazard waste container.
		•	Removed gloves and sanitized hands.
		•	Charted the results correctly.
		✶	Completed the procedure within 5 minutes.
			TOTALS

CHART	
Date	

Evaluation of Student Performance

EVALUATION CRITERIA			COMMENTS
Symbol	Category	Point Value	
✶	Critical Step	16 points	
•	Essential Step	6 points	
▷	Theory Question	2 points	
Score calculation: 100 points – ____ points missed ____ Score Satisfactory score: 85 or above			

AAMA/CAAHEP Competency Achieved:

☑ III. C. 3. b. (3) (c) (v): Perform microbiology testing.
☑ III. C. 3. c. (4) (d): Use methods of quality control.

Copyright © 2008, 2004, 2000, 1995, 1990 by Saunders, an imprint of Elsevier Inc. All rights reserved.

EVALUATION OF COMPETENCY

Procedure 16-8: Performing a Urine Pregnancy Test

Name: ______________________________ Date: ______________

Evaluated By: ______________________________ Score: ______________

Performance Objective

Outcome: Perform a urine pregnancy test.

Conditions: Given the following: disposable gloves, urine pregnancy testing kit, first-voided morning urine specimen, waste container.

Standards: Time: 5 minutes. Student completed procedure in ____ minutes.

Accuracy: Satisfactory score on the Performance Evaluation Checklist.

Performance Evaluation Checklist

Trial 1	*Trial 2*	*Point Value*	*Performance Standards*
		•	Sanitized hands.
		•	Assembled equipment.
		•	Checked the expiration date on the pregnancy test.
		▷	Explained why the expiration date should be checked.
		•	If necessary, ran controls on the pregnancy test.
		▷	Stated when controls should be run.
		•	Applied gloves.
		•	Mixed the urine specimen.
		•	Removed the test cassette from its pouch.
		•	Placed the test cassette on a clean, dry, level surface.
		•	Added 3 drops of urine to the well on the test cassette.
		•	Disposed of the pipet in a regular waste container.
		•	Waited 3 minutes and read the results.
		•	Interpreted the test results.
		*	The results were identical to the evaluator's results.
		▷	Described the appearance of a positive and a negative test result.
		▷	Explained what should be done if a blue control line does not appear.
		•	Disposed of the test cassette in a regular waste container.
		•	Removed gloves and sanitized hands.

Copyright © 2008, 2004, 2000, 1995, 1990 by Saunders, an imprint of Elsevier Inc. All rights reserved.

		•	Charted the results correctly.
		✶	Completed the procedure within 5 minutes.
			TOTALS

CHART	
Date	

Evaluation of Student Performance

EVALUATION CRITERIA			COMMENTS
Symbol	Category	Point Value	
✶	Critical Step	16 points	
•	Essential Step	6 points	
▷	Theory Question	2 points	
Score calculation: 100 points –_____ points missed ____ Score Satisfactory score: 85 or above			

AAMA/CAAHEP Competency Achieved:

☑ III. C. 3. b. (4) (i): Screen and follow-up test results.
☑ III. C. 3. c. (4) (d): Use methods of quality control.

Copyright © 2008, 2004, 2000, 1995, 1990 by Saunders, an imprint of Elsevier Inc. All rights reserved.

17

Phlebotomy

CHAPTER ASSIGNMENTS

√ After Completing	Date Due	Textbook Page(s)	TEXTBOOK ASSIGNMENTS	Possible Points	Points You Earned
		628-673	Read Chapter 17: Phlebotomy		
		636 670	Read Case Study 1 Case Study 1 questions	5	
		639 670	Read Case Study 2 Case Study 2 questions	5	
		652 670	Read Case Study 3 Case Study 3 questions	5	
		671-672	Apply Your Knowledge questions	10	
			TOTAL POINTS		
√ After Completing	**Date Due**	**Study Guide Page(s)**	**STUDY GUIDE ASSIGNMENTS (CTA: Critical Thinking Activity)**	**Possible Points**	**Points You Earned**
		717	Pretest	10	
		718	Key Term Assessment	16	
		719-722	Evaluation of Learning questions	33	
		722	CTA A: Antecubital Veins	5	
			CD Activity: Chapter 17 Got Blood? (Record points earned)		
		722-723	CTA B: Venipuncture-Vacuum Tube Method	15	
		724	CTA C: Venipuncture Situations	7	
		724-725	CTA D: Separating Serum	6	
		725	CTA E: Skin Puncture	8	
		726	CTA F: Crossword Puzzle	21	
		717	Posttest	10	

Copyright © 2008, 2004, 2000, 1995, 1990 by Saunders, an imprint of Elsevier Inc. All rights reserved.

√ After Completing	Date Due	Study Guide Page(s)	STUDY GUIDE ASSIGNMENTS (CTA: Critical Thinking Activity)	Possible Points	Points You Earned
			ADDITIONAL ASSIGNMENTS		
			TOTAL POINTS		

Copyright © 2008, 2004, 2000, 1995, 1990 by Saunders, an imprint of Elsevier Inc. All rights reserved.

√ When Assigned By Your Instructor	Study Guide Page(s)	Practices Required	LABORATORY ASSIGNMENTS (Procedure Number and Name)	*Score
	727-728	5	**Practice for Competency** 17-1: Venipuncture—Vacuum Tube Method Textbook reference: pp. 641-645	
	729-731		**Evaluation of Competency** 17-1: Venipuncture—Vacuum Tube Method	*
	727-728	5	**Practice for Competency** 17-2: Venipuncture—Butterfly Method Textbook reference: pp. 647-651	
	733-736		**Evaluation of Competency** 17-2: Venipuncture—Butterfly Method	*
	727-728	5	**Practice for Competency** 17-3: Venipuncture—Syringe Method Textbook reference: pp. 653-655	
	737-739		**Evaluation of Competency** 17-3: Venipuncture—Syringe Method	*
	727-728	3	**Practice for Competency** 17-4: Separating Serum from Whole Blood Textbook reference: pp. 659-660	
	741-742		**Evaluation of Competency** 17-4: Separating Serum from Whole Blood	*
	727-728	3	**Practice for Competency** 17-5: Skin Puncture—Disposable Semiautomatic Lancet Device Textbook reference: pp. 664-666	
	743-744		**Evaluation of Competency** 17-5: Skin Puncture—Disposable Semiautomatic Lancet Device	*
	727-728	3	**Practice for Competency** 17-6: Skin Puncture—Reusable Semiautomatic Lancet Device Textbook reference: pp. 667-669	
	745-746		**Evaluation of Competency** 17-6: Skin Puncture—Reusable Semiautomatic Lancet Device	*
			ADDITIONAL ASSIGNMENTS	

Copyright © 2008, 2004, 2000, 1995, 1990 by Saunders, an imprint of Elsevier Inc. All rights reserved.

Notes

Copyright © 2008, 2004, 2000, 1995, 1990 by Saunders, an imprint of Elsevier Inc. All rights reserved.

Name ______________________________ Date ______________

PRETEST

True or False

_____ 1. An individual who collects blood specimens is known as a vampire.

_____ 2. The purpose of applying a tourniquet when performing venipuncture is to make the patient's veins stand out.

_____ 3. The tourniquet should be left on the patient's arm for at least 2 minutes before performing a venipuncture.

_____ 4. Serum is obtained from whole blood that has been centrifuged.

_____ 5. A 25-gauge needle is recommended for performing venipuncture.

_____ 6. The size of the evacuated tube used to obtain a venous blood specimen depends on the size of the patient's veins.

_____ 7. A correct order of draw for the vacuum-tube method of venipuncture is red, lavender, gray, and green.

_____ 8. Veins are most likely to collapse in patients with large veins and thick walls.

_____ 9. Hemolysis of a blood specimen results in inaccurate test results.

_____ 10. When obtaining a capillary specimen, the first drop of blood should be used for the test.

POSTTEST

True or False

_____ 1. Venous reflux can be prevented by filling the evacuated tube to the exhaustion of the vacuum.

_____ 2. If the tourniquet is applied too tightly, inaccurate test results may occur.

_____ 3. The median cubital vein is the best vein to use for venipuncture.

_____ 4. Upon standing, a blood specimen to which an anticoagulant has been added separates into plasma, buffy coat, and blood cells.

_____ 5. Whole blood is obtained by using a tube containing an anticoagulant.

_____ 6. An evacuated glass tube with a lavender stopper contains EDTA.

_____ 7. A red-stoppered tube is used to collect a blood specimen for most blood chemistries.

_____ 8. Not filling a tube to the exhaustion of the vacuum can result in hemolysis of the blood specimen.

_____ 9. If the needle is removed from the arm before removing the tourniquet, the evacuated tube will not fill completely.

_____ 10. If a fibrin clot forms in the serum layer of a blood specimen, it will lead to inaccurate test results.

Copyright © 2008, 2004, 2000, 1995, 1990 by Saunders, an imprint of Elsevier Inc. All rights reserved.

Term KEY TERM ASSESSMENT

Directions: Match each medical term with its definition.

_____ 1. Antecubital space

_____ 2. Anticoagulant

_____ 3. Buffy coat

_____ 4. Evacuated tube

_____ 5. Hematoma

_____ 6. Hemoconcentration

_____ 7. Hemolysis

_____ 8. Osteochondritis

_____ 9. Osteomyelitis

_____ 10. Phlebotomist

_____ 11. Phlebotomy

_____ 12. Plasma

_____ 13. Serum

_____ 14. Venipuncture

_____ 15. Venous reflux

_____ 16. Venous stasis

A. The liquid part of blood, consisting of a clear, yellowish fluid that makes up approximately 55% of the total blood volume
B. A substance that inhibits blood clotting
C. A health professional trained in the collection of blood specimens
D. The breakdown of blood cells
E. A closed glass or plastic tube that contains a premeasured vacuum
F. The temporary cessation or slowing of the venous blood flow
G. A thin, light-colored layer of white blood cells and platelets that lays between a top layer of plasma and a bottom layer of red blood cells when an anticoagulant has been added to a blood specimen
H. The surface of the arm in front of the elbow
I. Inflammation of bone and cartilage
J. An increase in the concentration of the nonfilterable blood components
K. Plasma from which the clotting factor fibrinogen has been removed
L. Incision of a vein for the removal or withdrawal of blood
M. Inflammation of the bone due to bacterial infection
N. A swelling or mass of coagulated blood caused by a break in a blood vessel
O. Puncturing of a vein
P. The backflow of blood (from an evacuated tube) into the patient's vein

Copyright © 2008, 2004, 2000, 1995, 1990 by Saunders, an imprint of Elsevier Inc. All rights reserved.

EVALUATION OF LEARNING

Directions: Fill in each blank with the correct answer.

1. List the three major areas of blood collection included in phlebotomy.

   ____

   ____

2. What is the purpose of performing a venipuncture?

   ____

   ____

3. List the three methods that can be used to perform a venipuncture.

   ____

   ____

   ____

4. What are the advantages of using the vacuum tube method of venipuncture?

   ____

   ____

5. When would the butterfly method of venipuncture be preferred over the vacuum tube method?

   ____

   ____

   ____

6. Explain how to prevent venous reflux.

   ____

   ____

7. What is the purpose of the tourniquet?

   ____

   ____

8. After locating a suitable vein for venipuncture, what three qualities should be determined with respect to the vein?

   ____

   ____

9. Why are the antecubital veins preferred for performing a venipuncture?

   ____

   ____

   ____

10. List four techniques that can be used to make veins more prominent.

   ____

   ____

   ____

   ____

Copyright © 2008, 2004, 2000, 1995, 1990 by Saunders, an imprint of Elsevier Inc. All rights reserved.

11. Why should the veins of the hand be used only as a last resort when performing a venipuncture?

____

____

____

12. How is a serum specimen obtained?

____

____

13. How is a whole blood specimen obtained?

____

____

14. List the three layers into which blood separates when it is mixed with an anticoagulant.

____

____

15. List the layers into which blood separates when an anticoagulant is not added to it.

____

____

16. List four OSHA safety precautions that must be followed when performing a venipuncture and separating serum or plasma from whole blood.

____

____

17. What is the range for the gauge and size of the needle used for the vacuum tube method of venipuncture?

____

____

18. What is the purpose of the flange on the plastic holder of the vacuum tube system?

____

____

19. What type of additive is present in each of the following evacuated tubes?

Red ______________________________

Lavender ______________________________

Gray ______________________________

Light blue ______________________________

Green ______________________________

20. What color stopper must be used to collect the blood specimen for each of the tests listed below?

Complete blood count ______________________________

Prothrombin time ______________________________

Glucose tolerance test ______________________________

Copyright © 2008, 2004, 2000, 1995, 1990 by Saunders, an imprint of Elsevier Inc. All rights reserved.

Most blood chemistry tests ____________________

Blood gas determinations ____________________

21. Why is it important to use the correct order of draw when performing a venipuncture?

22. Why is it important to mix a tube containing an anticoagulant immediately after drawing it?

23. What is the range for the gauge and size of needle used for the butterfly method of venipuncture?

24. List four ways to prevent a blood specimen from becoming hemolyzed.

25. List examples of dissolved substances contained in the serum of blood.

26. What is the purpose of performing laboratory tests on serum?

27. List the proper size tube that must be used to obtain the following serum specimens.

    2 ml of serum ____________________

    6 ml of serum ____________________

    4 ml of serum ____________________

28. What is a fibrin clot and why should it be avoided in a serum specimen?

29. How does a serum separator tube function in the collection of a serum specimen?

Copyright © 2008, 2004, 2000, 1995, 1990 by Saunders, an imprint of Elsevier Inc. All rights reserved.

30. List four types of solutes contained in plasma.

____

____

____

____

31. What is the preferred site for a skin puncture for the following individuals?
    a. Adult ______________________________
    b. Infant ______________________________

32. List two examples of microcollection devices.

____

____

33. Why should a finger puncture not be performed on the index finger?

____

____

CRITICAL THINKING ACTIVITIES

A. ANTECUBITAL VEINS

Practice palpating the antecubital veins on at least five classmates. Use a tourniquet applied to each person's arm and ask the individual to clench his or her fist. Record the individual's name and which vein would be considered the best to use on each person when performing venipuncture.

	NAME	SUITABLE VEIN
1.		
2.		
3.		
4.		
5.		

B. VENIPUNCTURE—VACUUM TUBE METHOD

Using the principles outlined in the vacuum tube venipuncture procedure, state what might happen under the following circumstances:

1. An evacuated tube is used that is past its expiration date.

____

____

2. The vacuum tube is not labeled.

____

____

3. The tourniquet is not applied tightly enough.

____

____

Copyright © 2008, 2004, 2000, 1995, 1990 by Saunders, an imprint of Elsevier Inc. All rights reserved.

4. The tourniquet is left on for more than 1 minute.

5. The area that has just been cleansed with an antiseptic is not allowed to dry before the venipuncture is made.

6. The evacuated tube is inserted past the indentation in the plastic holder before the vein is entered.

7. An angle of less than 15 degrees is used when performing venipuncture.

8. An angle of more than 15 degrees is used when performing venipuncture.

9. The needle is moved after inserting it.

10. Venous reflux occurs when using an EDTA evacuated tube.

11. The vacuum tube is not allowed to fill to the exhaustion of the vacuum.

12. The needle is removed from the arm before the tourniquet has been removed.

13. A gauze pad is not placed over the puncture site before removing the needle.

14. The patient bends the arm at the elbow after the needle is removed.

15. The patient lifts a heavy object after the procedure.

Copyright © 2008, 2004, 2000, 1995, 1990 by Saunders, an imprint of Elsevier Inc. All rights reserved.

C. VENIPUNCTURE SITUATIONS

You are responsible for performing the venipunctures in your medical office. In the space provided, explain what you would do in each of the following situations:

1. The patient asks you if the venipuncture will hurt.

____

____

2. Upon palpating the patient's vein, you find that it feels stiff and hard.

____

____

3. You have attempted one venipuncture in a patient with small veins using the vacuum tube method of venipuncture; however, the vein collapsed and you were unable to obtain blood.

____

____

4. The patient moves during the procedure, causing the needle to come out of his arm.

____

____

5. You have inserted the needle in the vein, but notice a sudden swelling around the puncture site.

____

____

6. You inadvertently puncture the brachial artery after inserting the needle.

____

____

7. The patient begins to sweat and tells you that he or she feels warm and light-headed.

____

____

D. SEPARATING SERUM

Explain why the following guidelines must be observed while separating serum from whole blood.

1. Label the transfer tube with the word serum.

____

____

2. Place the tube in an upright position for 30 to 45 minutes.

____

____

3. Do not allow the specimen to stand for more than 1 hour before centrifuging it.

____

____

Copyright © 2008, 2004, 2000, 1995, 1990 by Saunders, an imprint of Elsevier Inc. All rights reserved.

4. Make sure the tube is stoppered during centrifugation.

____

____

5. Wear personal protective equipment when transferring serum from whole blood.

____

____

6. Do not disturb the cell layer while pipetting the serum.

____

____

E. SKIN PUNCTURE

The medical assistant is performing a skin puncture on an adult patient in order to obtain a capillary blood specimen for a hemoglobin test. For each of the following situations, write **C** if the technique is correct and **I** if the technique is incorrect. If the technique is correct, explain the rationale for performing it that way; if incorrect, explain what might happen if the technique were performed in the incorrect manner.

_______ 1. Before making the puncture, the medical assistant asks the patient to rinse his hand in warm water.

____

____

_______ 2. The puncture is made with the patient in a standing position.

____

____

_______ 3. The site is allowed to dry thoroughly after it is cleansed with an antiseptic wipe.

____

____

_______ 4. The specimen is collected from the lateral part of the tip of the ring finger.

____

____

_______ 5. The puncture is made perpendicular to the lines of the fingerprint.

____

____

_______ 6. The depth of the puncture is 4 mm.

____

____

_______ 7. The first drop of blood is wiped away.

____

____

_______ 8. The puncture site is squeezed in order to obtain the blood specimen.

____

____

Copyright © 2008, 2004, 2000, 1995, 1990 by Saunders, an imprint of Elsevier Inc. All rights reserved.

F. CROSSWORD PUZZLE

Phlebotomy

Directions: Complete the crossword puzzle using the clues presented below.

ACROSS

2 PT tube
4 Transports nutrients
7 Bad bruise
11 No additive tube
14 Best VP vein
15 EDTA tube
18 Outdated tube problem
20 Fluoride/oxalate tube
21 Collects blood

DOWN

1 Contains a "separating" gel
3 For small veins
5 Inhibits blood clotting
6 WBCs and platelets
8 In front of the elbow
9 Backflow of blood
10 What BP does during fainting
12 Faint position
13 Rolling vein
16 Broken RBCs
17 Last choice veins
19 Fainting warning signal

Copyright © 2008, 2004, 2000, 1995, 1990 by Saunders, an imprint of Elsevier Inc. All rights reserved.

PRACTICE FOR COMPETENCY

Procedure 17-1: Venipuncture Vacuum Tube Method. Practice the procedure for collecting a venous blood specimen using the vacuum tube method. Record the procedure in the chart provided.

Procedure 17-2: Venipuncture Butterfly Method. Practice the procedure for collecting a venous blood specimen using the butterfly method. Record the procedure in the chart provided.

Procedure 17-3: Venipuncture Syringe Method. Practice the procedure for collecting a venous blood specimen using the syringe method. Record the procedure in the chart provided.

Procedure 17-4: Separating Serum from Whole Blood. Separate serum from whole blood and record the procedure in the chart provided.

Procedure 17-5: Disposable Lancet. Obtain a capillary blood specimen using a disposable semiautomatic lancet device.

Procedure 17-6: Reusable Lancet. Obtain a capillary blood specimen using a reusable semiautomatic lancet.

CHART	
Date	

Copyright © 2008, 2004, 2000, 1995, 1990 by Saunders, an imprint of Elsevier Inc. All rights reserved.

CHART

Date	

Copyright © 2008, 2004, 2000, 1995, 1990 by Saunders, an imprint of Elsevier Inc. All rights reserved.

EVALUATION OF COMPETENCY

Procedure 17-1: Venipuncture—Vacuum Tube Method

Name: ______________________________ Date: ______________

Evaluated By: ______________________________ Score: ______________

Performance Objective

Outcome: Perform a venipuncture using the vacuum tube method.

Conditions: Given the following: disposable gloves, tourniquet, antiseptic wipe, double-pointed needle, plastic holder, evacuated tubes with labels, gauze pad, adhesive bandage, biohazard sharps container, biohazard specimen bag, and a laboratory request form.

Standards: Time: 10 minutes. Student completed procedure in ____ minutes.

Accuracy: Satisfactory score on the Performance Evaluation Checklist.

Performance Evaluation Checklist

Trial 1	*Trial 2*	*Point Value*	*Performance Standards*
		•	Sanitized hands.
		•	Greeted the patient and introduced yourself.
		•	Identified the patient.
		•	Asked patient if he or she prepared properly.
			Prepared the Equipment.
		•	Assembled equipment.
		•	Selected the proper evacuated tubes.
		•	Checked the expiration date of the tubes.
		▷	Stated the purpose of checking the expiration date.
		•	Labeled the evacuated tubes.
		•	Completed a laboratory request form, if necessary.
		•	Screwed the plastic holder onto the Luer adapter and tightened securely.
		•	Opened the gauze packet.
		•	Positioned the evacuated tubes in the correct order of draw.
		•	Tapped evacuated tubes with a powdered additive below the stopper.
		▷	Stated the purpose for tapping the tube.
		•	Placed the first tube loosely in the plastic holder.
			Prepared the Patient.
		•	Explained the procedure to the patient and reassured patient.
		•	Performed a preliminary assessment of both arms.

Copyright © 2008, 2004, 2000, 1995, 1990 by Saunders, an imprint of Elsevier Inc. All rights reserved.

Trial 1	Trial 2	Point Value	Performance Standards
		•	Correctly applied the tourniquet.
		•	Asked patient to clench fist.
		▷	Stated the purpose of the tourniquet and clenched fist.
		•	Assessed the veins of both arms.
		•	Determined the best vein to use.
		•	Positioned the patient's arm correctly.
		•	Thoroughly palpated the selected vein.
		•	Did not leave the tourniquet on for more than 1 minute.
		▷	Explained why the tourniquet should not be left on for more than 1 minute.
		•	Removed tourniquet and cleansed the puncture site.
		•	Allowed puncture site to air dry.
		▷	Explained why the site should be allowed to air dry.
		•	Did not touch the site after cleansing.
		•	Placed supplies within comfortable reach of the nondominant hand.
		•	Reapplied tourniquet and applied gloves.
			Performed the Venipuncture.
		•	Correctly positioned safety shield and removed cap from the needle.
		•	Properly held the venipuncture setup (bevel up) with the dominant hand.
		•	Positioned the tube with the label facing downward.
		▷	Explained why the label should face downward.
		•	Grasped the patient's arm and anchored the vein correctly.
		•	Positioned the venipuncture setup at a 15-degree angle to the arm, with the needle pointing in the same direction as the vein to be entered.
		•	Positioned the needle approximately ⅛-inch below the place where the vein is to be entered.
		•	Told the patient that a small stick will be felt.
		•	With one continuous motion, entered the skin and then the vein.
		•	Stabilized the vacuum tube setup.
		▷	Stated why the vacuum tube setup should be stabilized.
		•	Pushed the tube forward slowly to the end of the holder using the flange.
		•	Allowed evacuated tube to fill to the exhaustion of the vacuum.
		▷	Explained why the tube should be allowed to fill to the exhaustion of the vacuum.
		•	Removed the tube from the plastic holder using the flange.
		•	Immediately and gently inverted tube 8 to 10 times if it contained an additive.
		•	Inserted the next tube into the holder using the flange.
		•	Continued until the last tube was filled.
		*	Removed the tourniquet and asked the patient to unclench fist.
		•	Removed the last tube from the holder.

Copyright © 2008, 2004, 2000, 1995, 1990 by Saunders, an imprint of Elsevier Inc. All rights reserved.

Trial 1	Trial 2	Point Value	Performance Standards
		▷	Stated why the last tube should be removed.
		•	Placed gauze pad slightly above puncture site and withdrew the needle slowly and at the same angle as that for penetration.
		•	Immediately moved gauze over puncture site and applied pressure.
		•	Pushed safety shield forward with thumb until audible click is heard.
		•	Properly disposed of holder and needle in a biohazard sharps container.
		•	Instructed patient to apply pressure with the gauze pad for 1 to 2 minutes.
		▷	Stated why pressure should be applied.
		•	Applied adhesive bandage to puncture site.
		•	Removed gloves and sanitized hands.
		•	Charted the procedure correctly.
		•	Tested specimen or prepared specimen for transport according to medical office policy.
		*	Completed the procedure within 10 minutes.
			TOTALS

CHART	
Date	

Evaluation of Student Performance

EVALUATION CRITERIA			COMMENTS
Symbol	Category	Point Value	
*	Critical Step	16 points	
•	Essential Step	6 points	
▷	Theory Question	2 points	
Score calculation: 100 points – ____ points missed ____ Score Satisfactory score: 85 or above			

AAMA/CAAHEP Competency Achieved:

☑ III. C. 3. b. (2) (a): Perform venipuncture.

Copyright © 2008, 2004, 2000, 1995, 1990 by Saunders, an imprint of Elsevier Inc. All rights reserved.

Notes

Copyright © 2008, 2004, 2000, 1995, 1990 by Saunders, an imprint of Elsevier Inc. All rights reserved.

EVALUATION OF COMPETENCY

Procedure 17-2: Venipuncture—Butterfly Method

Name: ______________________________ Date: ______________

Evaluated By: ______________________________ Score: ______________

Performance Objective

Outcome: Perform a venipuncture using the butterfly method.

Conditions: Given the following: disposable gloves, tourniquet, antiseptic wipe, winged infusion set, plastic holder, evacuated tubes with labels, gauze pad, adhesive bandage, biohazard sharps container, biohazard specimen bag, and a laboratory request form.

Standards: Time: 10 minutes. Student completed procedure in ____ minutes.

Accuracy: Satisfactory score on the Performance Evaluation Checklist.

Performance Evaluation Checklist

Trial 1	Trial 2	Point Value	*Performance Standards*
		•	Sanitized hands.
		•	Greeted the patient and introduced yourself.
		•	Identified patient.
		▷	Stated why the patient must be correctly identified.
		•	Asked patient if he or she prepared properly.
		▷	Explained why it is important for the patient to prepare properly.
			Prepared the Equipment.
		•	Assembled equipment.
		•	Selected the proper evacuated tubes.
		•	Checked the expiration date of the tubes.
		•	Labeled the evacuated tubes.
		•	Completed a laboratory request form, if necessary.
		•	Removed the winged infusion set from its package.
		•	Extended the tubing to its full length and stretched it.
		▷	Explained why the tubing should be extended and stretched.
		•	Screwed the plastic holder onto the Luer adapter and tightened it securely.
		•	Opened the gauze packet.
		•	Positioned the evacuated tubes in the correct order of draw.
		•	Tapped evacuated tubes with a powdered additive below the stopper.
		▷	Stated why tubes with powdered additives must be tapped.
		•	Placed the first tube loosely in the plastic holder with the label facing downward.

Copyright © 2008, 2004, 2000, 1995, 1990 by Saunders, an imprint of Elsevier Inc. All rights reserved.

Trial 1	Trial 2	Point Value	Performance Standards
		▷	Explained why the label should be facing downward.
			Prepared the Patient.
		•	Explained the procedure to the patient and reassured patient.
		•	Performed a preliminary assessment of both arms.
		•	Correctly applied the tourniquet and asked patient to clench fist.
		•	Assessed the veins of both arms.
		•	Determined the best vein to use.
		•	Positioned the patient's arm correctly.
		▷	Stated why arm must be positioned correctly.
		•	Thoroughly palpated the selected vein.
		▷	Stated the purpose of palpating the vein.
		•	Did not leave the tourniquet on for more than 1 minute.
		•	Removed tourniquet and cleansed puncture site.
		•	Allowed puncture site to air dry.
		•	Did not touch the site after cleansing.
		•	Placed supplies within comfortable reach.
		•	Reapplied tourniquet and applied gloves.
			Performed the Venipuncture.
		•	Grasped the winged infusion set correctly.
		•	Removed the protective shield.
		•	Positioned the needle with the bevel up.
		▷	Explained why the bevel should be up.
		•	Grasped patient's arm and anchored the vein correctly.
		•	Positioned the needle at a 15-degree angle to arm, with needle pointing in the same direction as the vein to be entered.
		•	Positioned the needle approximately ⅛-inch below the place where the vein is to be entered.
		•	Told the patient that a small stick will be felt.
		•	With one continuous motion, entered the skin and then the vein.
		▷	Explained why a continuous motion should be used.
		•	Decreased the angle of the needle to 5 degrees.
		•	Seated the needle.
		▷	Stated the purpose of seating the needle.
		•	Opended the butterfly wings and rested them flat against the skin.
		•	Kept the tube and holder in a downward position.
		•	Slowly pushed the tube forward to the end of the plastic holder.
		•	Allowed evacuated tube to fill to the exhaustion of the vacuum.
		▷	Explained why the tube should be filled to the exhaustion of the vacuum.

Copyright © 2008, 2004, 2000, 1995, 1990 by Saunders, an imprint of Elsevier Inc. All rights reserved.

Trial 1	Trial 2	Point Value	*Performance Standards*
		•	Removed the tube from the plastic holder.
		•	Immediately and gently inverted evacuated tube 8 to 10 times if it contained an additive.
		▷	Explained why a tube with an additive must be inverted immediately.
		•	Inserted the next tube into the holder.
		•	Continued until the last tube was filled.
		*	Removed the tourniquet and asked the patient to unclench fist.
		▷	Stated why the tourniquet must be removed before the needle.
		•	Removed the last tube from the holder.
		•	Placed gauze pad slightly above puncture site. Grasped the setup just below the wings and withdrew the needle slowly and at the same angle as that for penetration.
		•	Immediately moved gauze over puncture site and applied pressure.
		•	Instructed the patient to apply pressure with the gauze.
		•	Activated the safety shield on the needle.
		•	Properly disposed of the winged infusion set and plastic holder in a biohazard sharps container.
		•	Continued to apply pressure for 1 to 2 minutes.
		•	Applied adhesive bandage.
		•	Removed gloves and sanitized hands.
		•	Charted the procedure correctly.
		•	Tested specimen or prepared specimen for transport according to medical office policy.
		*	Completed the procedure within 10 minutes.
			TOTALS

CHART	
Date	

Copyright © 2008, 2004, 2000, 1995, 1990 by Saunders, an imprint of Elsevier Inc. All rights reserved.

Evaluation of Student Performance

EVALUATION CRITERIA			COMMENTS
Symbol	**Category**	**Point Value**	
∗	Critical Step	16 points	
•	Essential Step	6 points	
▷	Theory Question	2 points	
Score calculation: 100 points – _____ points missed ____ Score Satisfactory score: 85 or above			

AAMA/CAAHEP Competency Achieved:

☑ III. C. 3. b. (2) (a): Perform venipuncture.

Copyright © 2008, 2004, 2000, 1995, 1990 by Saunders, an imprint of Elsevier Inc. All rights reserved.

EVALUATION OF COMPETENCY

Procedure 17-3: Venipuncture—Syringe Method

Name: ______________________________ Date: ______________

Evaluated By: ______________________________ Score: ______________

Performance Objective

Outcome: Perform a venipuncture using the syringe method.

Conditions: Given the following: disposable gloves, tourniquet, antiseptic wipe, syringe and needle, evacuated tubes with labels, needleless blood transfer tube, test tube rack, sterile gauze pad, adhesive bandage, biohazard sharps container, biohazard specimen bag, and a laboratory request form.

Standards: Time: 10 minutes. Student completed procedure in ____ minutes.

Accuracy: Satisfactory score on the Performance Evaluation Checklist.

Performance Evaluation Checklist

Trial 1	Trial 2	Point Value	*Performance Standards*
		•	Sanitized hands.
		•	Greeted the patient and introduced yourself.
		•	Identified the patient.
		•	Asked patient if he or she prepared properly.
			Prepared the Equipment.
		•	Assembled equipment.
		•	Selected the proper evacuated tubes.
		•	Checked the expiration date of the tubes.
		•	Labeled the evacuated tubes.
		•	Completed a laboratory request form, if necessary.
		•	Prepared the needle and syringe.
		•	Broke the seal on the syringe.
		•	Checked to make sure the tube was screwed tightly into the syringe.
		•	Placed evacuated tubes in a test tube rack in the correct order to be filled.
		•	Tapped evacuated tubes with a powdered additive below the stopper.
		•	Opened the gauze packet.
			Prepared the Patient.
		•	Explained the procedure to the patient and reassured patient.
		•	Performed a preliminary assessment of both arms.
		•	Correctly applied the tourniquet and asked patient to clench fist.

Copyright © 2008, 2004, 2000, 1995, 1990 by Saunders, an imprint of Elsevier Inc. All rights reserved.

Trial 1	Trial 2	Point Value	Performance Standards
		•	Assessed the veins of both arms.
		•	Determined the best vein to use.
		•	Positioned the patient's arm correctly.
		•	Thoroughly palpated the selected vein.
		•	Did not leave the tourniquet on for more than 1 minute.
		•	Removed tourniquet and cleansed puncture site.
		•	Allowed puncture site to dry.
		•	Did not touch the site after cleansing.
		•	Placed supplies within comfortable reach.
		•	Reapplied tourniquet and applied gloves.
			Performed the Venipuncture.
		•	Removed cap from the needle.
		•	Properly held the syringe (bevel up).
		•	Grasped patient's arm and anchored the vein correctly.
		•	Positioned the needle at a 15-degree angle to arm, with needle pointing in the same direction as the vein to be entered.
		▷	Explained what would happen if an angle of less than 15 degrees or more than 15 degrees was used.
		•	Positioned the needle approximately ⅛-inch below the place where the vein is to be entered.
		•	Told the patient that a small stick will be felt.
		•	With one continuous motion, entered the skin and then the vein.
		•	Stabilized the syringe.
		•	Removed the desired amount of blood by slowly pulling back the plunger.
		▷	Explained why the blood should be withdrawn slowly.
		*	Removed the tourniquet and asked patient to unclench fist.
		▷	Explained why the tourniquet should be removed before the needle.
		•	Placed gauze pad slightly above puncture site and withdrew the needle slowly and at the same angle as that for penetration.
		•	Immediately moved gauze over puncture site and applied pressure.
		•	Activated safety shield on needle.
		•	Instructed the patient to apply pressure with the gauze pad for 1 to 2 minutes.
		▷	Stated the reason for applying pressure.
		•	Transferred the blood to the evacuated tube as soon as possible using a needleless transfer device.
		▷	Stated why a needleless transfer device must be used.
		▷	Explained why the blood should be transferred as soon as possible.
		•	Immediately and gently inverted the collection tube 8 to 10 times if it contained an additive.

Copyright © 2008, 2004, 2000, 1995, 1990 by Saunders, an imprint of Elsevier Inc. All rights reserved.

Trial 1	Trial 2	Point Value	Performance Standards
		▷	Explained why the blood should be handled carefully and gently.
		•	Properly disposed of the needle and syringe in a biohazard sharps container.
		•	Applied adhesive bandage.
		•	Removed gloves and sanitized hands.
		•	Charted the procedure correctly.
		•	Tested specimen or prepared specimen for transport according to medical office policy.
		*	Completed the procedure within 10 minutes.
			TOTALS

CHART	
Date	

Evaluation of Student Performance

EVALUATION CRITERIA			COMMENTS
Symbol	Category	Point Value	
*	Critical Step	16 points	
•	Essential Step	6 points	
▷	Theory Question	2 points	
Score calculation: 100 points –______ points missed _____ Score Satisfactory score: 85 or above			

AAMA/CAAHEP Competency Achieved:

☑ III. C. 3. b. (2) (a): Perform venipuncture.

Copyright © 2008, 2004, 2000, 1995, 1990 by Saunders, an imprint of Elsevier Inc. All rights reserved.

Notes

Copyright © 2008, 2004, 2000, 1995, 1990 by Saunders, an imprint of Elsevier Inc. All rights reserved.

EVALUATION OF COMPETENCY

Procedure 17-4: Separating Serum from Whole Blood

Name: ______________________________ Date: ______________

Evaluated By: ______________________________ Score: ______________

Performance Objective

Outcome: Separate serum from whole blood.

Conditions: Given the following: red-stoppered evacuated tube venipuncture setup, test tube rack, disposable pipet, transfer tube and label, disposable gloves, face shield or mask and eye protection device, centrifuge, and a biohazard sharps container.

Standards: Time: 20 minutes. Student completed procedure in ____ minutes.

Accuracy: Satisfactory score on the Performance Evaluation Checklist.

Performance Evaluation Checklist

Trial 1	*Trial 2*	*Point Value*	*Performance Standards*
		•	Collected the blood specimen by performing a venipuncture.
		▷	Stated why a red-stoppered tube should be used.
		•	Placed specimen tube in an upright position for 30 to 45 minutes at room temperature, keeping stopper on specimen tube.
		▷	Explained why specimen tube must be placed in an upright position.
		•	Placed specimen tube in the centrifuge, with stopper end up.
		▷	Stated why the stopper must remain on the specimen tube.
		•	Balanced the specimen with the same type and weight of tube.
		▷	Stated the purpose for balancing the centrifuge.
		•	Centrifuged the specimen for 10 to 15 minutes.
		▷	Explained the purpose of centrifugation.
		•	Put on a face shield or a mask and an eye protection device and applied gloves.
		▷	Stated the purpose of wearing personal protective equipment.
		•	Removed specimen tube from centrifuge without disturbing the contents.
		▷	Explained what must be done if the contents of the tube are disturbed.
		•	Carefully removed the stopper from the tube.
		•	Squeezed bulb of the pipet and placed tip of the pipet against the side of specimen tube approximately ¼-inch above the cell layer.
		▷	Explained why the bulb should be squeezed before inserting pipet into serum.
		•	Released bulb to suction serum into the pipet.

Copyright © 2008, 2004, 2000, 1995, 1990 by Saunders, an imprint of Elsevier Inc. All rights reserved.

Trial 1	Trial 2	Point Value	Performance Standards
		•	Transferred serum to transfer tube.
		•	Did not disturb the cell layer.
		•	Continued pipetting until as much serum as possible was removed.
		•	Capped specimen tube tightly and held it up to the light to examine it for hemolysis.
		▷	Explained what should be done if hemolysis is present in the specimen.
		•	Made sure that the proper amount of serum was obtained.
		•	Properly disposed of equipment.
		•	Removed gloves and sanitized hands.
		•	Tested the specimen or prepared specimen for transport to an outside laboratory according to medical office policy.
		✶	Completed the procedure within 20 minutes.
			TOTALS

Evaluation of Student Performance

EVALUATION CRITERIA			COMMENTS
Symbol	Category	Point Value	
✶	Critical Step	16 points	
•	Essential Step	6 points	
▷	Theory Question	2 points	

Score calculation: 100 points
– _____ points missed
_____ Score
Satisfactory score: 85 or above

AAMA/CAAHEP Competency Achieved:
☑ III. C. 3. b. (2) (a): Perform venipuncture.

Copyright © 2008, 2004, 2000, 1995, 1990 by Saunders, an imprint of Elsevier Inc. All rights reserved.

EVALUATION OF COMPETENCY

Procedure 17-5: Skin Puncture—Disposable Semiautomatic Lancet Device

Name: ______________________________ Date: ______________

Evaluated By: ______________________________ Score: ______________

Performance Objective

Outcome:	Obtain a capillary blood specimen.
Conditions:	Given the following: disposable gloves, antiseptic wipe, Microtainer lancet, gauze pad, and a biohazard sharps container.
Standards:	Time: 5 minutes. Student completed procedure in ____ minutes.
	Accuracy: Satisfactory score on the Performance Evaluation Checklist.

Performance Evaluation Checklist

Trial 1	*Trial 2*	*Point Value*	*Performance Standards*
		•	Sanitized hands.
		•	Greeted the patient and introduced yourself.
		•	Identified the patient.
		•	Asked patient if he or she prepared properly.
		•	Assembled equipment.
		•	Opened sterile gauze packet.
		•	Explained the procedure to the patient and reassured patient.
		•	Seated patient in chair.
		•	Extended the palmar surface of patient's hand facing up.
		•	Selected a puncture site.
		•	Warmed site if needed.
		▷	Explained why the site should be warmed.
		•	Cleansed puncture site and allowed it to air dry.
		▷	Explained why the site should be allowed to air dry.
		•	Did not touch the site after cleansing.
		•	Applied gloves.
		•	Firmly grasped patient's finger.
		•	Positioned the lancet firmly on the fingertip slightly to the side of center.
		•	Depressed the activation button without moving the lancet or finger.
		▷	Stated why the lancet and finger should not be moved.

Copyright © 2008, 2004, 2000, 1995, 1990 by Saunders, an imprint of Elsevier Inc. All rights reserved.

Trial 1	Trial 2	Point Value	Performance Standards
		•	Disposed of lancet in biohazard sharps container.
		•	Waited a few seconds to allow blood flow to begin.
		•	Wiped away the first drop of blood with a gauze pad.
		▷	Stated why the first drop of blood should be wiped away.
		•	Allowed a second large, well-rounded drop of blood to form.
		•	Did not squeeze finger to obtain blood.
		•	Collected the blood specimen on a test strip or in the appropriate microcollection device.
		•	Instructed patient to hold a gauze pad over puncture site with pressure.
		•	Remained with patient until bleeding stopped.
		•	Applied an adhesive bandage if needed.
		•	Tested the blood specimen following the manufacturer's instructions.
		•	Removed gloves.
		•	Sanitized hands.
		✶	Completed the procedure within 5 minutes.
			TOTALS

Evaluation of Student Performance

EVALUATION CRITERIA			COMMENTS
Symbol	Category	Point Value	
✶	Critical Step	16 points	
•	Essential Step	6 points	
▷	Theory Question	2 points	
Score calculation: 100 points – ______ points missed ____ Score Satisfactory score: 85 or above			

AAMA/CAAHEP Competency Achieved:

☑ III. C. 3. b. (2) (b): Perform capillary puncture.

Copyright © 2008, 2004, 2000, 1995, 1990 by Saunders, an imprint of Elsevier Inc. All rights reserved.

EVALUATION OF COMPETENCY

Procedure 17-6: Skin Puncture—Reusable Semiautomatic Lancet Device

Name: ______________________________ Date: ______________

Evaluated By: ______________________________ Score: ______________

Performance Objective

Outcome: Obtain a capillary blood specimen.

Conditions: Given the following: disposable gloves, antiseptic wipe, Glucolet II lancet device, sterile lancet/endcap, gauze pad, and a biohazard sharps container.

Standards: Time: 10 minutes. Student completed procedure in ____ minutes.

Accuracy: Satisfactory score on the Performance Evaluation Checklist.

Performance Evaluation Checklist

Trial 1	Trial 2	Point Value	*Performance Standards*
		•	Sanitized hands.
		•	Greeted the patient and introduced yourself.
		•	Identified patient.
		•	Asked patient if he or she prepared properly.
		•	Assembled equipment.
		•	Pushed the transparent barrel toward the release button until it clicked into place.
		•	Inserted lancet/endcap onto the lancet device.
		•	Opened sterile gauze packet.
		•	Explained the procedure to the patient and reassured patient.
		•	Seated patient in chair.
		•	Extended the palmar surface of patient's hand facing up.
		•	Selected a puncture site.
		•	Warmed site if needed.
		▷	Explained how patient's finger can be warmed.
		•	Cleansed puncture site and allowed it to air dry.
		•	Applied gloves.
		•	Twisted off plastic post from the endcap.
		•	Firmly grasped patient's finger.
		•	Placed the endcap firmly on the fingertip slightly to the side of center.
		•	Depressed the activation button without moving the Glucolet or finger.

Copyright © 2008, 2004, 2000, 1995, 1990 by Saunders, an imprint of Elsevier Inc. All rights reserved.

Trial 1	Trial 2	Point Value	*Performance Standards*
		•	Wiped away the first drop of blood with a gauze pad.
		•	Allowed a second large, well-rounded drop of blood to form.
		▷	Explained why the finger should not be squeezed.
		•	Collected the blood specimen on a test strip or in the appropriate microcollection device.
		•	Instructed patient to hold a gauze pad over puncture site with pressure.
		•	Remained with patient until bleeding stopped.
		•	Applied an adhesive bandage if needed.
		•	Removed the endcap from the lancet device.
		•	Discarded the endcap in a biohazard waste container.
		•	Tested the blood specimen following the manufacturer's instructions.
		•	Removed gloves.
		•	Sanitized hands.
		•	Sanitized and disinfected the Glucolet.
		•	Stored Glucolet in its resting position.
		✶	Completed the procedure within 5 minutes.
			TOTALS

Evaluation of Student Performance

EVALUATION CRITERIA			COMMENTS
Symbol	Category	Point Value	
✶	Critical Step	16 points	
•	Essential Step	6 points	
▷	Theory Question	2 points	
Score calculation: 100 points – ____ points missed ____ Score Satisfactory score: 85 or above			

AAMA/CAAHEP Competency Achieved:

☑ III. C. 3. b. (2) (b): Perform capillary puncture.

Copyright © 2008, 2004, 2000, 1995, 1990 by Saunders, an imprint of Elsevier Inc. All rights reserved.

18

Hematology

CHAPTER ASSIGNMENTS

√ After Completing	Date Due	Textbook Page(s)	TEXTBOOK ASSIGNMENTS	Possible Points	Points You Earned
		674-690	Read Chapter 18: Hematology		
		682 686-687	Read Case Study 1 Case Study 1 questions	5	
		682 687	Read Case Study 2 Case Study 2 questions	5	
		684 687	Read Case Study 3 Case Study 3 questions	5	
		687-688	Apply Your Knowledge questions	10	
			TOTAL POINTS		

√ After Completing	Date Due	Study Guide Page(s)	STUDY GUIDE ASSIGNMENTS (CTA: Critical Thinking Activity)	Possible Points	Points You Earned
		751	Pretest	10	
		752	Key Term Assessment	12	
		753-755	Evaluation of Learning questions	25	
		755	CTA A: Diseases	40	
		759	CTA B: Hematocrit	5	
		759	CTA C: Iron Content of Food	10	
		760	CTA D: Iron-Deficiency Anemia	20	
		762	CTA E: Dear Gabby	10	
		764	CTA F: Find It! Game (Team Players) (Record points earned)		
			CD Activity: Chapter 18 Name That Cell (Individual Player) (Record points earned)		

Copyright © 2008, 2004, 2000, 1995, 1990 by Saunders, an imprint of Elsevier Inc. All rights reserved.

√ After Completing	Date Due	Study Guide Page(s)	STUDY GUIDE ASSIGNMENTS (CTA: Critical Thinking Activity)	Possible Points	Points You Earned
		767	CTA G: Hematology Laboratory Report (5 points each)	30	
		768	CTA H: Crossword Puzzle	23	
			CD Activity: Chapter 18 Time for a Test (Record points earned)		
			CD Activity: Chapter 18 Animations	20	
		751	Posttest	10	
			ADDITIONAL ASSIGNMENTS		
			TOTAL POINTS		

Copyright © 2008, 2004, 2000, 1995, 1990 by Saunders, an imprint of Elsevier Inc. All rights reserved.

√ When Assigned By Your Instructor	Study Guide Page(s)	Practices Required	LABORATORY ASSIGNMENTS (Procedure Number and Name)	*Score
	769-770	3	**Practice for Competency** 18-A: Hemoglobin Determination Textbook reference: pp. 678-679	
	771-772		**Evaluation of Competency** 18-A: Hemoglobin Determination	*
	769-770	3	**Practice for Competency** 18-1: Hematocrit Textbook reference: pp. 680-681	
	773-775		**Evaluation of Competency** 18-1: Hematocrit	*
	769-770	10	**Practice for Competency** 18-2: Preparation of a Blood Smear for a Differential Cell Count Textbook reference: pp. 684-686	
	777-778		**Evaluation of Competency** 18-2: Preparation of a Blood Smear for a Differential Cell Count	*
			ADDITIONAL ASSIGNMENTS	

Copyright © 2008, 2004, 2000, 1995, 1990 by Saunders, an imprint of Elsevier Inc. All rights reserved.

Notes

Copyright © 2008, 2004, 2000, 1995, 1990 by Saunders, an imprint of Elsevier Inc. All rights reserved.

Name ______________________________ Date ______________

PRETEST

True or False

_____ 1. Plasma makes up approximately 55% of the blood volume.

_____ 2. A mature erythrocyte is biconcave in shape and contains a nucleus.

_____ 3. Erythrocytes are responsible for defending the body against infection.

_____ 4. The life span of a red blood cell is 120 days.

_____ 5. The function of hemoglobin is to assist in blood clotting.

_____ 6. Leukocytosis is an abnormal increase in the number of leukocytes.

_____ 7. Another name for a thrombocyte is a platelet.

_____ 8. A low hemoglobin reading occurs with polycythemia.

_____ 9. A neutrophil is classified as a granular leukocyte.

_____ 10. An increase in neutrophils occurs during an acute infection.

POSTTEST

True or False

_____ 1. A function of the plasma is to transport antibodies, enzymes, and hormones.

_____ 2. The red bone marrow of the sternum produces red blood cells in the adult.

_____ 3. The normal range for a red blood cell count for an adult female is 4 to 5.5 million.

_____ 4. The normal range for hemoglobin for an adult male is 12 to 16 g/dL.

_____ 5. The normal adult range for a white blood cell count is 4,500 to 11,000.

_____ 6. Leukocytes do their work in the tissues.

_____ 7. Bilirubin is an orange-colored pigment that is produced through the breakdown of hemoglobin.

_____ 8. Leukopenia occurs when a patient has appendicitis.

_____ 9. An immature form of a neutrophil is known as a seg.

_____ 10. The primary function of a neutrophil is to form antibodies.

Copyright © 2008, 2004, 2000, 1995, 1990 by Saunders, an imprint of Elsevier Inc. All rights reserved.

KEY TERM ASSESSMENT

Directions: Match each medical term with its definition.

_____ 1. Ameboid movement
_____ 2. Anemia
_____ 3. Bilirubin
_____ 4. Diapedesis
_____ 5. Hematology
_____ 6. Hemoglobin
_____ 7. Hemolysis
_____ 8. Leukocytosis
_____ 9. Leukopenia
_____ 10. Oxyhemoglobin
_____ 11. Phagocytosis
_____ 12. Polycythemia

A. An abnormal decrease in the number of white blood cells (below 4,500 per cubic millimeter of blood)
B. The breakdown of erythrocytes with the release of hemoglobin into the plasma
C. Movement used by leukocytes that permits them to propel themselves from the capillaries to the tissues
D. The ameboid movement of blood cells (especially leukocytes) through the wall of a capillary and into the tissues
E. A disorder in which there is an increase in the red cell mass
F. A condition in which there is a decrease in the number of erythrocytes or in the amount of hemoglobin in the blood
G. Hemoglobin that has combined with oxygen
H. The study of blood and blood-forming tissues
I. An abnormal increase in the number of white blood cells (above 11,000 per cubic millimeter of blood)
J. An orange-colored bile pigment produced by the breakdown of heme from the hemoglobin molecule
K. The engulfing and destruction of foreign particles, such as bacteria, by special cells called phagocytes
L. The iron-containing pigment of erythrocytes that transports oxygen in the body

Copyright © 2008, 2004, 2000, 1995, 1990 by Saunders, an imprint of Elsevier Inc. All rights reserved.

EVALUATION OF LEARNING

Directions: Fill in each blank with the correct answer.

1. List the tests generally included in a CBC.

____

____

2. What is the function of plasma?

____

____

3. Where are erythrocytes formed in the adult?

____

____

4. Describe the shape of an erythrocyte and explain how it acquires this shape.

____

____

5. Describe the normal appearance of arterial and venous blood.

____

____

6. What is the average lifespan of a red blood cell?

____

7. What is the function of leukocytes?

____

____

8. Where do leukocytes do their work?

____

9. What is the function of platelets?

____

10. What is the normal range for platelets in an adult?

____

11. What is the normal hemoglobin range?

    a. Adult female: ____

    b. Adult male: ____

12. List five conditions that cause a decrease in the hemoglobin level.

____

____

____

Copyright © 2008, 2004, 2000, 1995, 1990 by Saunders, an imprint of Elsevier Inc. All rights reserved.

13. What is the purpose of the hematocrit?

____

____

14. What is the normal hematocrit range?
    a. Adult female: ______________________________
    b. Adult male: ______________________________

15. What is the normal range for the white blood count for an adult?

____

16. List examples of conditions that may result in leukocytosis.

____

____

17. What is the normal range for the red blood count for an adult?
    a. Adult female: ______________________________
    b. Adult male: ______________________________

18. List the five types of white blood cells and the normal adult range for each.

____

____

____

19. Why must the white blood cells be stained when performing a differential cell count?

____

____

20. The least numerous white blood cell is the ______________________________

21. Why are neutrophils also known as "segs"?

____

____

22. What is a band?

____

23. The largest of the white blood cells is the ______________________________

24. What is the function of lymphocytes?

____

____

Copyright © 2008, 2004, 2000, 1995, 1990 by Saunders, an imprint of Elsevier Inc. All rights reserved.

25. List the abbreviation for each of the following tests:
    a. Hematocrit ______
    b. Hemoglobin ______
    c. Differential cell count ______
    d. White blood cell count ______
    e. Red blood cell count ______

CRITICAL THINKING ACTIVITIES

A. DISEASES

1. You and your classmates work at a large clinic. It is National Disease Awareness Week. The physicians at your clinic ask you to develop informative, creative, and colorful brochures for patients relating to diseases. Choose a condition below and design a brochure using the blank FAQ (Frequently Asked Questions) brochure provided on the following page. Each student in the class should select a different disease. On a separate sheet of paper, write three true/false questions relating to the information in your brochure.
2. Present your brochure to the class. After all the brochures have been presented, each student should ask their three questions to the entire class to see how well the class understands the diseases that were presented. (Note: You can take notes during the presentations and refer to them when answering the questions.)

Diseases

1. Addison's disease
2. Amyotrophic lateral sclerosis
3. Aplastic anemia
4. Bell's palsy
5. Cirrhosis
6. Crohn's disease
7. Cushing's syndrome
8. Cystic fibrosis
9. Degenerative disc disease
10. Epilepsy
11. Hemolytic anemia
12. Hemophilia
13. Hernia
14. Hodgkin's disease
15. Hyperthyroidism
16. Hypothyroidism
17. Leukemia
18. Lupus erythematosus
19. Multiple sclerosis
20. Muscular dystrophy
21. Parkinson's disease
22. Peptic ulcer
23. Pernicious anemia
24. Polycythemia
25. Sickle-cell anemia
26. Ulcerative colitis

Copyright © 2008, 2004, 2000, 1995, 1990 by Saunders, an imprint of Elsevier Inc. All rights reserved.

Notes

Copyright © 2008, 2004, 2000, 1995, 1990 by Saunders, an imprint of Elsevier Inc. All rights reserved.

FAQ on:

Q:

A:

Q:

A:

Q:

A:

Q:

A:

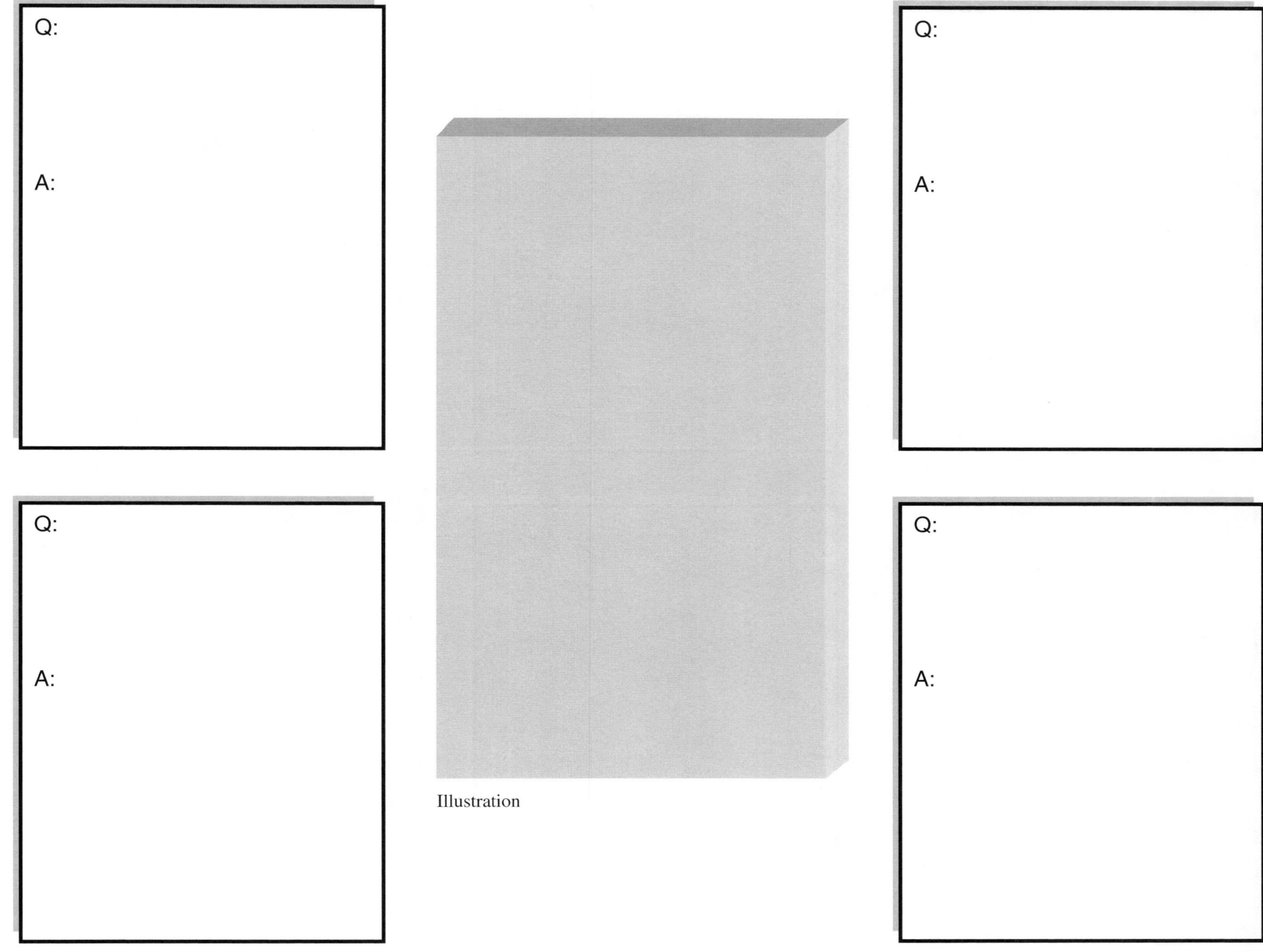

Illustration

B. HEMATOCRIT

Label the layers of this microhematocrit capillary tube that has been centrifuged. Place an arrow at the point where you would take the hematocrit reading.

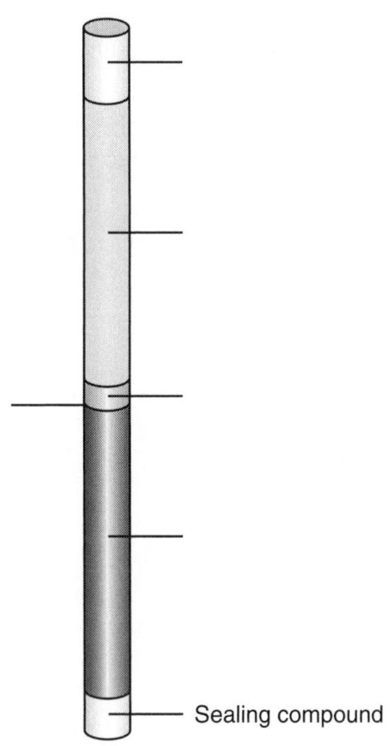

C. IRON CONTENT OF FOOD

Consuming food that is high in iron helps to prevent the development of iron-deficiency anemia. To become familiar with foods that are high in iron content and foods that contain little or no iron, plan the following two meals. One meal should be as high as possible in iron content and the other meal should not contain any iron at all.

Meal 1

____

____

____

____

____

Meal 2

____

____

____

____

____

Copyright © 2008, 2004, 2000, 1995, 1990 by Saunders, an imprint of Elsevier Inc. All rights reserved.

D. IRON-DEFICIENCY ANEMIA

Create a profile of an individual who has iron-deficiency anemia following these guidelines:

1. Using colored pencils, crayons, or markers, draw a figure of an individual exhibiting iron-deficiency anemia. Be as creative as possible.
2. Do not use any text on your drawing, other than to label items you have drawn in your picture. (A picture is worth a thousand words!)
3. Try to include all of the symptoms of iron-deficiency anemia in your drawing. The Iron-Deficiency Anemia Patient Teaching Box in your textbook can be used as a reference source.
4. In the classroom, find a partner and trade drawings. Identify the symptoms of iron-deficiency anemia in your partner's drawing. With your partner, discuss what treatment is recommended and also what this person could do to prevent iron-deficiency anemia.

Copyright © 2008, 2004, 2000, 1995, 1990 by Saunders, an imprint of Elsevier Inc. All rights reserved.

IRON-DEFICIENCY ANEMIA

Copyright © 2008, 2004, 2000, 1995, 1990 by Saunders, an imprint of Elsevier Inc. All rights reserved.

E. DEAR GABBY

Gabby is attending her class reunion and wants you to fill in for her. In the space provided, respond to the following letter.

Dear Gabby,

I am a housewife with two adorable children, ages 2 and 4. I have been feeling run-down and tired lately, so I bought some vitamin pills at the drug store. They came individually packaged in foil and plastic. They are hard to open, so I cut each package and transferred the iron pills to a little plastic baggie. When I told my mother about what I thought was a great idea, she got very upset. She told me that I could possibly be putting my children at danger. She said that iron is poisonous to children and that I should not do that. Gabby, my mom has always been overprotective. Is this just another one of her episodes?

Signed,

Curious in Kansas

____

____

____

____

____

____

____

____

____

____

____

Copyright © 2008, 2004, 2000, 1995, 1990 by Saunders, an imprint of Elsevier Inc. All rights reserved.

Notes

Copyright © 2008, 2004, 2000, 1995, 1990 by Saunders, an imprint of Elsevier Inc. All rights reserved.

F. FIND IT! GAME

Object: The object of the game is to identify the different types of blood cells.

Directions:

1. Cut out the game cards on the following page.
2. Refer to Figure 18-3 in your textbook.
3. Using colored pencils, draw the appropriate blood cell types on the blank side of the card.
4. Get into a group of three students.
5. Hold your game cards with the cells facing you.
6. In turn, each player "names" a blood cell. All players should place a blood cell on the table with the cell side facing up.
7. When all players have placed a card on the table, turn the cards over.
8. Award yourself 5 points if you have correctly determined the proper blood cell. If you have a question regarding the correct answer, consult your instructor.
9. In turn, each player can earn an additional 5 points by stating a fact about that blood cell.
10. Keep track of your points on the score card provided below.
11. Continue the game until all of the game cards have been used.

FIND IT!
SCORE CARD

Name: ______________________________

Recording Points:
Cross off a number each time you properly sequence a game card (starting with 5 and continuing in sequence). Cross off another number if you are able to state a fact about the blood cell. Your points will be equal to the last number you crossed off. Record this number in the space provided and determine the knowledge level you attained.

Points:	
5	75
10	80
15	85
20	90
25	95
30	100
35	105
40	110
45	115
50	120
55	125
60	130
65	135
70	140

TOTAL POINTS: ______

LEVEL OF KNOWLEDGE: ______

- ☐ 70 to 80 points: **No Signs of Anemia**
- ☐ 55 to 65 points: **A Little Anemic**
- ☐ 50 points and below: **Better Take Some Iron**

Copyright © 2008, 2004, 2000, 1995, 1990 by Saunders, an imprint of Elsevier Inc. All rights reserved.

Red Blood Cell	Platelets
Neutrophil	Neutrophilic Band
Eosinophil	Basophil
Lymphocyte	Monocyte

G. HEMATOLOGY LABORATORY REPORT

The following terms may appear on hematology laboratory reports that describe changes in the shape, size, and staining reaction of erythrocytes. Using a reference source, define each in the space provided.

a. Anisocytosis

____

____

____

b. Macrocyte

____

____

____

c. Microcyte

____

____

____

d. Poikilocyte

____

____

____

e. Hypochromia

____

____

____

f. Hyperchromia

____

____

____

Copyright © 2008, 2004, 2000, 1995, 1990 by Saunders, an imprint of Elsevier Inc. All rights reserved.

H. CROSSWORD PUZZLE
Hematology

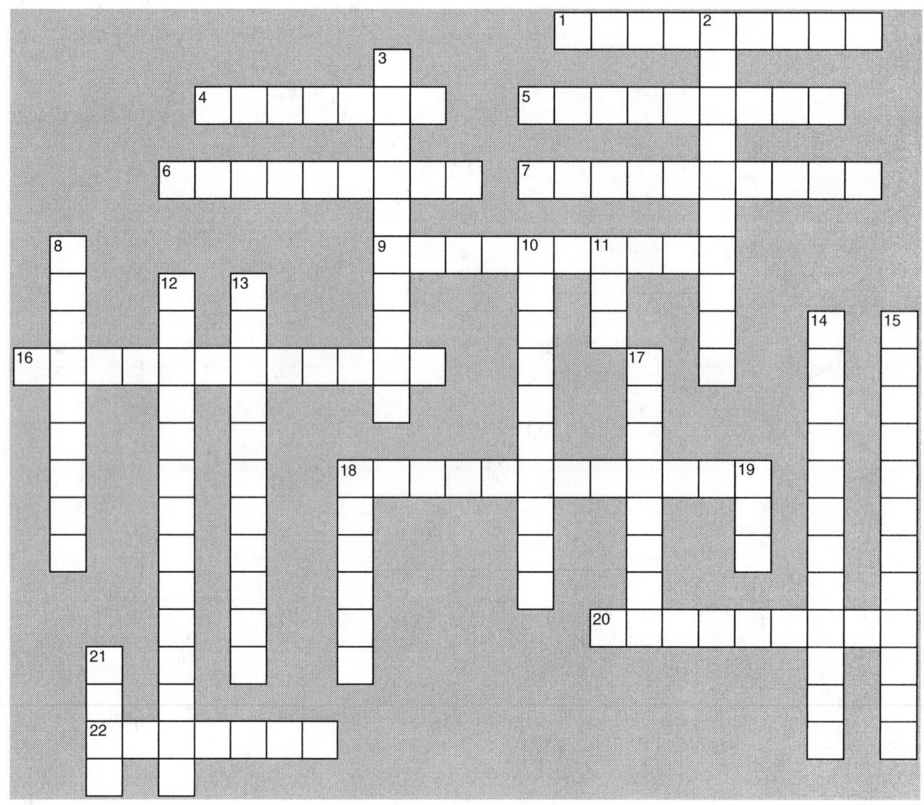

Directions: Complete the crossword puzzle using the clues presented below.

ACROSS

1 Broken RBC
4 WBCs work here
5 Orange bile pigment
6 Platelets and WBCs
7 Study of blood
9 Produces antibodies
16 Above 11,000 WBCs
18 Engulfing pathogens
20 White blood cell
22 Not in a RBC

DOWN

2 Below 4,500 WBCs
3 Carries oxygen
8 Symptom of anemia
10 To separate blood
11 Common hematology test
12 Common cause of anemia
13 Red blood cell
14 Clots blood
15 Condition of too many RBCs
17 Largest WBC
18 Liquid part of blood
19 Neutrophil's other name
21 Immature neutrophil

Copyright © 2008, 2004, 2000, 1995, 1990 by Saunders, an imprint of Elsevier Inc. All rights reserved.

PRACTICE FOR COMPETENCY

Procedure 18-A: Hemoglobin Determination. Perform a hemoglobin determination using an automated blood analyzer and record results in the chart provided. Circle any values falling outside of normal range.

Procedure 18-1: Hematocrit Determination. Perform a hematocrit determination in duplicate and record results in the chart provided. Circle any values falling outside of normal range.

Procedure 18-2: Preparation of a Blood Smear for a Differential Cell Count. Prepare a blood smear for a differential white blood cell count.

CHART	
Date	

Copyright © 2008, 2004, 2000, 1995, 1990 by Saunders, an imprint of Elsevier Inc. All rights reserved.

CHART	
Date	

Copyright © 2008, 2004, 2000, 1995, 1990 by Saunders, an imprint of Elsevier Inc. All rights reserved.

EVALUATION OF COMPETENCY

Procedure 18-A: Hemoglobin Determination

Name: ______________________ Date: __________

Evaluated By: ______________________ Score: __________

Performance Objective

Outcome: Perform a hemoglobin determination.

Conditions: Using a hemoglobin meter and operating manual.

Given the following: disposable gloves, antiseptic wipe, lancet, gauze pad, test cards, cod key, control solutions, quality control log, and a biohazard sharps container.

Standards: Time: 10 minutes. Student completed procedure in ____ minutes.

Accuracy: Satisfactory score in the Performance Evaluation Checklist.

Performance Evaluation Checklist

Trial 1	*Trial 2*	*Point Value*	*Performance Standards*
		•	Sanitized hands.
		•	Assembled equipment.
		•	Checked expiration date of test cards.
		•	Calibrated the hemoglobin meter.
		▷	Stated the purpose of calibrating the meter.
		•	Checked expiration date of control solution.
		•	Applied gloves and ran a low and high control.
		▷	Stated the purpose of running controls.
		•	Removed gloves and sanitized hands.
		•	Recorded control results in the quality control log.
		•	Greeted the patient and introduced yourself.
		•	Identified the patient and explained the procedure.
		•	Turned on the hemoglobin meter and checked the code number.
		•	Inserted a test card into the meter.
		•	Opened gauze packet.
		•	Cleansed puncture site and allowed it to air dry.
		▷	Stated what happens to the blood drop if the site is not dry.
		•	Applied gloves and performed a finger puncture.
		•	Wiped away the first drop of blood.

Copyright © 2008, 2004, 2000, 1995, 1990 by Saunders, an imprint of Elsevier Inc. All rights reserved.

Trial 1	*Trial 2*	*Point Value*	*Performance Standards*
		•	Collected the blood specimen.
		•	Placed a gauze pad over puncture site and applied pressure.
		•	Applied blood specimen to test card.
		•	Waited while hemoglobin meter analyzed the blood specimen.
		•	Read results on the display screen.
		▷	Stated the normal hemoglobin range for a female (12-16 g/dL) and a male (14-18 g/dL).
		•	Removed test card from meter.
		•	Properly disposed of test card in a biohazard waste container..
		• •	Checked puncture site and applied adhesive bandage, if needed. Removed gloves.
		•	Sanitized hands.
		•	Charted the test results correctly.
		*	The hemoglobin recording was identical to the reading on the digital display screen.
		*	Completed the procedure within 10 minutes.
			TOTALS

CHART	
Date	

Evaluation of Student Performance

EVALUATION CRITERIA			COMMENTS
Symbol	**Category**	**Point Value**	
*	Critical Step	16 points	
•	Essential Step	6 points	
▷	Theory Question	2 points	
Score calculation: 100 points – ______ points missed ____ Score Satisfactory score: 85 or above			

AAMA/CAAHEP Competency Achieved:

☑ III. C. 3. b. (3) (c) (ii): Perform hematology testing.
☑ III. C. 3. c. (4) (d): Use methods of quality control.

Copyright © 2008, 2004, 2000, 1995, 1990 by Saunders, an imprint of Elsevier Inc. All rights reserved.

EVALUATION OF COMPETENCY

Procedure 18-1: Hematocrit

Name: ______________________ Date: ____________

Evaluated By: ______________________ Score: ____________

Performance Objective

Outcome: Perform a hematocrit determination.

Conditions: Given the following: microhematocrit centrifuge, disposable gloves, lancet, antiseptic wipe, gauze pad, capillary tubes, sealing compound, biohazard specimen bag, laboratory request form, and a biohazard sharps container.

Standards: Time: 10 minutes. Student completed procedure in ____ minutes.

Accuracy: Satisfactory score in the Performance Evaluation Checklist.

Performance Evaluation Checklist

Trial 1	*Trial 2*	*Point Value*	*Performance Standards*
		•	Sanitized hands.
		•	Greeted the patient and introduced yourself.
		•	Identified the patient and explained the procedure.
		•	Assembled equipment.
		•	Opened gauze packet.
		•	Cleansed site with an antiseptic wipe and allowed it to air dry.
		•	Applied gloves.
		•	Performed a finger puncture and discarded the lancet in a biohazard sharps container.
		•	Wiped away the first drop of blood.
		•	Massaged finger until large blood drop forms.
		•	Held one end of capillary tube horizontally, but slightly downward next to the free-flowing puncture.
		•	Kept the tip of the pipet in the blood, but did not allow it to press against the skin of the patient's finger.
		▷	Explained why the capillary tube should be kept in the blood specimen.
		•	Filled capillary tube (calibrated tubes filled to the calibration line; uncalibrated tubes filled approximately ¾ full).
		▷	Explained why a tube with air bubbles is unacceptable.
		•	Filled a second capillary tube.
		▷	Stated why 2 capillary tubes must be filled.

Copyright © 2008, 2004, 2000, 1995, 1990 by Saunders, an imprint of Elsevier Inc. All rights reserved.

Trial 1	Trial 2	Point Value	*Performance Standards*
		•	Placed gauze pad over puncture site and applied pressure.
		•	Sealed one end of each capillary tube.
		•	Checked puncture site and applied adhesive bandage, if needed.
		•	Placed capillary tubes in the microhematocrit centrifuge with the sealed end facing toward the outside.
		▷	Explained why the sealed end must face toward the outside.
		•	Balanced one tube with the other tube placed opposite it.
		•	Placed the cover over the capillary tubes and locked it securely.
		•	Centrifuged blood specimen for 3 to 5 minutes.
		▷	Explained the reason for centrifuging the blood specimen.
		•	Allowed centrifuge to come to a complete stop.
		•	Removed the protective cover from the capillary tubes.
		•	Read the results using the appropriate reading device.
		•	Determined if the results agreed within 4 percentage points.
		▷	Explained what to do if the results are not within 4 percentage points.
		•	Averaged the values of the two tubes together to derive the test results.
		*	The results were within ± 1% of the evaluator's results.
		▷	Stated the normal hematocrit range for a female (37% to 47%) and a male (40% to 54%).
		•	Properly disposed of capillary tubes in a biohazard sharps container.
		•	Removed gloves.
		•	Sanitized hands.
		•	Charted the test results correctly.
		•	Returned equipment.
		*	Completed the procedure within 10 minutes.
			TOTALS

CHART	
Date	

Copyright © 2008, 2004, 2000, 1995, 1990 by Saunders, an imprint of Elsevier Inc. All rights reserved.

Evaluation of Student Performance

EVALUATION CRITERIA			COMMENTS
Symbol	Category	Point Value	
✶	Critical Step	16 points	
•	Essential Step	6 points	
▷	Theory Question	2 points	
Score calculation: 100 points – ______ points missed ____ Score Satisfactory score: 85 or above			

AAMA/CAAHEP Competency Achieved:

☑ III. C. 3. b. (3) (c) (ii): Perform hematology testing.
☑ III. C. 3. c. (4) (d): Use methods of quality control.

Copyright © 2008, 2004, 2000, 1995, 1990 by Saunders, an imprint of Elsevier Inc. All rights reserved.

Notes

Copyright © 2008, 2004, 2000, 1995, 1990 by Saunders, an imprint of Elsevier Inc. All rights reserved.

EVALUATION OF COMPETENCY

Procedure 18-2: Preparation of a Blood Smear for a Differential Cell Count

Name: ______________________ Date: ____________

Evaluated By: ______________________ Score: ____________

Performance Objective

Outcome:	Prepare a blood smear for a differential white blood cell count.
Conditions:	Given the following: disposable gloves, supplies to perform a finger puncture or venipuncture, slides with a frosted edge, slide container, biohazard specimen bag, laboratory request form, and a biohazard sharps container.
Standards:	Time: 10 minutes. Student completed procedure in ____ minutes. Accuracy: Satisfactory score in the Performance Evaluation Checklist.

Performance Evaluation Checklist

Trial 1	*Trial 2*	*Point Value*	*Performance Standards*
		•	Sanitized hands.
		•	Greeted the patient and introduced yourself.
		•	Identified the patient and explained the procedure.
		•	Assembled equipment.
		•	Labeled slides.
		•	Cleansed puncture site.
		•	Applied gloves.
		•	Performed a venipuncture or finger puncture.
		•	Placed a drop of blood in the middle of each slide approximately ¼ inch from the frosted edge of the slide.
		•	Held a spreader slide at a 30-degree angle to first slide in front of the drop of blood.
		▷	Stated what occurs if the angle is more than 30 degrees or less than 30 degrees.
		•	Moved the spreader slide until it touched the drop of blood.
		•	Spread the blood thinly and evenly across slide using the spreader slide.
		•	Prepared the second blood smear.
		•	Disposed of the spreader slide in a biohazard sharps container.
		•	Laid the blood smears on a flat surface and allowed them to dry.
		▷	Explained why the blood smears should be dried immediately.
		•	The length of the smear was approximately 1½ inches.
		•	The smear was smooth and even with no ridges, holes, lines, streaks, or clumps.

Copyright © 2008, 2004, 2000, 1995, 1990 by Saunders, an imprint of Elsevier Inc. All rights reserved.

Trial 1	Trial 2	Point Value	*Performance Standards*
		•	The smear was not too thick or too thin.
		•	There was a feathered edge at the thin end of the smear.
		•	There was a margin on all sides of the smear.
		•	Placed the slides in a protective slide container.
		•	Prepared blood tube and slides for transport to outside laboratory.
		•	Removed gloves and sanitized hands.
		•	Charted the procedure correctly.
		✶	Completed the procedure within 10 minutes.
			TOTALS

CHART	
Date	

Evaluation of Student Performance

EVALUATION CRITERIA			COMMENTS
Symbol	Category	Point Value	
✶	Critical Step	16 points	
•	Essential Step	6 points	
▷	Theory Question	2 points	
Score calculation: 100 points – ______ points missed ____ Score Satisfactory score: 85 or above			

AAMA/CAAHEP Competency Achieved:

☑ III. C. 3. c. (4) (d): Use methods of quality control.

Copyright © 2008, 2004, 2000, 1995, 1990 by Saunders, an imprint of Elsevier Inc. All rights reserved.

19

Blood Chemistry and Serology

CHAPTER ASSIGNMENTS

√ After Completing	Date Due	Textbook Page(s)	TEXTBOOK ASSIGNMENTS	Possible Points	Points You Earned
		691-720	Read Chapter 19: Blood Chemistry and Serology		
		698 716	Read Case Study 1 Case Study 1 questions	5	
		701 716	Read Case Study 2 Case Study 2 questions	5	
		704 716	Read Case Study 3 Case Study 3 questions	5	
		717-718	Apply Your Knowledge questions	20	
			TOTAL POINTS		
√ After Completing	**Date Due**	**Study Guide Page(s)**	**STUDY GUIDE ASSIGNMENTS (CTA: Critical Thinking Activity)**	**Possible Points**	**Points You Earned**
		783	Pretest	10	
		784	Key Term Assessment	17	
		785-789	Evaluation of Learning questions	50	
		789	CTA A: Coronary Heart Disease	20	
		791	CTA B: Cholesterol and Saturated Fat (5 points each)	15	
		791	CTA C: Glucose Tolerance Test (2 points each)	10	
		792	CTA D: Rh Incompatibility (2 points each)	20	

Copyright © 2008, 2004, 2000, 1995, 1990 by Saunders, an imprint of Elsevier Inc. All rights reserved.

√ After Completing	Date Due	Study Guide Page(s)	STUDY GUIDE ASSIGNMENTS (CTA: Critical Thinking Activity)	Possible Points	Points You Earned
		792	CTA E: Type 2 Diabetes Brochure	40	
			CD Activity: Chapter 19 The Right Chemistry (Record points earned)		
		795	CTA F: Crossword Puzzle	24	
			CD Activity: Chapter 19 Serologic Tests (Record points earned)		
			CD Activity: Chapter 19 Animations	20	
		783	Posttest	10	
			ADDITIONAL ASSIGNMENTS		
			TOTAL POINTS		

Copyright © 2008, 2004, 2000, 1995, 1990 by Saunders, an imprint of Elsevier Inc. All rights reserved.

√ When Assigned By Your Instructor	Study Guide Page(s)	Practices Required	LABORATORY ASSIGNMENTS (Procedure Number and Name)	*Score
	797-798	3	**Practice for Competency** 19-A: Performing a Blood Chemistry Test Textbook reference: pp. 697-700	
	799-801		**Evaluation of Competency** 19-A: Performing a Blood Chemistry Test	*
	797-798	3	**Practice for Competency** 19-1: Blood Glucose Measurement Using the Accu-Check Advantage Glucose Meter Textbook reference: pp. 708-710	
	803-805		**Evaluation of Competency** 19-1: Blood Glucose Measurement Using the Accu-Check Advantage Glucose Meter	*
	797-798	3	**Practice for Competency** 19-B: Rapid Mononucleosis Testing (Quick Vue + Mono Test) Textbook reference: p. 712	
	807-808		**Evaluation of Competency** 19-B: Rapid Mononucleosis Testing (Quick Vue + Mono Test)	*
			ADDITIONAL ASSIGNMENTS	

Copyright © 2008, 2004, 2000, 1995, 1990 by Saunders, an imprint of Elsevier Inc. All rights reserved.

Notes

Copyright © 2008, 2004, 2000, 1995, 1990 by Saunders, an imprint of Elsevier Inc. All rights reserved.

Name ______________________________ Date ______________

PRETEST

True or False

_____ 1. Most of the cholesterol found in the blood comes from the intake of dietary cholesterol.

_____ 2. The primary use of the cholesterol test is to screen for the presence of coronary heart disease.

_____ 3. LDL picks up cholesterol from ingested fats and the liver and carries it to the cells.

_____ 4. The function of glucose in the body is to build and repair tissue.

_____ 5. Insulin is required for normal utilization of glucose in the body.

_____ 6. An abnormally low level of glucose in the body is known as hypoglycemia.

_____ 7. The hemoglobin A_{1C} test measures the average amount of blood glucose over a 3-month period.

_____ 8. An antibody is a substance that is capable of combining with an antigen.

_____ 9. Mononucleosis is transmitted through coughing and sneezing.

_____ 10. Blood antigens (A, B, Rh) are located on the surface of red blood cells.

POSTTEST

True or False

_____ 1. Serum is required for most blood chemistry tests.

_____ 2. The buildup of plaque (due to high cholesterol) on the walls of arteries is known as thrombophlebitis.

_____ 3. An HDL cholesterol level greater than 50 mg/dL is a risk factor for coronary heart disease.

_____ 4. The triglyceride test requires that the patient not eat or drink for 12 hours before the test.

_____ 5. The normal range for a fasting blood sugar is 120 to 160 mg/dL.

_____ 6. The glucose tolerance test is used to assist in the diagnosis of diabetes mellitus.

_____ 7. Before meals, it is recommended that the blood glucose level for a diabetic patient fall between 60 to 80 mg/dL.

_____ 8. The recommended A_{1C} level for an individual with diabetes is 4% to 6%.

_____ 9. The RPR test is a screening test for syphilis.

_____ 10. The varicella virus causes infectious mononucleosis.

Copyright © 2008, 2004, 2000, 1995, 1990 by Saunders, an imprint of Elsevier Inc. All rights reserved.

KEY TERM ASSESSMENT

Directions: Match each medical term with its definition.

_______ 1. Agglutination

_______ 2. Antibody

_______ 3. Antigen

_______ 4. Antiserum

_______ 5. Blood antibody

_______ 6. Blood antigen

_______ 7. Donor

_______ 8. Gene

_______ 9. Glycogen

_______ 10. HDL cholesterol

_______ 11. Hyperglycemia

_______ 12. Hypoglycemia

_______ 13. In vitro

_______ 14. In vivo

_______ 15. LDL cholesterol

_______ 16. Lipoprotein

_______ 17. Recipient

A. An abnormally high level of glucose in the blood
B. A complex molecule consisting of protein and a lipid fraction such as cholesterol
C. The form in which carbohydrate is stored in the body
D. A lipoprotein consisting of protein and cholesterol that removes excess cholesterol from the cells
E. An abnormally low level of glucose in the blood
F. A lipoprotein, consisting of protein and cholesterol, that picks up cholesterol and delivers it to the cells
G. A substance that is capable of combining with an antigen resulting in an antigen-antibody reaction
H. A substance capable of stimulating the formation of antibodies
I. One who receives something, such as a blood transfusion, from a donor
J. Clumping of blood cells
K. A protein present on the surface of red blood cells that determines a person's blood type
L. Occurring in the living body or organism
M. A unit of heredity
N. A serum that contains antibodies
O. One who furnishes something such as blood, tissue, or organs to be used in another person
P. Occurring in glass; refers to tests performed under artificial conditions, as in the laboratory
Q. A protein present in the blood plasma that is capable of combining with its corresponding antigen to produce an antigen-antibody reaction

Copyright © 2008, 2004, 2000, 1995, 1990 by Saunders, an imprint of Elsevier Inc. All rights reserved.

EVALUATION OF LEARNING

Directions: Fill in each blank with the correct answer.

1. What type of specimen is required for most blood chemistry tests?

 ____

2. What is the purpose of quality control?

 ____

 ____

3. What is the purpose of calibrating a blood chemistry analyzer?

 ____

 ____

4. List two reasons why a control may not fall within its normal range.

 ____

 ____

5. What is cholesterol?

 ____

 ____

6. List the two main sources of cholesterol in the blood.

 ____

 ____

7. What is atherosclerosis and why is it a health risk?

 ____

 ____

8. Why is LDL cholesterol referred to as "bad" cholesterol and HDL referred to as "good" cholesterol?

 ____

 ____

9. What does a total cholesterol test measure?

 ____

 ____

10. List the ranges for each of the following cholesterol categories:
 a. Desirable cholesterol level ______________________________
 b. Borderline cholesterol level ______________________________
 c. High cholesterol level ______________________________

11. At what level is HDL cholesterol considered a risk factor for coronary heart disease?

 ____

 ____

Copyright © 2008, 2004, 2000, 1995, 1990 by Saunders, an imprint of Elsevier Inc. All rights reserved.

12. What type of patient preparation is required for a triglyceride test?

____

____

13. What is the primary use of the cholesterol test?

____

____

14. What is the purpose of performing a BUN?

____

____

15. What is the function of glucose in the body?

____

____

16. Explain the function of insulin in the body.

____

____

17. List the abbreviation for each of the following tests:
    a. Fasting blood sugar _______________
    b. Two-hour postprandial glucose _______________
    c. Glucose tolerance test _______________

18. What type of patient preparation is required for a fasting blood sugar?

____

____

19. What is the normal range for a fasting blood sugar?

____

20. List two reasons for performing a fasting blood sugar.

____

21. What type of patient preparation is required for a 2-hour postprandial glucose test?

____

____

22. Describe the procedure for performing a 2-hour postprandial glucose test.

____

____

23. What is the purpose of the glucose tolerance test?

____

____

Copyright © 2008, 2004, 2000, 1995, 1990 by Saunders, an imprint of Elsevier Inc. All rights reserved.

24. What type of patient preparation is required for the glucose tolerance test?

25. Describe the procedure for a glucose tolerance test.

26. Define hypoglycemia and list three conditions that may cause it to occur.

27. Why is it important for an insulin-dependent diabetic to perform SMBG?

28. What is the ideal insulin testing schedule for SMBG?

29. What type of damage can occur to the body from prolonged high blood glucose levels?

30. List three advantages of blood glucose monitoring at home.

31. What is the recommended blood glucose level for a diabetic during the following times of the day:

a. Before meals __________

b. One to two hours after meals __________

c. At bedtime __________

32. What information is provided by a hemoglobin A_{1C} test?

33. What is the normal A_{1C} range for an individual without diabetes?

34. What is the recommended A_{1C} percentage for an individual with diabetes?

35. What are the storage requirements for blood glucose reagent strips?

Copyright © 2008, 2004, 2000, 1995, 1990 by Saunders, an imprint of Elsevier Inc. All rights reserved.

36. What is the definition of serology?

37. List three examples of antigens.

38. What is the purpose of performing each of the following serologic tests?
   a. Rheumatoid factor
   b. Antistreptolysin test
   c. C-reactive protein
   d. ABO and Rh blood typing

39. How is infectious mononucleosis transmitted?

40. What are the symptoms of infectious mononucleosis?

41. What happens when a blood antigen and antibody combine?

42. Where are the A, B, and Rh antigens located?

43. What is the term used to describe "in glass"?

44. Why is agglutination of blood in vivo a threat to life?

Copyright © 2008, 2004, 2000, 1995, 1990 by Saunders, an imprint of Elsevier Inc. All rights reserved.

45. If a person has type A blood, what antigens and antibodies will be present?

____

____

____

46. If a person has type B blood, what antigens and antibodies will be present?

____

____

47. If a person has type AB blood, what antigens and antibodies will be present?

____

48. If a person has type O blood, what antigens and antibodies will be present?

____

49. What is the difference between Rh-positive and Rh-negative blood?

____

____

50. What term is used to describe the breakdown of blood?

____

CRITICAL THINKING ACTIVITIES

A. CORONARY HEART DISEASE

Create a profile of an individual who is at risk for developing coronary heart disease (CHD) following these guidelines:

1. Using colored pencils, crayons, or markers, draw a figure of an an individual exhibiting risk factors for CHD. Be as creative as possible.

2. Do not use any text on your drawing, other than to label items you have drawn in your picture. (A picture is worth a thousand words!)

3. Try to include at least eight risk factors for CHD in your drawing. The *Highlight on Coronary Heart Disease* box in your textbook can be used as a reference source.

4. In the classroom, find a partner and trade drawings. Identify the risk factors for CHD in your partner's drawing. With your partner, discuss what this person could do to lower his or her chances of developing coronary heart disease.

Copyright © 2008, 2004, 2000, 1995, 1990 by Saunders, an imprint of Elsevier Inc. All rights reserved.

AT RISK FOR CHD

Copyright © 2008, 2004, 2000, 1995, 1990 by Saunders, an imprint of Elsevier Inc. All rights reserved.

B. CHOLESTEROL AND SATURATED FAT

Using a reference source, complete the following activities:

1. Create a dinner meal that is as high as possible in saturated fat and cholesterol.

2. Create a dinner meal that is as low as possible in saturated fat and cholesterol.

3. Choose a fast-food restaurant and plan a meal that is as low as possible in saturated fat and cholesterol.

C. GLUCOSE TOLERANCE TEST

Marty Wolf has arrived at your office for a glucose tolerance test. What should you tell her regarding the following? Explain the reason for each answer.

1. Consumption of food and fluid

2. Water consumption

3. Smoking

4. Leaving the test site

5. Activity

Copyright © 2008, 2004, 2000, 1995, 1990 by Saunders, an imprint of Elsevier Inc. All rights reserved.

D. Rh INCOMPATIBILITY

Erythroblastosis fetalis is a blood disorder of the newborn, usually due to incompatibility between the infant's blood and the mother's blood. Using a reference source, answer the following questions regarding this condition in the space provided:

1. Explain how Rh incompatibility between the mother and infant can cause this condition to occur.

2. Describe the symptoms associated with erythroblastosis fetalis.

3. Explain the treatment used for this condition.

4. How can this condition be prevented?

E. TYPE 2 DIABETES

You are working for a physician specializing in internal medicine. Your physician is concerned about the increase in the numbers of patients developing type 2 diabetes mellitus. He asks you to design a colorful, creative, and informative brochure on type 2 diabetes using the brochure provided on the following page. This brochure will be published and placed in the waiting room to provide patients with education on type 2 diabetes. The diabetes Internet sites listed under **On the Web** at the end of Chapter 19 in your textbook can be used to complete this activity.

Copyright © 2008, 2004, 2000, 1995, 1990 by Saunders, an imprint of Elsevier Inc. All rights reserved.

FAQ on:

Q:

A:

Q:

A:

Q:

A:

Q:

A:

Copyright © 2008, 2004, 2000, 1995, 1990 by Saunders, an imprint of Elsevier Inc. All rights reserved.

Q:

A:

Q:

A:

Illustration

Q:

A:

Q:

A:

Copyright © 2008, 2004, 2000, 1995, 1990 by Saunders, an imprint of Elsevier Inc. All rights reserved.

F. CROSSWORD PUZZLE
Blood Chemistry and Serology

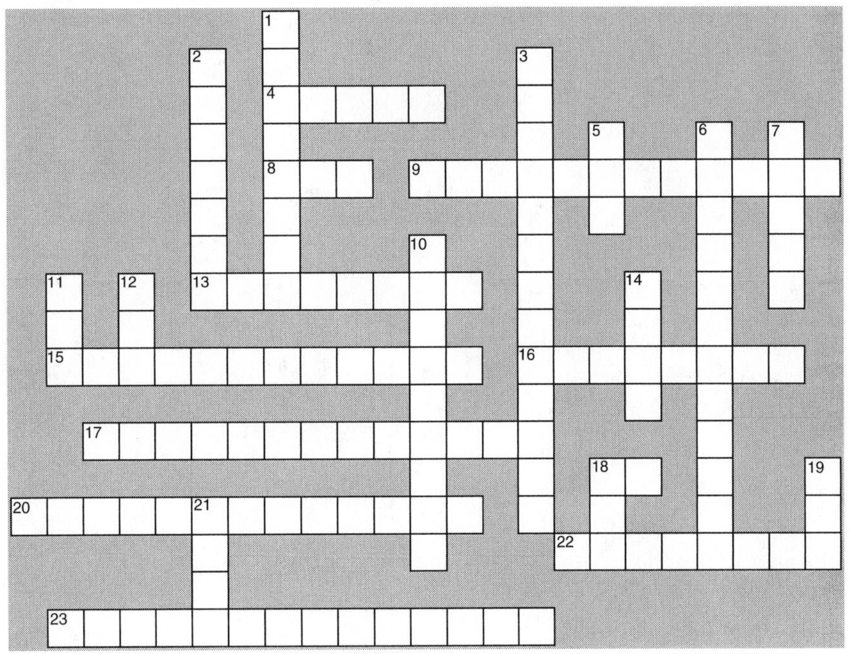

Directions: Complete the crossword puzzle using the clues presented below.

ACROSS

4 Assesses thyroid functioning
8 Detects renal disease
9 Low BS
13 Stored glucose
15 Raises chol
16 Increases HDL chol
17 Normal: <150 mg/dL
18 Assists in confirming an MI
20 High BS
22 Unsaturated fat (ex)
23 Chol: 200-239

DOWN

1 Combines with an antigen
2 Increases risk of CHD
3 Kissing disease
5 Detects liver disease
6 #1 killer in U.S.
7 Makes cholesterol
10 Blood donor disqualifier
11 70-110 mg/dL
12 Series of glucose tests
14 Syphilis test
18 Bad cholesterol
19 Good cholesterol
21 Unit of heredity

Copyright © 2008, 2004, 2000, 1995, 1990 by Saunders, an imprint of Elsevier Inc. All rights reserved.

Notes

Copyright © 2008, 2004, 2000, 1995, 1990 by Saunders, an imprint of Elsevier Inc. All rights reserved.

PRACTICE FOR COMPETENCY

Procedure 19-A: Blood Chemistry Test. Perform a blood chemistry test and record results in the chart provided. Examples of Blood Chemistry Tests: Cholesterol, Triglycerides, Hemoglobin A1C, BUN

Procedure 19-1: Blood Glucose Measurement. Perform a fasting blood sugar and record results in the chart provided.
Procedure 19-B: Rapid Mononucleosis Test. Perform a rapid mononucleosis test and record results in the chart provided.

CHART	
Date	

Copyright © 2008, 2004, 2000, 1995, 1990 by Saunders, an imprint of Elsevier Inc. All rights reserved.

CHART	
Date	

Copyright © 2008, 2004, 2000, 1995, 1990 by Saunders, an imprint of Elsevier Inc. All rights reserved.

EVALUATION OF COMPETENCY

Procedure 19-A: Performing a Blood Chemistry Test

Name: ______________________________ Date: ____________

Evaluated By: ______________________________ Score: ____________

Performance Objective

Outcome:	Perform a blood chemistry test.
Conditions:	Given the following: disposable gloves, an antiseptic wipe, a lancet, gauze pad, quality control log, and a biohazard sharps container. Using an automated blood chemistry analyzer and operating manual.
Standards:	Time: 10 minutes. Student completed procedure in ____ minutes.
	Accuracy: Satisfactory score in the Performance Evaluation Checklist.

Performance Evaluation Checklist

Trial 1	Trial 2	Point Value	*Performance Standards*
		•	Sanitized hands.
		•	Assembled equipment.
		•	Calibrated the blood chemistry analyzer.
		•	Applied gloves and ran controls.
		•	Recorded results in the quality control log.
		•	Sanitized hands. Greeted the patient and introduced yourself.
		•	Identified patient and explained the procedure.
		•	Applied gloves.
		•	Performed a finger puncture.
		•	Collected the specimen according to manufacturer's instructions.
		•	Placed a gauze pad over the puncture site and applied pressure.
		•	Inserted the specimen into blood chemistry analyzer according to manufacturer's instructions.
		•	Operated the blood chemistry analyzer according to manufacturer's instructions.
		•	Read the results on digital display screen.
		•	Properly disposed of used materials.
		•	Checked puncture site and applied adhesive bandage if needed.
		•	Removed gloves.
		•	Sanitized hands.

Copyright © 2008, 2004, 2000, 1995, 1990 by Saunders, an imprint of Elsevier Inc. All rights reserved.

		•	Charted the test results correctly.
		*	The recording was identical to the reading on the digital display screen.
		*	Completed the procedure within 10 minutes.
			TOTALS

CHART

Date	

Copyright © 2008, 2004, 2000, 1995, 1990 by Saunders, an imprint of Elsevier Inc. All rights reserved.

Evaluation of Student Performance

EVALUATION CRITERIA			COMMENTS
Symbol	Category	Point Value	
✶	Critical Step	16 points	
●	Essential Step	6 points	
▷	Theory Question	2 points	
Score calculation: 100 points – ______ points missed ____ Score Satisfactory score: 85 or above			

AAMA/CAAHEP Competency Achieved:

☑ III. C. 3. b. (3) (c) (iii): Perform chemistry testing.

☑ III. C. 3. c. (4) (d): Use methods of quality control.

Copyright © 2008, 2004, 2000, 1995, 1990 by Saunders, an imprint of Elsevier Inc. All rights reserved.

Notes

Copyright © 2008, 2004, 2000, 1995, 1990 by Saunders, an imprint of Elsevier Inc. All rights reserved.

EVALUATION OF COMPETENCY

Procedure 19-1: Blood Glucose Measurement Using the Accu-Check Advantage Glucose Meter

Name: ______________________________ Date: ______________

Evaluated By: ______________________________ Score: ______________

Performance Objective

Outcome: Perform a fasting blood sugar.

Conditions: Given the following: disposable gloves, ACU-Chek Advantage glucose meter, reagent strips, check strip, code key, control solutions, lancet, antiseptic wipe, gauze pad, quality control log, and a biohazard sharps container.

Standards: Time: 10 minutes. Student completed procedure in ____ minutes.

Accuracy: Satisfactory score in the Performance Evaluation Checklist.

Performance Evaluation Checklist

Trial 1	Trial 2	Point Value	*Performance Standards*
		•	Sanitized hands.
		•	Assembled equipment.
		•	Checked the expiration date on container of reagent strips.
		•	Calibrated the meter using the code key.
		▷	Stated the purpose of calibrating the meter.
		•	Ran a low and high control.
		▷	Stated the purpose for running controls.
		•	Recorded results in the quality control log.
		•	Sanitized hands. Greeted the patient and introduced yourself.
		•	Identified the patient and explained the procedure.
		•	Asked the patient if he or she prepared properly.
		▷	Stated the preparation required for a fasting blood sugar.
		•	Removed a test strip from the container.
		•	Immediately replaced the lid of the container.
		▷	Explained why the lid should be replaced immediately.
		•	Gently inserted the test strip into the test strip guide.
		•	The yellow target area was facing up.
		•	Turned on the meter (if the meter does not turn on automatically).
		•	Checked the code number.
		•	Opened gauze packet.
		•	Cleansed the puncture site with an antiseptic wipe and allowed it to dry.
		•	Applied gloves.

Copyright © 2008, 2004, 2000, 1995, 1990 by Saunders, an imprint of Elsevier Inc. All rights reserved.

Trial 1	*Trial 2*	*Point Value*	*Performance Standards*
		•	Performed a finger puncture.
		•	Disposed of the lancet in the biohazard sharps container.
		•	Wiped away the first drop of blood with a gauze pad.
		▷	Explained why the first drop of blood should be wiped away.
		•	Placed the patient's hand in a dependent position and gently massaged finger until a large drop of blood formed.
		•	Applied the drop of blood to the yellow target area of the test strip.
		•	Completely covered the yellow target area with blood.
		▷	Explained what to do if the yellow area is not completely covered
		•	Placed a gauze pad over puncture site and applied pressure.
		•	Observed the digital display of the test results.
		▷	Stated the normal range for a fasting blood glucose (70 to 110 mg/dL).
		•	Removed the test strip from the meter and discarded it in a biohazard waste container.
		•	Turned off the meter.
		•	Checked puncture site and applied adhesive bandage, if needed.
		•	Removed gloves and sanitized hands.
		•	Charted the test results correctly.
		✶	The recording was identical to the reading on the digital display screen.
		•	Properly stored the glucose meter.
		✶	Completed the procedure within 10 minutes.
			TOTALS

CHART

Date	

Copyright © 2008, 2004, 2000, 1995, 1990 by Saunders, an imprint of Elsevier Inc. All rights reserved.

Evaluation of Student Performance

EVALUATION CRITERIA			COMMENTS
Symbol	**Category**	**Point Value**	
✶	Critical Step	16 points	
●	Essential Step	6 points	
▷	Theory Question	2 points	
Score calculation: 100 points – ______ points missed ____ Score Satisfactory score: 85 or above			

AAMA/CAAHEP Competency Achieved:

☑ III. C. 3. b. (3) (c) (iii): Perform chemistry testing.

☑ III. C. 3. c. (4) (d): Use methods of quality control.

Copyright © 2008, 2004, 2000, 1995, 1990 by Saunders, an imprint of Elsevier Inc. All rights reserved.

Notes

Copyright © 2008, 2004, 2000, 1995, 1990 by Saunders, an imprint of Elsevier Inc. All rights reserved.

EVALUATION OF COMPETENCY

Procedure 19-3: Rapid Mononucleosis Testing (Quick Vue + Mono Test)

Name: ______________________________ Date: ______________

Evaluated By: ______________________________ Score: ______________

Performance Objective

Outcome: Perform a rapid mononucleosis test.

Conditions: Given the following: personal protective equipment including gloves, the supplies needed to perform a finger puncture, a mononucleosis testing kit, and a biohazard waste container.

Standards: Time: 10 minutes. Student completed procedure in ____ minutes.

Accuracy: Satisfactory score in the Performance Evaluation Checklist.

Performance Evaluation Checklist

Trial 1	*Trial 2*	*Point Value*	*Performance Standards*
		•	Sanitized hands.
		•	Assembled equipment.
		•	Checked the expiration date on the testing kit.
		•	Applied gloves and ran a positive and a negative control, if necessary.
		•	Removed gloves and recorded results in the quality control log.
		•	Greeted the patient and introduced yourself.
		•	Identified the patient and explained the procedure.
		•	Cleansed the puncture site and allowed it to air dry.
		•	Applied gloves.
		•	Performed a finger puncture.
		•	Disposed of the lancet in a biohazard sharps container.
		•	Wiped away the first drop of blood.
		•	Collected the blood specimen with a capillary tube.
		•	Placed a gauze pad over puncture site and applied pressure.
		•	Dispensed the blood specimen into the add well on the test cassette.
		•	Added 5 drops of developing solution to the add well.
		•	Waited 5 minutes and read the results.
		▷	Described the appearance of a positive and negative test result.
		•	Disposed of the test cassette in a biohazard waste container.
		•	Checked puncture site and applied adhesive bandage, if needed.
		•	Removed gloves.

Copyright © 2008, 2004, 2000, 1995, 1990 by Saunders, an imprint of Elsevier Inc. All rights reserved.

Trial 1	Trial 2	Point Value	Performance Standards
		•	Sanitized hands.
		•	Charted the results correctly.
		•	The results were identical to the evaluator's results.
		•	Completed the procedure within 10 minutes.
			TOTALS

	CHART
Date	

Evaluation of Student Performance

EVALUATION CRITERIA			COMMENTS
Symbol	Category	Point Value	
∗	Critical Step	16 points	
•	Essential Step	6 points	
▷	Theory Question	2 points	
Score calculation: 100 points – ______ points missed ____ Score Satisfactory score: 85 or above			

AAMA/CAAHEP Competency Achieved:

☑ III. C. 3. b. (3) (c) (iv): Perform immunology testing.
☑ III. C. 3. c. (4) (d): Use methods of quality control.

Copyright © 2008, 2004, 2000, 1995, 1990 by Saunders, an imprint of Elsevier Inc. All rights reserved.

20

Medical Microbiology

CHAPTER ASSIGNMENTS

√ After Completing	Date Due	Textbook Page(s)	TEXTBOOK ASSIGNMENTS	Possible Points	Points You Earned
		721-744	Read Chapter 20: Medical Microbiology		
		724 741	Read Case Study 1 Case Study 1 questions	5	
		732 741	Read Case Study 2 Case Study 2 questions	5	
		738 741	Read Case Study 3 Case Study 3 questions	5	
		742	Apply Your Knowledge questions	10	
			TOTAL POINTS		

√ After Completing	Date Due	Study Guide Page(s)	STUDY GUIDE ASSIGNMENTS (CTA: Critical Thinking Activity)	Possible Points	Points You Earned
		813	Pretest	10	
		814	Key Term Assessment	15	
		815-818	Evaluation of Learning questions	25	
		818-819	CTA A: Stages of an Infectious Disease	20	
			CD Activity: Chapter 20 Under the Microscope (Record points earned)		
		821-822	CTA B: Choose-a-Clue (Record points earned)		
		827	CTA C: Disease and Infection Control	10	
		827	CTA D: Sensitivity Testing	12	
		828	CTA E: Crossword Puzzle	21	
			CD Activity: Chapter 20 Animations	20	

Copyright © 2008, 2004, 2000, 1995, 1990 by Saunders, an imprint of Elsevier Inc. All rights reserved.

√ After Completing	Date Due	Study Guide Page(s)	STUDY GUIDE ASSIGNMENTS (CTA: Critical Thinking Activity)	Possible Points	Points You Earned
		813	Posttest	10	
			ADDITIONAL ASSIGNMENTS		
			TOTAL POINTS		

Copyright © 2008, 2004, 2000, 1995, 1990 by Saunders, an imprint of Elsevier Inc. All rights reserved.

√ When Assigned By Your Instructor	Study Guide Page(s)	Practices Required	LABORATORY ASSIGNMENTS (Procedure Number and Name)	*Score
	829-830	3	**Practice for Competency** 20-1: Using the Microscope Textbook reference: pp. 728-730	
	831-833		**Evaluation of Competency** 20-1: Using the Microscope	*
	829-830	3	**Practice for Competency** 20-2: Collecting a Specimen for a Throat Culture Textbook reference: p. 733	
	835-837		**Evaluation of Competency** 20-2: Collecting a Specimen for a Throat Culture	*
	829-830	3	**Practice for Competency** 20-A: Rapid Strep Testing Textbook reference: p. 735	
	839-841		**Evaluation of Competency** 20-A: Rapid Strep Testing	*
	829-830		**Practice for Competency** 20-3: Preparing a Smear Textbook reference: pp. 739-740	
	843-844		**Evaluation of Competency** 20-3: Preparing a Smear	*
			ADDITIONAL ASSIGNMENTS	

Copyright © 2008, 2004, 2000, 1995, 1990 by Saunders, an imprint of Elsevier Inc. All rights reserved.

Notes

Copyright © 2008, 2004, 2000, 1995, 1990 by Saunders, an imprint of Elsevier Inc. All rights reserved.

Name ______________________________ Date ______________

PRETEST

True or False

_____ 1. Microbiology is the scientific study of microorganisms and their activities.

_____ 2. A disease that can be spread from one person to another is known as an infectious disease.

_____ 3. Droplet infection is the transfer of pathogens from a fine spray emitted from a person already infected with the disease.

_____ 4. Streptococci are round bacteria that grow in pairs.

_____ 5. Chickenpox is caused by a virus.

_____ 6. The course adjustment on a microscope is used to obtain precise focusing of an object.

_____ 7. The purpose of transport media is to provide nutrients for the multiplication of the specimen.

_____ 8. A throat specimen should be collected from the tonsillar area and posterior pharynx.

_____ 9. A wet mount is used to examine microorganisms in the living state.

_____ 10. A smear is material spread on a slide for microscopic examination.

POSTTEST

True or False

_____ 1. Microorganisms that reside in the body but do not cause disease are known as transient flora.

_____ 2. The invasion of the body by a pathogenic microorganism is known as infection.

_____ 3. The interval of time between the invasion by a pathogen and the first symptoms of disease is known as the prodromal period.

_____ 4. Staphylococcal infections usually result in pus formation.

_____ 5. *E. coli* normally reside in the urinary tract.

_____ 6. The high-power objective has a magnification of 40X.

_____ 7. Examination of urine sediment requires the use of the oil immersion objective.

_____ 8. A mixed culture contains two or more types of microorganisms.

_____ 9. The purpose of sensitivity testing is to identify the type of microorganism present.

_____ 10. When viewed under a microscope, gram-positive bacteria appear pink or red in color.

Copyright © 2008, 2004, 2000, 1995, 1990 by Saunders, an imprint of Elsevier Inc. All rights reserved.

KEY TERM ASSESSMENT

Directions: Match each medical term with its definition.

_______ 1. Bacilli

_______ 2. Cocci

_______ 3. Contagious

_______ 4. Culture

_______ 5. Culture medium

_______ 6. Incubate

_______ 7. Incubation period

_______ 8. Infectious disease

_______ 9. Inoculate

_______ 10. Microbiology

_______ 11. Normal flora

_______ 12. Sequelae

_______ 13. Smear

_______ 14. Specimen

_______ 15. Spirilla

A. A disease caused by a pathogen that produces harmful effects on its host

B. Capable of being transmitted directly or indirectly from one person to another

C. To introduce microorganisms into a culture medium for growth and multiplication

D. Round bacteria

E. The scientific study of microorganisms and their activities

F. Material spread on a slide for microscopic examination

G. A morbid (secondary) condition occurring as a result of a less serious primary infection

H. A mixture of nutrients in which microorganisms are grown in the laboratory

I. The interval of time between invasion by a pathogenic microorganism and the appearance of the first symptoms of the disease

J. Bacteria that have a spiral or curved shape

K. Harmless, nonpathogenic microorganisms that normally reside in many parts of the body

L. Rod-shaped bacteria

M. The propagation of a mass of microorganisms in a laboratory culture medium

N. In microbiology, the act of placing a culture in a chamber that provides optimal growth requirements for the multiplication of the organisms, such as the proper temperature, humidity, and darkness

O. A small sample taken from the body to show the nature of the whole

Copyright © 2008, 2004, 2000, 1995, 1990 by Saunders, an imprint of Elsevier Inc. All rights reserved.

EVALUATION OF LEARNING

Directions: Fill in each blank with the correct answer.

1. Explain what happens when a pathogen invades the body.

____

____

2. How does droplet infection contribute to the transmission of infectious disease?

____

____

3. What occurs during the prodromal period of an infectious disease?

____

____

4. List three infectious diseases caused by *Staphylococcus aureus*.

____

____

5. List three infectious diseases caused by different types of streptococci.

____

____

6. List three infectious diseases caused by different types of bacilli.

____

____

7. In what part of the body does *Escherichia coli* normally reside?

____

8. List four infectious diseases caused by different types of viruses.

____

____

9. Explain the purpose of each of the following parts of a microscope:

   Stage

   ____

   ____

   Substage condenser

   ____

   ____

Copyright © 2008, 2004, 2000, 1995, 1990 by Saunders, an imprint of Elsevier Inc. All rights reserved.

Iris diaphragm

Coarse adjustment

Fine adjustment

Ocular lens

10. Describe the function of each of the following objective lenses:

Low-power

High-power

Oil-immersion

11. What is the purpose of using oil with the oil-immersion objective?

12. List five guidelines that should be followed for proper care of the microscope.

13. List five common areas of the body from which a microbiologic specimen may be obtained.

Copyright © 2008, 2004, 2000, 1995, 1990 by Saunders, an imprint of Elsevier Inc. All rights reserved.

14. List two ways to prevent contamination of a specimen with extraneous microorganisms.

____

____

15. List two precautions a medical assistant should take to prevent infecting herself or himself with a microbiologic specimen.

____

____

16. Why should a specimen be processed as soon as possible after it is collected?

____

17. What is the purpose of culturing microorganisms?

____

____

18. What is the name given to the type of culture that contains two or more types of microorganisms?

____

19. Why is it important to diagnose streptococcal pharyngitis as early as possible?

____

____

20. What type of reaction is used to identify streptococcus with the direct antigen rapid streptococcus test?

____

21. When performing a hemolytic reaction and bacitracin susceptibility test, what is observed on the blood agar medium if a patient has streptococcal pharyngitis?

____

____

22. What is the purpose of performing a sensitivity test on a bacterial culture?

____

23. List two reasons for examining a microorganism in the living state.

____

____

Copyright © 2008, 2004, 2000, 1995, 1990 by Saunders, an imprint of Elsevier Inc. All rights reserved.

24. What is the purpose of staining a smear?

____

____

25. What color does gram-positive bacteria exhibit in a gram-stained smear?

____

CRITICAL THINKING ACTIVITIES

A. STAGES OF AN INFECTIOUS DISEASE

Your physician wants you to design a poster to hang in the office outlining the stages of an infectious disease. Complete this project using the following diagram in your study guide.

Copyright © 2008, 2004, 2000, 1995, 1990 by Saunders, an imprint of Elsevier Inc. All rights reserved.

STAGES OF INFECTIOUS DISEASE

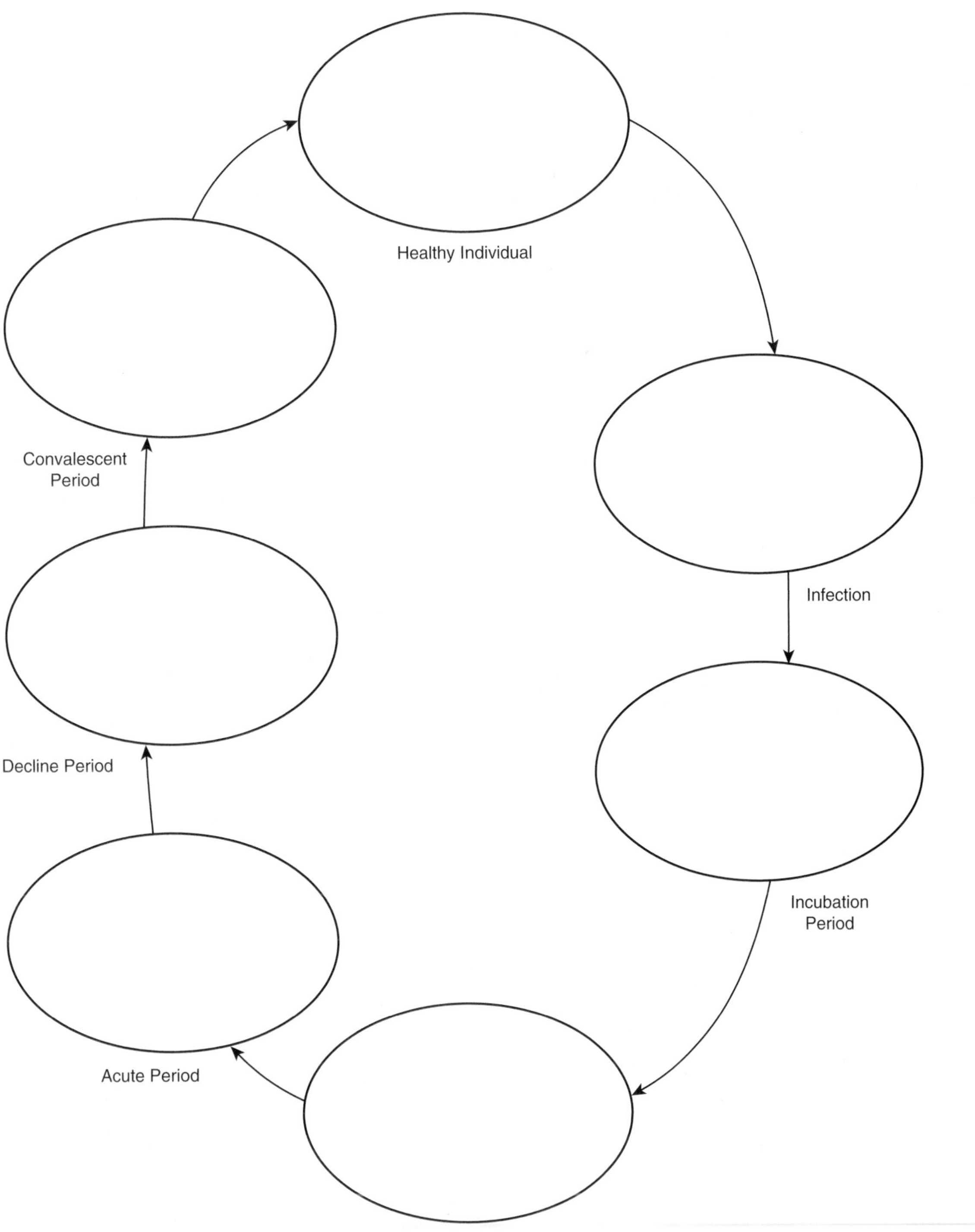

Copyright © 2008, 2004, 2000, 1995, 1990 by Saunders, an imprint of Elsevier Inc. All rights reserved.

Notes

Copyright © 2008, 2004, 2000, 1995, 1990 by Saunders, an imprint of Elsevier Inc. All rights reserved.

B. CHOOSE-A-CLUE

Object: The object of the game is to become familiar with infectious diseases.

Directions:

1. Cut out the game cards on the following pages.
2. List three clues for each condition specified on the reverse of the card. Your clues should include information on symptoms, prevention, and treatment. The name of the disease must not be written on this side of the card.
3. Use the game cards as flash cards to study the diseases.
4. Get into a group of three students.
5. Place your game cards on the table in front of you with the clues facing up.
6. One of the players should name the first disease on the list presented below.
7. Each player places the appropriate game card in the middle of the table with the clues facing upward.
8. When all players have placed a card on the table, turn the cards over.
9. Award yourself 5 points if you have correctly determined the disease.
10. Review the information each player listed on his or her game card.
11. Keep track of your points on the score card provided below.

Good Internet reference sources to help you find clues include:

www.merck.com
www.kidshealth.org

Conditions

1. Botulism
2. Chronic Fatigue Syndrome
3. Common Cold
4. Diphtheria
5. Gonorrhea
6. Infectious mononucleosis
7. Poliomyelitis
8. Rabies
9. Rheumatic fever
10. Rubella
11. Rubeola
12. Salmonella food poisoning
13. Smallpox
14. Staphylococcal food poisoning
15. Syphilis
16. Tetanus

Copyright © 2008, 2004, 2000, 1995, 1990 by Saunders, an imprint of Elsevier Inc. All rights reserved.

CHOOSE-A-CLUE
SCORE CARD

Name: ____

Recording Points:
Cross off a number each time you properly identify a disease (starting with 5 and continuing in sequence). Your total points will be equal to the last number you crossed off. Record this number in the space provided and determine the knowledge level you attained.

Points:	
5	75
10	80
15	85
20	90
25	95
30	100
35	105
40	110
45	115
50	120
55	125
60	130
65	135
70	140

TOTAL POINTS: ________

LEVEL: ________

☐ 75 points and above: **Free from Infection**
☐ 65 to 70 points: **Putting Up a Good Fight**
☐ 55 to 60 points: **Susceptible**
☐ 50 points and under: **Infected**

Copyright © 2008, 2004, 2000, 1995, 1990 by Saunders, an imprint of Elsevier Inc. All rights reserved.

Botulism

Chronic fatigue syndrome

Common cold

Diptheria

Gonorrhea

Infectious mononucleosis

Poliomyelitis

Rabies

Sym:

Prev:

Tx:

Sym:

Prev:

Tx:.

Sym:

Prev:

Tx:

Sym:

Prev:

Tx:

Sym:

Prev:

Tx:

Sym:

Prev:

Tx:

Sym:

Prev:

Tx:

Sym:

Prev:

Tx:

Rheumatic fever

Rubella

Rubeola

Salmonella food poisoning

Smallpox

Staphylococcal food poisoning

Syphilis

Tetanus

Sym:

Prev:

Tx:

Sym:

Prev:

Tx:

Sym:

Prev:

Tx:

Sym:

Prev:

Tx:

Sym:

Prev:

Tx:

Sym:

Prev:

Tx:

Sym:

Prev:

Tx:

Sym:

Prev:

Tx:

C. DISEASE AND INFECTION CONTROL

Obtain a current journal article on disease and infection control. The Internet sites listed under **On the web** at the end of chapter 20 in your textbook can be used to locate an article. List the important parts of your article below.

____

____

____

____

____

____

____

____

____

____

____

____

D. SENSITIVITY TESTING

Refer to Figure 20-9 in your textbook. Place a check mark next to each antibiotic that is effective against the pathogen growing on the culture medium in the Petri plate.

_____ 1. azithromycin
_____ 2. cephalothin
_____ 3. ciprofloxacin
_____ 4. cefprozil
_____ 5. clarithromycin
_____ 6. doxycycline
_____ 7. erythromycin
_____ 8. nitrofurantoin
_____ 9. norflaxin
_____ 10. penicillin
_____ 11. sulfisoxazole
_____ 12. tetracycline

Copyright © 2008, 2004, 2000, 1995, 1990 by Saunders, an imprint of Elsevier Inc. All rights reserved.

E. CROSSWORD PUZZLE
Medical Microbiology

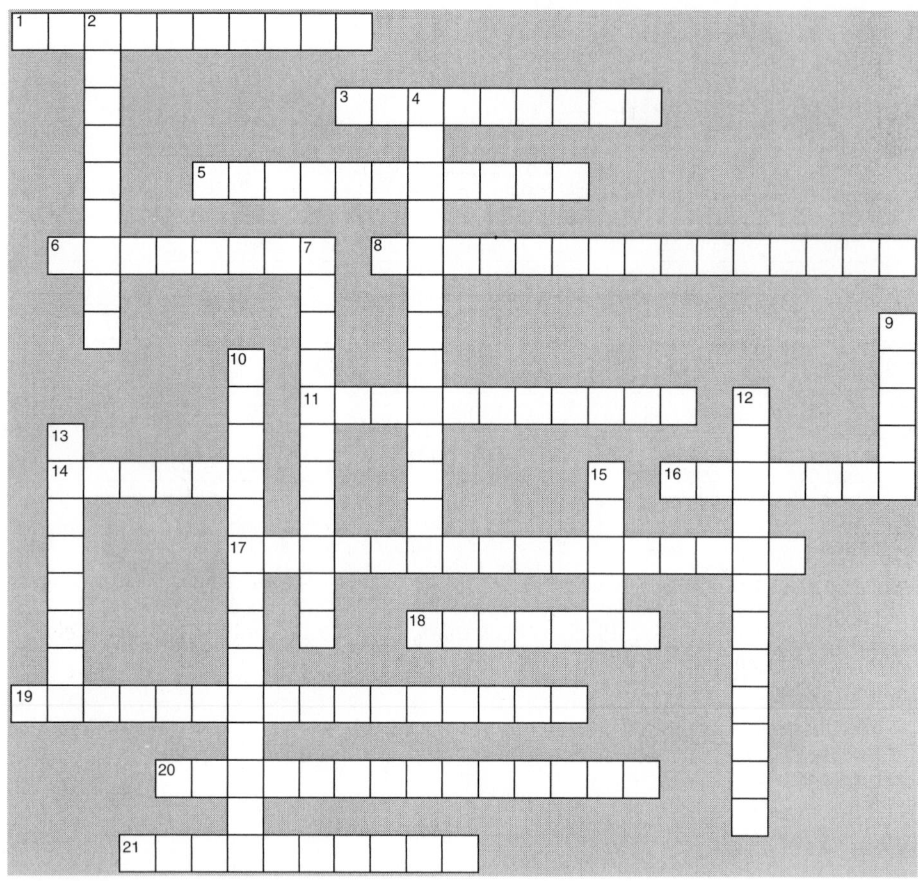

Directions: Complete the crossword puzzle using the clues presented below.

ACROSS

1 It is everywhere!
3 Invasion by pathogens
5 Only 1 MO growing
6 Disease producing MO
8 Which antibiotic?
11 Tx for strep throat
14 Color of gram + bacteria
16 Rod-shaped bacteria
17 Way to transmit pathogens
18 Mass of MOs on a medium
19 Between invasion and first sym
20 Sequela to strep throat
21 Can catch it!

DOWN

2 Introduce MOs to a culture
4 Not really present
7 Harmless MOs
9 Round bacteria
10 For precise focusing
12 Study of MOs
13 Sample of the body
15 Material spread on a slide

Copyright © 2008, 2004, 2000, 1995, 1990 by Saunders, an imprint of Elsevier Inc. All rights reserved.

PRACTICE FOR COMPETENCY

Procedure 20-1: Using the Microscope. Practice using a microscope.
Procedure 20-2: Collecting a Specimen for a Throat Culture. Obtain a specimen for a throat culture using a sterile cotton swab and/or a collection and transport system. Record the procedure in the chart provided.
Procedure 20-A: Rapid Strep Testing. Perform a strep test using a rapid strep testing kit and record results in the chart provided.
Procedure 20-3: Preparing a Smear. Prepare a microbiologic smear.

Chart	
Date	

Copyright © 2008, 2004, 2000, 1995, 1990 by Saunders, an imprint of Elsevier Inc. All rights reserved.

Copyright © 2008, 2004, 2000, 1995, 1990 by Saunders, an imprint of Elsevier Inc. All rights reserved.

EVALUATION OF COMPETENCY

Procedure 20-1: Using the Microscope

Name: ______________________ Date: ____________

Evaluated By: ______________________ Score: ____________

Performance Objective

Outcome:	Use a microscope.
Conditions:	Given a microscope, lens paper, specimen slide, tissue or gauze, immersion oil, xylene, and a soft cloth.
Standards:	Time: 15 minutes. Student completed procedure in ____ minutes.
	Accuracy: Satisfactory score on the Performance Evaluation Checklist.

Performance Evaluation Checklist

Trial 1	*Trial 2*	*Point Value*	*Performance Standards*
		•	Cleaned the ocular and objective lenses with lens paper.
		•	Turned on the light source.
		•	Rotated the nosepiece to the low-power objective.
		•	Used the coarse adjustment to provide sufficient working space for placing the slide on the stage.
		•	Placed the slide on the stage specimen side up and secured it.
		•	Positioned the low-power objective until it almost touched the slide using the coarse adjustment.
		•	Observed this step.
		▷	Explained why this step should be observed.
		•	Looked through the ocular.
		•	Brought the specimen into coarse focus using the coarse adjustment knob.
		•	Observed the specimen until it came into coarse focus.
		•	Used the fine adjustment knob to bring the specimen into a sharp, clear focus.
		•	Adjusted the light as needed using the iris diaphragm.
		•	Rotated the nosepiece to the high-power objective.
		•	Used the fine adjustment knob to bring the specimen into a precise focus.
		•	Did not use the coarse adjustment to focus the high-power objective.
		▷	Explained why the coarse adjustment should not be used for focusing at this point.
		•	Examined the specimen as required by the test or procedure being performed.
		•	Turned off the light after use.

Copyright © 2008, 2004, 2000, 1995, 1990 by Saunders, an imprint of Elsevier Inc. All rights reserved.

Trial 1	Trial 2	Point Value	Performance Standards
		•	Removed the slide from the stage.
		•	Cleaned the stage with a tissue or gauze.
		•	Properly cared for and stored the microscope.
			Using the Oil-Immersion Objective:
		•	Rotated the nosepiece to the oil-immersion objective.
		•	Placed the objective to one side.
		•	Placed a drop of immersion oil on the slide directly over the center opening in the stage.
		•	Moved the oil-immersion objective into place.
		•	Made sure the objective did not touch the stage or slide.
		•	Used the coarse adjustment to position the oil-immersion objective.
		•	Brought the objective down until the lens touched the oil but did not come in contact with the slide.
		•	Looked through the eyepiece.
		•	Focused slowly using the coarse objective until the object was visible.
		•	Used the fine adjustment to bring the object into sharp focus.
		•	Adjusted the light as needed using the iris diaphragm.
		•	Examined the specimen as required by the test or procedure being performed.
		•	Turned off the light after use.
		•	Removed the slide from the stage.
		•	Cleaned the oil-immersion objective with lens paper.
		▷	Explained why the lens must be cleaned immediately.
		•	Cleaned the oil from the slide by immersing it in xylene and wiping it with a soft cloth.
		*	Completed the procedure within 15 minutes.
			TOTALS

Copyright © 2008, 2004, 2000, 1995, 1990 by Saunders, an imprint of Elsevier Inc. All rights reserved.

Evaluation of Student Performance

EVALUATION CRITERIA			COMMENTS
Symbol	Category	Point Value	
★	Critical Step	16 points	
●	Essential Step	6 points	
▷	Theory Question	2 points	
Score calculation: 100 points – ______ points missed ______ Score Satisfactory score: 85 or above			

AAMA/CAAHEP Competency Achieved:

☑ III. C. 3. b. (3) (c) (v): Perform microbiology testing.

Copyright © 2008, 2004, 2000, 1995, 1990 by Saunders, an imprint of Elsevier Inc. All rights reserved.

Notes

Copyright © 2008, 2004, 2000, 1995, 1990 by Saunders, an imprint of Elsevier Inc. All rights reserved.

EVALUATION OF COMPETENCY

Procedure 20-2: Collecting a Specimen for a Throat Culture

Name: ______________________________ Date: ______________

Evaluated By: ______________________________ Score: ______________

Performance Objective

Outcome: Collect a specimen for a throat culture.

Conditions: Given the following: disposable gloves, tongue depressor, sterile swab, collection and transport system, laboratory request form, and a biohazard specimen bag.

Standards: Time: 5 minutes. Student completed procedure in ____ minutes.

Accuracy: Satisfactory score on the Performance Evaluation Checklist.

Performance Evaluation Checklist

Trial 1	*Trial 2*	*Point Value*	*Performance Standards*
			Throat Specimen—Sterile Swab for Strep Testing in Medical Office
		•	Sanitized hands.
		•	Assembled equipment.
		•	Greeted the patient and introduced yourself.
		•	Identified the patient and explained the procedure.
		•	Positioned patient and adjusted light.
		•	Applied gloves.
		•	Removed the sterile swab from its peel-apart package, being careful not to contaminate it.
		•	Depressed patient's tongue with tongue depressor.
		•	Placed swab at the back of patient's throat and firmly rubbed it over lesions or white or inflamed areas of the tonsillar area and posterior pharynx.
		▷	Explained why swab should be rubbed over these types of areas.
		•	Constantly rotated swab as the specimen was being obtained.
		▷	Described why a rotating motion should be used.
		•	Did not allow swab to touch any area other than throat.
		▷	Explained why swab should not be allowed to touch any areas other than throat.
		•	Kept patient's tongue depressed and withdrew swab and removed tongue depressor.
		•	Disposed of the tongue depressor.
		•	Performed the rapid strep test according to the directions accompanying the rapid strep testing kit.
		•	Removed gloves and sanitized hands.
		•	Charted the test results correctly.

Copyright © 2008, 2004, 2000, 1995, 1990 by Saunders, an imprint of Elsevier Inc. All rights reserved.

Trial 1	Trial 2	Point Value	Performance Standards
		▷	Completed the procedure within 5 minutes.
			Throat Specimen—Collection and Transport System
		•	Sanitized hands.
		•	Greeted the patient and introduced yourself.
		•	Identified the patient and explained the procedure.
		•	Positioned patient and adjusted light.
		•	Applied gloves.
		•	Checked the expiration date on the peel-apart package.
		•	Peeled open the package and removed the cap from the collection tube.
		•	Removed the cap/swab unit from the peel-apart package.
		•	Depressed the patient's tongue with tongue depressor.
		•	Placed swab at the back of patient's throat and firmly rubbed it over lesions or white or inflamed areas of the tonsillar area and posterior pharynx.
		•	Constantly rotated swab as the specimen was being obtained.
		•	Did not allow swab to touch any area other than the collection site.
		•	Kept patient's tongue depressed and withdrew swab and removed tongue depressor.
		•	Disposed of the tongue depressor.
		•	Inserted swab into the collection tube.
		•	Pushed cap/swab in as far as it will go.
		•	Made sure the cap was tightly in place.
		•	Removed gloves and sanitized hands.
		•	Labeled tube.
		•	Completed a laboratory request form.
		•	Placed tube in a biohazard specimen transport bag.
		•	Placed laboratory request in outside pocket of bag.
		•	Charted the procedure.
		•	Transported specimen to the laboratory within 24 hours.
		▷	Explained why the specimen must be transported within 24 hours.
		✶	Completed the procedure within 5 minutes.
			TOTALS

CHART	
Date	

Copyright © 2008, 2004, 2000, 1995, 1990 by Saunders, an imprint of Elsevier Inc. All rights reserved.

Evaluation of Student Performance

EVALUATION CRITERIA			COMMENTS
Symbol	Category	Point Value	
★	Critical Step	16 points	
●	Essential Step	6 points	
▷	Theory Question	2 points	
Score calculation: 100 points – ____ points missed ____ Score Satisfactory score: 85 or above			

AAMA/CAAHEP Competency Achieved:

☑ III. C. 3. b. (2) (c): Obtain specimens for microbiological testing.

Copyright © 2008, 2004, 2000, 1995, 1990 by Saunders, an imprint of Elsevier Inc. All rights reserved.

Notes

Copyright © 2008, 2004, 2000, 1995, 1990 by Saunders, an imprint of Elsevier Inc. All rights reserved.

EVALUATION OF COMPETENCY

Procedure 20-A: Rapid Strep Testing

Name: ______________________ Date: __________

Evaluated By: ______________________ Score: __________

Performance Objective

Outcome:	Perform a rapid strep test.
Conditions:	Given the following: disposable gloves, tongue blade, a Quick Vue rapid strep testing kit, controls, manufacturer's instructions, quality control log, and a biohazard sharps container.
Standards:	Time: 10 minutes. Student completed procedure in ____ minutes.
	Accuracy: Satisfactory score on the Performance Evaluation Checklist.

Performance Evaluation Checklist

Trial 1	*Trial 2*	*Point Value*	*Performance Standards*
		•	Sanitized hands.
		•	Assembled equipment.
		•	Checked the expiration date on the testing kit.
		•	Applied gloves and ran a positive and negative control, if needed.
		▷	Stated when controls should be run.
		•	Disposed of test cassettes and swabs in a biohazard waste container.
		•	Removed gloves and sanitized hands.
		•	Recorded results in the quality control log.
		•	Greeted the patient and introduced yourself.
		•	Identified the patient and explained the procedure.
		•	Positioned patient and adjusted light.
		•	Sanitized hands and applied gloves.
		•	Removed test cassette from its foil pouch and placed it on a clean, dry, level surface.
		•	Removed the sterile swab from its peel-apart package.
		•	Depressed patient's tongue with tongue depressor.
		•	Placed swab at the back of patient's throat and firmly rubbed it over lesions or white or inflamed areas of the tonsillar area and posterior pharynx.
		•	Constantly rotated swab as the specimen was being obtained.
		▷	Stated why the swab should be rotated.
		•	Did not allow swab to touch any area other than throat.
		•	Kept patient's tongue depressed and withdrew swab.
		•	Removed tongue depressor and discarded it.

Copyright © 2008, 2004, 2000, 1995, 1990 by Saunders, an imprint of Elsevier Inc. All rights reserved.

Trial 1	*Trial 2*	*Point Value*	*Performance Standards*
		•	Inserted the swab completely into the swab chamber.
		•	Squeezed the extraction bottle once to break the glass ampule.
		•	Vigorously shake the extraction bottle 5 times.
		•	Filled the swab chamber to the rim. Started the timer.
		•	Waited 5 minutes and read the results.
		▷	Described the appearance of a positive and negative result.
		▷	Described the appearance of an invalid result.
		▷	Explained what to do if an invalid result occurs.
		✶	The results were identical to the evaluator's results.
		•	Disposed of the test cassette and swab in a biohazard waste container.
		•	Removed gloves and sanitized hands.
		•	Recorded results in patient's chart.
		✶	Completed the procedure within 10 minutes.
			TOTALS

CHART	
Date	

Copyright © 2008, 2004, 2000, 1995, 1990 by Saunders, an imprint of Elsevier Inc. All rights reserved.

Evaluation of Student Performance

EVALUATION CRITERIA			COMMENTS
Symbol	Category	Point Value	
★	Critical Step	16 points	
●	Essential Step	6 points	
▷	Theory Question	2 points	
Score calculation: 100 points – ______ points missed ____ Score Satisfactory score: 85 or above			

AAMA/CAAHEP Competency Achieved:

☑ III. C. 3. b. (3) (c) (v): Perform microbiology testing.
☑ III. C. 3. c. (4) (d): Use methods of quality control.

Copyright © 2008, 2004, 2000, 1995, 1990 by Saunders, an imprint of Elsevier Inc. All rights reserved.

Notes

Copyright © 2008, 2004, 2000, 1995, 1990 by Saunders, an imprint of Elsevier Inc. All rights reserved.

EVALUATION OF COMPETENCY

Procedure 20-3: Preparing a Smear

Name: ______________________ Date: ____________

Evaluated By: ______________________ Score: ____________

Performance Objective

Outcome:	Prepare a microbiologic smear.
Conditions:	Given the following: disposable gloves, Bunsen burner, clean glass slide, microbiologic specimen, slide forceps, sterile swab, and a biohazard waste container.
Standards:	Time: 15 minutes. Student completed procedure in ____ minutes.
	Accuracy: Satisfactory score on the Performance Evaluation Checklist.

Performance Evaluation Checklist

Trial 1	*Trial 2*	*Point Value*	*Performance Standards*
		•	Sanitized hands.
		•	Assembled equipment.
		•	Labeled slide.
		•	Applied gloves and held the edge of slide between thumb and index finger.
		•	Started at the right side of slide, used a rolling motion, and gently and evenly spread the material from the specimen over slide.
		▷	Explained why the material should not be rubbed over slide.
		•	Allowed the smear to air-dry.
		▷	Explained why heat should not be applied at this point.
		•	Held slide with slide forceps and heat-fixed the smear.
		•	Stated the purpose of heat-fixing the smear.
		•	Allowed the slide to cool completely.
		•	Prepared the slide for examination by the physician under the microscope.
		✶	Completed the procedure within 15 minutes.
			TOTALS

Copyright © 2008, 2004, 2000, 1995, 1990 by Saunders, an imprint of Elsevier Inc. All rights reserved.

Evaluation of Student Performance

EVALUATION CRITERIA			COMMENTS
Symbol	Category	Point Value	
★	Critical Step	16 points	
●	Essential Step	6 points	
▷	Theory Question	2 points	
Score calculation: 100 points – ______ points missed ____ Score Satisfactory score: 85 or above			

AAMA/CAAHEP Competency Achieved:

☑ III. C. 3. b. (3) (c) (v): Perform microbiology testing.

Copyright © 2008, 2004, 2000, 1995, 1990 by Saunders, an imprint of Elsevier Inc. All rights reserved.

21

Emergency Medical Procedures

CHAPTER ASSIGNMENTS

√ After Completing	Date Due	Textbook Page(s)	TEXTBOOK ASSIGNMENTS	Possible Points	Points You Earned
		745-773	Read Chapter 21: Emergency Medical Procedures		
		763 769	Read Case Study 1 Case Study 1 questions	 5	
		764 770	Read Case Study 2 Case Study 2 questions	 5	
		767 770	Read Case Study 3 Case Study 3 questions	 5	
		770-771	Apply Your Knowledge questions	10	
			TOTAL POINTS		
√ After Completing	**Date Due**	**Study Guide Page(s)**	**STUDY GUIDE ASSIGNMENTS (CTA: Critical Thinking Activity)**	**Possible Points**	**Points You Earned**
		847	Pretest	10	
		848	Key Term Assessment	16	
		849-853	Evaluation of Learning questions	27	
		853	CTA A: First Aid Kit	10	
		853	CTA B: EMD Information	5	
		854	CTA C: Emergency Care (2 points each)	6	
		854-856	CTA D: Emergency Situations (3 points each)	55	
		847	Posttest	10	
			ADDITIONAL ASSIGNMENTS		
			TOTAL POINTS		

Copyright © 2008, 2004, 2000, 1995, 1990 by Saunders, an imprint of Elsevier Inc. All rights reserved.

Notes

Copyright © 2008, 2004, 2000, 1995, 1990 by Saunders, an imprint of Elsevier Inc. All rights reserved.

Name ______________________ Date ____________

PRETEST

True or False

_____ 1. A specially equipped cart for holding and transporting medications, equipment, and supplies needed in an emergency is known as a crash cart.

_____ 2. Symptoms of an asthmatic attack include dyspnea and wheezing.

_____ 3. Symptoms of a heart attack include sudden weakness on one side of the body.

_____ 4. Another name for a stroke is a coronary occlusion.

_____ 5. Arterial bleeding is characterized by a slow and steady flow of blood that is dark red in color.

_____ 6. A laceration is an example of a closed wound.

_____ 7. Symptoms of a fracture include pain, swelling, deformity, and loss of function.

_____ 8. A sprain is a tearing of ligaments at a joint.

_____ 9. Heat stroke is a life-threatening emergency.

_____ 10. Insulin enables glucose to enter the body's cells and be converted to energy.

POSTTEST

True or False

_____ 1. When providing emergency care, you should make sure to obtain information as to what happened from bystanders.

_____ 2. Emphysema is a progressive lung disorder in which there is a loss of elasticity of the alveoli of the lungs.

_____ 3. Symptoms that may occur with hyperventilation include rapid and deep respirations and tachycardia.

_____ 4. The first priority for hypovolemic shock is to control bleeding.

_____ 5. Status asthmaticus is the type of shock caused by a reaction of the body to a substance to which an individual is highly allergic.

_____ 6. Another name for a nosebleed is epistaxis.

_____ 7. The type of fracture in which the broken ends of the bone are forcefully jammed together is a greenstick fracture.

_____ 8. The type of seizure in which the abnormal electrical activity is localized into very specific areas of the brain is a tonic-clonic seizure.

_____ 9. Chipmunks have a high incidence of rabies.

_____ 10. Emergency care for insulin shock is to give the patient sugar immediately.

Copyright © 2008, 2004, 2000, 1995, 1990 by Saunders, an imprint of Elsevier Inc. All rights reserved.

KEY TERM ASSESSMENT

Directions: Match each medical term with its definition.

_____ 1. Burn

_____ 2. Crash cart

_____ 3. Crepitus

_____ 4. Dislocation

_____ 5. Emergency medical services

_____ 6. First aid

_____ 7. Fracture

_____ 8. Hypothermia

_____ 9. Poison

_____ 10. Pressure point

_____ 11. Seizure

_____ 12. Shock

_____ 13. Splint

_____ 14. Sprain

_____ 15. Strain

_____ 16. Wound

A. A network of community resources, equipment, and personnel that provides care to victims of injury or sudden illness
B. Any substance that causes illness, injury, or death if it enters the body
C. An injury to the tissues caused by exposure to thermal, chemical, electrical, or radioactive agents
D. An orthopedic device used to immobilize, restrain, or support a part of the body
E. A grating sensation caused by fractured bone fragments rubbing against each other
F. A sudden episode of involuntary muscular contractions and relaxation, often accompanied by a change in sensation, behavior, and level of consciousness
G. A stretching or tearing of muscles or tendons caused by trauma
H. The immediate care that is administered to an individual who is injured or suddenly becomes ill before complete medical care can be obtained
I. A break in the continuity of an external or internal surface caused by physical means
J. A specially equipped cart for holding and transporting medications, equipment, and supplies needed for performing lifesaving procedures in an emergency
K. Any break in a bone
L. The failure of the cardiovascular system to deliver enough blood to all the vital organs of the body
M. An injury in which one end of a bone making up a joint is separated or displaced from its normal anatomic position
N. A life-threatening condition in which the temperature of the entire body falls to a dangerously low level
O. A site on the body where an artery lies close to the surface of the skin and can be compressed against an underlying bone to control bleeding
P. Trauma to a joint that causes tearing of ligaments

Copyright © 2008, 2004, 2000, 1995, 1990 by Saunders, an imprint of Elsevier Inc. All rights reserved.

EVALUATION OF LEARNING

Directions: Fill in each blank with the correct answer.

1. What is the purpose of first aid?

____

____

____

____

2. What is the purpose of the office crash cart?

____

____

____

____

3. What is the difference between an EMT-Basic and a paramedic?

____

____

____

4. What are the responsibilities of an emergency medical dispatcher?

____

____

____

5. List five OSHA Standards which should be followed when administering first aid.

____

____

____

____

____

6. What is the reason for performing each of the following during an emergency situation?

   a. Remaining calm and speaking in a normal tone of voice

   ____

   ____

   b. Making sure it is safe before approaching the patient

   ____

   ____

   c. Following OSHA Standards when providing emergency care

   ____

   ____

Copyright © 2008, 2004, 2000, 1995, 1990 by Saunders, an imprint of Elsevier Inc. All rights reserved.

d. Activating the emergency medical services

e. Not moving the patient unnecessarily

f. Checking the patient for a medical alert tag

7. What are the symptoms of asthma?

8. What is emphysema?

9. What are the symptoms of hyperventilation?

10. What are the symptoms of a heart attack?

11. What are the symptoms of a stroke?

12. What is the cause of the following types of shock?

a. Hypovolemic

b. Cardiogenic

c. Neurogenic

d. Anaphylactic

Copyright © 2008, 2004, 2000, 1995, 1990 by Saunders, an imprint of Elsevier Inc. All rights reserved.

e. Psychogenic

____

____

13. What are the characteristics of each of the following types of external bleeding?

a. Capillary

____

____

b. Venous

____

____

c. Arterial

____

____

14. What is the difference between an open wound and a closed wound?

____

____

15. What are the signs and symptoms of a fracture?

____

____

16. What are the characteristics of each of the following types of fractures?

a. Impacted

____

____

b. Greenstick

____

____

c. Transverse

____

____

d. Oblique

____

____

e. Comminuted

____

____

f. Spiral

____

____

Copyright © 2008, 2004, 2000, 1995, 1990 by Saunders, an imprint of Elsevier Inc. All rights reserved.

17. What are the characteristics of each of the following types of burns?
    a. Superficial

    ____

    ____

    b. Partial thickness

    ____

    ____

    c. Full thickness

    ____

    ____

18. What is the difference between a partial seizure and a generalized seizure?

    ____

    ____

19. List two examples of each of the following types of poisoning:
    a. Ingested

    ____

    ____

    b. Inhaled

    ____

    ____

    c. Absorbed

    ____

    ____

    d. Injected

    ____

    ____

20. What spiders (found in the United States) have bites that can result in serious or life-threatening reactions?

    ____

    ____

21. What species of snakes (found in the United States) are poisonous?

    ____

    ____

22. What animals tend to have a high incidence of rabies?

    ____

    ____

23. What factors place an individual at higher risk for developing heat- and cold-related injuries?

    ____

    ____

Copyright © 2008, 2004, 2000, 1995, 1990 by Saunders, an imprint of Elsevier Inc. All rights reserved.

24. What areas of the body are most susceptible to frostbite?

25. What is the difference between type 1 diabetes and type 2 diabetes?

26. What is insulin shock and what causes it to occur?

27. What is diabetic coma and what causes it to occur?

CRITICAL THINKING ACTIVITIES

A. FIRST AID KIT

You are assembling a first aid kit. What supplies should be included in your kit? Identify one use for each of the supplies you list.

B. EMD INFORMATION

Jeff Stickler suddenly develops weakness in his left arm and leg, has difficulty speaking, and has a severe headache and dizziness. You immediately call the EMS. What information should you be prepared to relay to the emergency medical dispatcher?

Copyright © 2008, 2004, 2000, 1995, 1990 by Saunders, an imprint of Elsevier Inc. All rights reserved.

C. EMERGENCY CARE

In which of the following emergency situations would you be legally permitted to administer first aid? Explain your answers.

1. A patient is unconscious and bleeding profusely.

____

____

2. You identify yourself and state your level of training and what you plan to do. You ask the patient if it is alright to administer emergency care. The patient responds by saying, "Yes, please help me."

____

____

3. You ask the patient if you can administer emergency care, but the patient refuses your help.

____

____

D. EMERGENCY SITUATIONS

Explain what you would do in each of the following situations.

1. Holly Murphy falls while roller skating. She comes down hard on her left arm, which begins to swell and discolor. Holly guards her arm and complains of intense pain.

____

____

____

____

2. John Phillips is mowing the grass and mows over a yellow jacket nest. He is stung twice and soon afterward starts complaining of intense itching and exhibits erythema and hives on his arms, torso, and face.

____

____

____

____

3. Steve Williams complains of severe indigestion and squeezing pain in the chest. He is short of breath and perspiring profusely.

____

____

____

____

4. Clara Miller is playing basketball and is accidentally hit in the face with the ball. Her nose begins bleeding profusely.

____

____

____

____

Copyright © 2008, 2004, 2000, 1995, 1990 by Saunders, an imprint of Elsevier Inc. All rights reserved.

5. Debbie Carter, age 4, finds some children's chewable vitamins that have been left open on a table. She eats about 10 of them.

6. Rita Preston accidentally cuts her finger with a knife while preparing dinner. Her finger begins bleeding profusely.

7. Jose Perez is jogging on a cinder track. He falls and scrapes his left knee on the cinders.

8. Charlotte Lambert is getting ready to perform a piano recital for her entire church congregation. Suddenly she starts breathing very rapidly and deeply and complains that she feels light-headed and dizzy.

9. Bruce Jones is a diabetic. He is in a hurry and forgets to eat breakfast. He begins exhibiting behavior similar to that of someone who is intoxicated.

10. Debra Murray is delivering newspapers and is bitten by a strange dog. The bite causes several puncture marks and slight bleeding.

Copyright © 2008, 2004, 2000, 1995, 1990 by Saunders, an imprint of Elsevier Inc. All rights reserved.

11. Tanya Howe is playing tennis on a hot and humid day and begins to feel weak and nauseous. Her skin feels cold and clammy, and she is sweating profusely and complains of dizziness.

Copyright © 2008, 2004, 2000, 1995, 1990 by Saunders, an imprint of Elsevier Inc. All rights reserved.

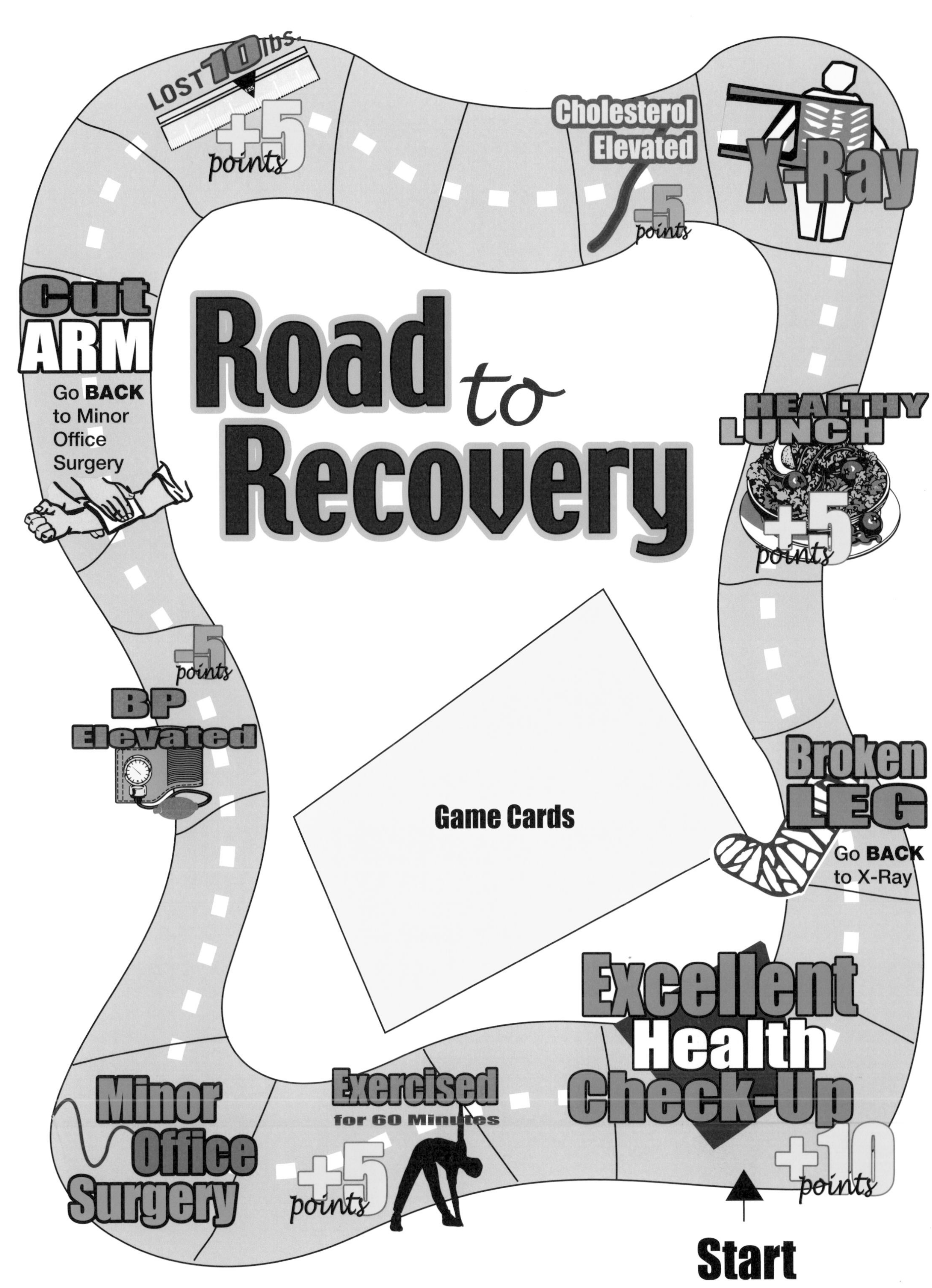
Road to Recovery
LOST 10 lbs.
+5 points
Cholesterol Elevated
-5 points
X-Ray
Cut ARM
Go BACK to Minor Office Surgery
HEALTHY LUNCH
+5 points
-5 points
BP Elevated
Game Cards
Broken LEG
Go BACK to X-Ray
Excellent Health Check-Up
+10 points
Minor Office Surgery
Exercised for 60 Minutes
+5 points
Start

Road *to* Recovery

DIRECTIONS:

1. Get into a group of 4 players. (Note: If needed the game can be played with less than 4 players).

2. To prepare for the game, each player should do the following:
   A. Name your token with the name of a "patient" and announce it to the other players. Write your patient's name in the space provided on your score card.
   B. Place your token on the square labeled START.

3. In turn each player should:
   A. Roll the dice and move your "patient" the specified number of spaces.
   B. Answer the required information on the game card. If the information is correct, you are awarded 5 points. If the information is incorrect, you receive no points.

4. Five points are awarded to a player's score when his/her "patient" lands on a healthy square (e.g., Healthy Lunch). These points are awarded regardless of whether the player answers the game card for his/her turn correctly or incorrectly.

5. Five points are deducted from a player's score when his/her "patient" lands on an unhealthy square (e.g., B/P Elevated).

6. If the "patient" is injured by landing on an injury box (e.g., Broken Leg), the "patient" must go back 4 spaces to the square to the square indicated; however the player is still permitted to answer the information on a game card.

7. Each time a "patient" lands on or passes over START square, the player is awarded 10 points for the patient's excellent health check-up.

8. Continue playing until all the cards have been used.

9. At the end of the game each player should do the following:
   A. Add up the total points on your score card.
   B. Compare your score with the other players.
   C. Determine which place your "patient" came in. In the case of a tie, more than one patient can be assigned to the same category.
   D. Determine how well your "patient" did on the ROAD TO RECOVERY using the information below.

Place	
1	Fully recovered
2	Almost recovered
3	Still recovering
4	Gasping for air